D0166404

PROVIDING HOME CARE
A Textbook for Home Health Aides

SECOND EDITION

William Leahy, MD
with Jetta Fuzy, RN, MS
and Julie Grafe, RN, BSN

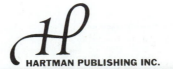

HARTMAN PUBLISHING INC.   *hartman*online.com

Managing Editor
Susan Alvare

Copy Editor
Kristin Calderon

Proofreaders
Suzanne Wegner
Joey Tulino
Yvonne Gillam

Cover and Interior Designer
Kirsten Browne

Illustrators
Thaddeus Castillo/Robert Christopher

Page Layout
Thaddeus Castillo

Photography
Art Clifton/Dick Ruddy/Susanita Marcos

Sales/Marketing
Gailynn Garberding/Debbie Rinker/Yvonne Gillam

Copyright Information
© 2004 by William Leahy, MD
Hartman Publishing, Inc.
8529 Indian School Road, NE
Albuquerque, NM 87112
(505) 291-1274
web: www.hartmanonline.com
e-mail: orders@hartmanonline.com

All rights reserved. No part of this book may be reproduced, in any form or by any means, without permission in writing from the publisher.

ISBN 1-888343-68-0

Notice to Readers
Though the guidelines and procedures contained in this text are based on consultations with healthcare professionals, they should not be considered absolute recommendations. The instructor and readers should follow employer, local, state, and federal guidelines concerning healthcare practices. These guidelines change, and it is the reader's responsibility to be aware of these changes and of the policies and procedures of her or his employer.

The publisher, author, editors, and reviewers cannot accept any responsibility for errors or omissions or for any consequences from application of the information in this book and make no warranty, expressed or implied, with respect to the contents of the book. The publisher does not warrant or guarantee any of the products described herein nor perform any analysis in connection with any of the product information contained herein.

Gender Usage
This textbook utilizes the pronouns he, his, she, and hers interchangeably to denote healthcare team members and clients.

Acknowledgments

All books need an author. Finding one who is passionate and knowledgeable is a publisher's most important work. William Leahy, MD became involved with home health aide education both out of an interest in the care his patients received and to give direction and meaning to the lives of young people in his community. After teaching the home health aide program at Bladensburg High School in suburban Maryland, he undertook the project of writing a better book. To his credit, he hired a registered nurse, working as a professional health journalist, to help craft the project. His vision was to have learning and teaching material that could be used by the program he founded and subsequently, to use the royalties from the project to ensure the program's continuance. All royalties from sales of this book fund a foundation formed to support young people studying healthcare careers.

Developing educational material for unlicensed healthcare workers demands the guidance of nurses who understand both educational theory and the practice of home health aide services. We found both in our experienced Consulting Editors, Jetta Fuzy, RN, MS, and Julie Grafe, RN, BSN.

During the years of creating and revising this text, many reviewers and customers guided us. A sincere thanks to each of them:

Betty Wolfe, RN
Susan Cutro, RN, BSN
Anna Blum, RN, MS
Betty J. Lipman
Barbara L. Haring
Inez Green, RN, C
Marti Pizzini
Mary Joan Greene
Maureen A. Williams, RN, C, MEd.
Linda Westerman, RN, MN
Delores Pederson, BSN

Table of Contents

Chapter 5
Infection Control and Standard Precautions

Chapter 6
Safety and Body Mechanics

Chapter 7
Emergency Care and Disaster Preparation

Section III

A Holistic Approach to Understanding Clients 95

Chapter 8
Physical, Psychological, and Social Health

Chapter 9
The Human Body in Health and Disease

Section IV

Developing Personal Care and Basic Healthcare Skills 138

Section V

Special Clients, Special Needs . . .232

Section VI

Practical Knowledge and Skills in Home Management 298

CHAPTER 21
Clean, Safe and Healthy Environments

CHAPTER 22
Clients' Nutritional Needs

CHAPTER 23
Meal Planning, Shopping, Preparation, and Storage

Procedure Index

Using this Book

This book will help you master what you need to know to provide excellent, compassionate care to clients with very different needs. It will also teach you to take care of yourself and your career.

Understanding how the book is organized will help you make the most of this resource.

Understanding Home Health Aide Services
Building a Foundation: Before Client Care
A Holistic Approach to Understanding Clients
Developing Personal Care and Basic Healthcare Skills
Special Clients, Special Needs
Practical Knowledge and Skills in Home Management
Where Do I Go From Here?

We have divided this book into seven sections and assigned each section its own colored tab. Each colored tab contains the chapter number and title, and you'll see them on the side of every page. At the top of every page, you'll find the name of the topic being taught.

1. List examples of legal and ethical behavior

Everything in this book, the student workbook, and your instructor's teaching material is organized around learning objectives. A learning objective is a very specific piece of knowledge or a very specific skill. After reading the text, if you can DO what the learning objective says, you know you have mastered the material.

intravenous *(in-trah-VEE-nus)*

Need help pronouncing a word? With each new word introduced in the text, the pronunciation is included.

Here are our rules for using the pronunciations:

Long vowels
A = AY
E = EE
I = EYE
O = Oh or O
U = oo or yoo

Short vowels
a = a as in "above"
e = e as in "bet"
i = i as in "sip"
o = o as in "not"
u = u as in "bud"

oo = oo as in "Sue"
yoo = as in "cute"
oy = as in "oil"

key terms

You'll find bold key terms throughout the text followed by their definitions.

Putting on gloves

All care procedures are highlighted by the same black bar for easy recognition.

Common disorders, guidelines, and observing and reporting are colored green for easy reference.

Chapter Review

Chapter-ending questions test your knowledge of the information found in the chapter. If you have trouble answering a question, you can return to the text and reread the material.

1

Home Care and the Healthcare System

1. Describe the structure of the healthcare system and describe ways it is changing

You are training to become a home health aide because you know that health care is a growing field. The healthcare system refers to all the different kinds of providers, facilities, and payers involved in delivering medical care. **Providers** are people or organizations that provide health care, including doctors, nurses, clinics, and agencies. **Facilities** are places where care is delivered or administered, including hospitals, long-term care facilities or nursing homes, and treatment centers. **Payers** are people or organizations paying for healthcare services. These include insurance companies, government programs like Medicare and Medicaid, and the individual patients or clients. Together, all these people, places, and organizations make up our healthcare system.

When you need health care you probably go to a doctor's office, a clinic, or an emergency room. Most of the time, you will be seen and treated by a physician (MD), a registered nurse (RN), a certified nurse practitioner (CNP), or a physician's assistant (PA). If you need further care or treatment, it may be provided by a specialist (MD), a physical therapist (PT), speech therapist (ST), or another kind of healthcare worker. People who need continuing care may spend time in a hospital, rehabilitation center, or a nursing home. Some people who need continuing care will be cared for in their homes (Fig. 1-1) by a home health aide (HHA) or other home care professional.

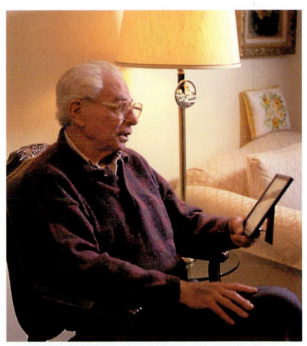

Fig. 1-1. Home health care is provided in a person's home.

Who will pay for your care may determine what kind of care you receive and where you receive it. Often payers control the amount and types of healthcare services people receive. **Traditional insurance companies** offer plans that pay for health care of plan members. Most people covered by traditional insurance are part of a plan at their place of work. The costs are paid for by the employer, the employee, or shared by both.

Traditional insurance plans usually provide excellent care for their members. However, the costs have risen greatly and many employers and employees can no longer afford to pay for traditional insurance plans.

As a reaction to the increased costs of traditional insurance plans, many employers and employees belong to **health maintenance organizations** (HMOs). If you belong to an HMO, you must use a particular doctor or group of doctors except in case of emergency. The doctors working for HMOs are paid to provide care while keeping costs down. Thus they may see more patients, order fewer tests, or cut costs in other ways.

Preferred provider organizations (PPOs) are another healthcare option used to reduce costs. A PPO is a network of providers that contract to provide health services to a group of people. Employees are given incentives to use network providers. Employers are given reduced, fee-for-service rates for getting employees to participate in the network. A person in a PPO may still get health care outside the network of providers, but must pay a higher portion of the cost.

If you become seriously ill, you may be admitted to a hospital. This decision is made by a doctor, and may have to be approved by your insurance company. The costs of hospital care have risen greatly. To make up for it, healthcare payers are controlling who can be admitted to a hospital and for how long.

After release from the hospital, many people need continuing care. This is particularly true as people are released after shorter hospital stays. Continuing care may be provided in a skilled nursing facility, a long-term care facility, a rehabilitation hospital, or by a home health agency. The type of care depends on the medical condition and needs of the patient or client.

Our healthcare system is constantly changing. As we develop new and better ways of caring for people, care becomes more expensive. Better health care helps people live longer, which leads

to a larger elderly population that may need additional health care. New discoveries and expensive equipment have also driven healthcare costs higher (Fig. 1-2).

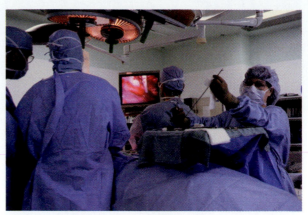

Fig. 1-2. Technology makes it possible to offer better health care, but drugs and equipment can be expensive.

HMOs and PPOs continue to replace traditional insurance plans. This affects the amount and quality of health care provided. These cost control strategies are often called **managed care**. In the past the goal of health care was to make sick people well. Today it is to get sick people well in the most efficient (least expensive) way possible. Home health care is in part a cost-controlling strategy because it is less expensive to care for someone in the home than in a facility. Shorter hospital stays, another cost-controlling strategy, have also increased the need for home health care.

2. Explain Medicare and Medicaid, and list when Medicare recipients may receive home care

Medicare was established in 1965 for people aged 65 or older. It now also covers people of any age with permanent kidney failure or certain disabilities. Medicare currently covers over 40 million people. Medicare pays for 28.4% of all home care. Medicare has two parts: Hospital Insurance (Part A), and Medical Insurance (Part B). Part A helps pay for care in a hospital or skilled nursing facility or for care from a home health agency or hospice. Part B helps pay for physician services and various other medical

services and equipment. Medicare will only pay for care it determines to be medically necessary. **Medicaid**, which pays for 18.5% of all home care, is a medical assistance program for low-income people.

Medicare pays for intermittent, not continuous, services provided by a certified home health agency. The agency must meet specific guidelines established by Medicare. To qualify for home health care, Medicare recipients must be unable to leave home, and their doctors must determine that they need home health care. Medicare will pay the full cost of most covered home healthcare services. However, Medicare will not pay for round-the-clock home health care. Home health care plays an important role when skilled care is needed on a part-time basis.

3. Explain the purpose of and need for home health care

Institutional health care delivered in hospitals and nursing homes is expensive. To reduce costs, hospitals have begun to discharge patients earlier. Many people who are discharged have not recovered their strength and stamina. Many require skilled assistance or monitoring. Others need only short-term assistance at home. Most insurance companies are willing to pay for a part of this care because it is less expensive than a long hospital or nursing home stay.

The growing numbers of older people and chronically ill people are also creating a demand for home care services. Family members who in the past would care for aging or ill relatives frequently leave home towns to live and work in distant areas. In addition, they often have other responsibilities or problems that interfere with their ability to provide care. For example, family members who work or who care for young children may be unable to look after aging relatives as they become frail and less functional.

Most people who need some medical care prefer the familiar surroundings of home to an institution. They choose to live alone or receive care from a relative or friend. Home health aides can provide assistance to the chronically ill, the elderly, and family caregivers who need relief from the physical and emotional stress of caregiving. Many home health aides also work in assisted living facilities. Assisted living facilities allow independent living in a home-like environment, with professional care available as needed.

As advances in medicine and technology extend the lives of people with chronic illnesses, the number of people needing health care will increase. Home services will be needed to provide continued care and assistance as chronic illnesses progress. For example, people with acquired immunodeficiency syndrome (AIDS), a chronic illness that is infecting more and more people throughout the world, will require in-home assistance (Fig. 1-3). They will also require disease-specific health care as their illnesses progress. Improvements in medications and better management of the disease have already shown that people with AIDS can live longer, with an improved quality of life.

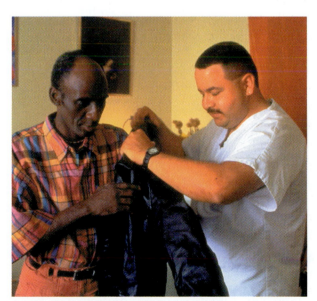

Fig. 1-3. Home health aides often provide care for people with chronic illnesses, such as AIDS.

One of the most important reasons for health care in the home is that most people who are ill or disabled feel more comfortable at home. Health care in familiar surroundings improves mental and physical well-being. It has proven to be a major factor in the healing process.

4. List key events in the history of home care services

The first home health aides were women hired to care for the homes and children of mothers who were sick or hospitalized in the early 1900s. During the Great Depression in the 1930s, women were hired as "housekeeping aides." They were paid by the government. When this government program was discontinued, some aides continued to work for local family and children's services, which provided services to families in need.

In 1959, a national conference on homemaker services was held. It was clear that there was a great need not only for homemaker or housekeeping services, but for personal, in-home care of sick people. Thus, the aide's role expanded to include personal care of the sick as well as care of the home and family.

In 1965, the Medicare program was created. Because many Medicare recipients need home care, home health services have been growing ever since. Medicare first began referring to homemakers as "home health aides."

Growth in the number of certified home health agencies, 1989 to 2000.

	Medicare Certified Home Health Agencies	Medicare Certified Hospice
1989	5,676	597
2000	7,830	2,255

Interest in home health care has increased for several reasons. Increased healthcare costs along with advances in capabilities have created a need for the affordable, continuing care that home care provides. The growing population of the elderly and people with chronic diseases, such as AIDS and Alzheimer's disease, has also created greater demand for home care.

Another reason home health care has grown is the use of **diagnostic related groups** (DRGs)

by Medicare and Medicaid. A DRG specifies the treatment cost Medicare or Medicaid will pay for various **diagnoses** (*dye-ag-NOH-seez*), or physicians' determinations of an illness. Because a flat fee is assigned for each diagnosis, hospitals lose money if a person's stay is longer than what is allotted in the DRG. Hospitals generally make money if a person's treatment is completed more quickly than specified in the DRG. Home health care has grown to take care of the needs of people who are discharged from the hospital earlier than they would have been in the past.

Today, the process of training and monitoring home health aides is changing. Many states are developing certification standards for programs that train aides.

The Centers for Medicare & Medicaid Services (CMS), formerly the Health Care Finance Administration (HCFA), is a federal agency within the U.S. Department of Health and Human Services. CMS runs the Medicare and Medicaid programs at the federal level. In 1999, CMS issued new rules for home health agencies that care for Medicare clients. These rules include criminal background checks for newly-hired aides, and they allow certified nursing assistants to work as home health aides.

5. Identify the basic methods of payment for home health services

Any of the following may pay for home health services (Fig. 1-4):

- Insurance company
- Health maintenance organization
- Medicare
- Medicaid
- Individual client or family

Medicare now pays agencies a fixed fee for a 60-day period of care based on a client's condition. If the cost of providing care exceeds the payment, the agency loses money. If the care provided costs less than the payment, they make

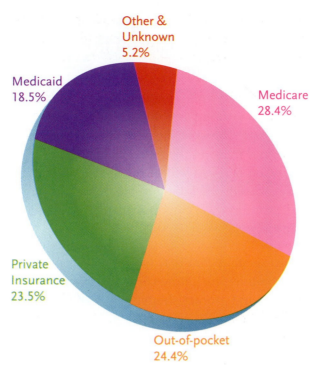

Fig. 1-4. Sources of payment for home health care.

Other &
Unknown
5.2%

Medicaid
18.5%

Medicare
28.4%

Private
Insurance
23.5%

Out-of-pocket
24.4%

money. For these reasons, home health agencies must pay great attention to costs. And because all payers monitor the quality of care provided, how work is documented or recorded is very important.

CMS's new payment system for home care is called the "Prospective Payment System." It works very much like the DRG system described earlier for hospitals.

6. Describe a typical home health agency

Many home health aides are employed by home health agencies. **Home health agencies** are businesses that provide health care and personal services in the home. Healthcare services provided by home health agencies may include nursing care, specialized therapy, specific medical equipment, pharmacy and intravenous (IV) products, and personal care. Personal care services may include housekeeping, shopping, help with activities of daily living, and cooking.

Clients who need home care are referred to a home health agency by their doctors. They can also be referred by a hospital discharge planner,

a social services agency, the state or local department of public health, the welfare office, a local agency on aging, or a senior center. Clients and family members can also choose an agency that meets their needs.

Once an agency is chosen and the doctor has made a referral, a staff member performs an assessment of the client. This determines how the care needs can best be met. The home environment will also be evaluated to determine whether it is safe for the client.

The services home health agencies provide depend on the size of the agency. Small agencies may provide basic nursing care, personal care, and housekeeping services. Larger agencies may provide speech, physical, and occupational therapies, and medical social work. Some common services are listed below. A brief description of each service is provided in chapter 2.

- physical therapy
- occupational therapy
- speech therapy
- medical-surgical nursing care, including management of clients with AIDS, diabetes (*dye-ah-BEE-teez*) management, instruction, care of different types of tubes, and catheterization (*kath-eh-ter-eye-ZAY-shun*)
- intravenous (*in-trah-VEE-nus*) infusion therapy
- maternal, pediatric (*pee-dee-A-trik*), and newborn nursing care
- nutrition therapy/dietary counseling
- medical social work
- personal care, including bathing; taking vital signs; skin, nail and hair care; meal preparation; light housekeeping; ambulation; and range of motion exercises
- homemaker/companion services
- medical equipment rental and service
- pharmacy (*FAHR-mah-see*) services
- hospice (*HAH-spiss*) services

All home health agencies have professional staff who make decisions about what services are needed. These professionals, who may be physicians, registered nurses, or other licensed professionals, also reassess clients' needs for service, write care plans, and schedule services.

Once staff determine the amount and types of care needed, assignments are given. A home health aide may be assigned to spend a certain number of hours each day or week with a client providing care and services. While the care plan and the assignments are developed by the supervisor or case manager, input from all members of the care team is needed. All HHAs are under the supervision of a skilled professional: either a registered nurse, a physical therapist, or a speech therapist. Figure 1-5 shows a typical home health agency organization chart. More information about the care team and how the members work together is in chapter 2.

7. Explain how working for a home health agency is different from working in other types of facilities

In some ways, working as a home health aide is similar to working as a nursing assistant or nurse's aide. Most of the basic medical procedures and many of the personal care procedures you perform will be the same. However, some aspects of working in the home are very different from working in a hospital or other care facility.

Housekeeping: You may have housekeeping responsibilities, including cooking, cleaning, laundry, and grocery shopping, for at least some of your clients.

Family contact: You may have a lot more contact with clients' families in the home than you would in a facility.

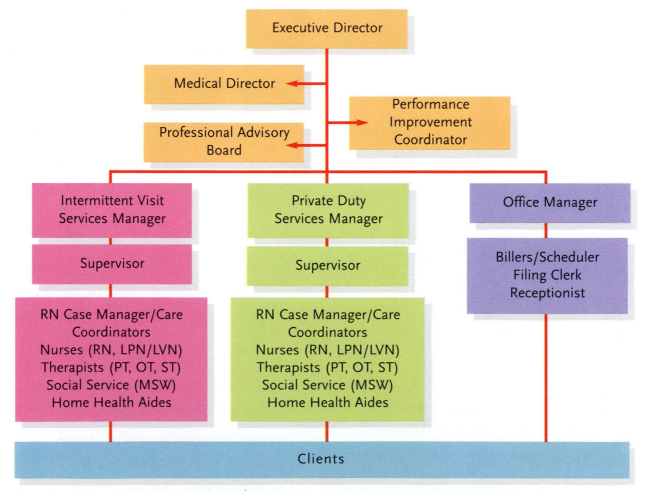

Fig. 1-5. **A typical home health agency organization chart.**

Independence: You will work independently as a home health aide. Your supervisor will monitor your work, but you will spend most of your hours working with clients without direct supervision. Thus you must be a responsible and independent worker.

Communication: Good written and verbal communication skills are important. Keep yourself informed of changes in the client care plan. You must keep others informed of changes you observe in the client and the client's environment.

Transportation: You will have to get yourself from one client's home to another. You will need to have a dependable car or know how to use public transportation. You may also face bad weather conditions. Clients need your care—rain, snow, or sleet.

Safety: Be aware of personal safety when you are traveling alone to visit clients. You may be visiting clients in high-crime areas. Be aware of your surroundings, walk confidently, and avoid dangerous situations, such as visits after dark.

Flexibility: Each client's home will be different. You will need to adapt to the changes in environment. In a care facility, you know what supplies will be available and what kind of cleanliness and organization to expect at work. In home care, you may not know until you get there.

Working environment: Nursing homes are built to make caregiving easier and safer. They have wide doors, large bathing facilities, and special equipment for transferring residents. If needed, other caregivers are close by and can help move a resident or answer questions you may have. In home care, the physical layout of rooms, stairs, lack of equipment, cramped bathrooms, rugs, clutter, and even pets can complicate caregiving.

Client's home: In a client's home, you are a guest. Be respectful of the client's property and customs (Fig. 1-6). The client is in control most of the time.

Clients' comfort: One of the best things about home care is that it allows clients to stay in the familiar and comfortable surroundings of their own homes. This can help most clients recover or adapt to their condition more quickly.

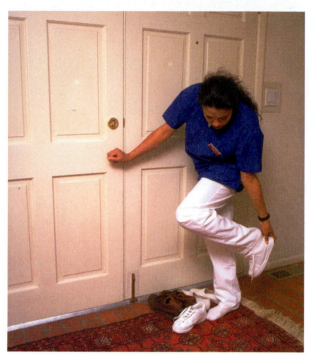

Fig. 1-6. As a home health aide, you are a guest in your clients' homes. Respect each client's property and customs. For example, removing shoes is a custom in some homes.

Chapter Review

1. Why is home health care a cost-controlling strategy?

2. How do Medicare recipients qualify for home health care?

3. Name three reasons for the increase in demand for home health care.

4. Why are the following years important: 1959, 1965, and 1999?

5. What are the three most common methods of payment for home health services?

6. List ten common services provided by a typical home health agency.

7. Which one of the many differences between working as an aide for a home health agency and working for a facility is most important to you?

2

The Home Health Aide and Care Team

1. Identify the role of each healthcare team member

You will work directly with clients and families in their homes. You will be part of a team of health professionals that includes physicians, nurses, social workers, therapists, and specialists. The team will work closely together to help clients recover from their illnesses. If full recovery is not possible, the team will help clients do as much as they can for themselves.

Your clients will have different needs and problems. Healthcare professionals with different kinds of education and experience will help care for them. Members of the healthcare team may include the following:

Home Health Aide (HHA): The **home health aide** performs delegated tasks, such as taking vital signs, and provides routine personal care, such as bathing clients or preparing meals. Home health aides spend more time with clients than other members of the healthcare team. That is why they act as the "eyes and ears" of the team. Observing and reporting changes in the client's condition or abilities is a very important role of the HHA (Fig. 2-1).

Case Manager or Supervisor: Usually a registered nurse, a case manager or supervisor is assigned to each client by the home health agency. The **case manager** or **supervisor**, with

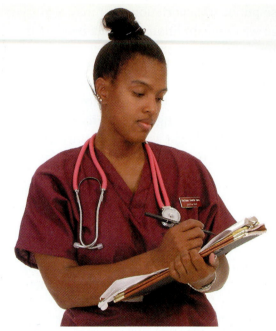

Fig. 2-1. Observing and reporting are some of the most important duties you'll have.

input from other team members, creates the basic care plan for the client. He or she monitors any changes that are observed and reported by the HHA. The case manager also makes changes in the client care plan when necessary.

Registered Nurse (RN): In a home health agency, a **registered nurse** coordinates, manages, and provides care. RNs also supervise and train home health aides. They develop the home health aide plan of care, or assignments. A registered nurse has graduated from a two- to four-year nursing program. RNs have diplomas

or college degrees and have passed a licensing examination administered by the state board of nursing. Registered nurses may have additional academic degrees or education in specialty areas.

Physician or Doctor (MD): A **doctor's** job is to diagnose disease or disability and prescribe treatment. Doctors have graduated from four-year medical schools, which they attended after receiving bachelor's degrees. Many doctors also attend specialized training programs after medical school. A doctor generally decides when patients need home health care and refers them to home health agencies (Fig. 2-2).

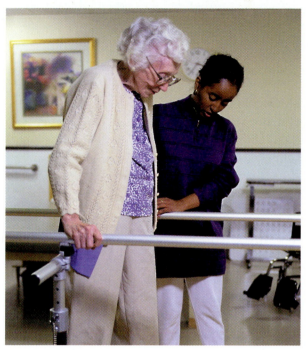
Fig. 2-3. A physical therapist will help restore specific abilities.

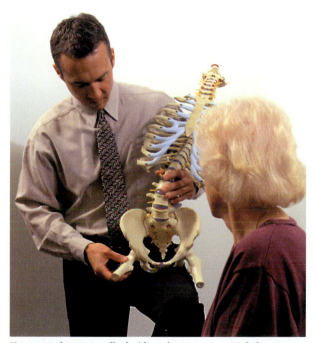
Fig. 2-2. A doctor usually decides when a person needs home health care.

Physical Therapist (PT): A **physical therapist** administers therapy in the form of heat, cold, massage, ultrasound, electricity, and exercise to muscles, bones, and joints. Goals of physical therapy include improving blood circulation, promoting healing, helping the client regain or maintain mobility, and easing pain (Fig. 2-3).

Speech Language Pathologist (*pa-THAH-loh-jist*) (SLP): A **speech language pathologist**, or **speech therapist**, identifies communication disorders in clients and addresses factors involved in recovery. An SLP develops a plan of

care to meet short- and long-term goals for recovery. An SLP teaches exercises that will help the client improve or overcome speech impediments. An SLP also evaluates a person's ability to swallow food and drink.

Occupational Therapist (OT): An **occupational therapist** helps clients understand and learn to compensate for disabilities. For clients in home care, an occupational therapist may assist in training clients to perform activities of daily living (ADLs), such as dressing, eating, and bathing. This often involves the use of special equipment called assistive or adaptive devices (Fig. 2-4). The OT evaluates the client's needs and develops a treatment program.

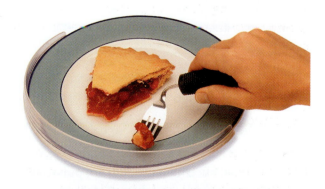
Fig. 2-4. An occupational therapist will help clients learn to use adaptive devices, such as this one for eating.

Registered Dietitian (RDT): A **registered dietitian** or **nutritionist** teaches clients and their families about special diets to improve their health and help manage their illness.

Medical Social Worker (MSW): A **medical social worker** determines clients' needs and helps them get support services, such as counseling, meal services, and financial assistance. An MSW holds a master's or bachelor's degree in social work.

2. Define the client care plan and explain its purpose

The client care plan is individualized for each client. It is developed to help achieve the goals of care (Fig. 2-5). It lists tasks healthcare providers, including home health aides, must perform. It states how often these tasks should be performed, and specifies how they should be carried out. For example, the care plan for a client who has had a stroke may list the following HHA responsibilities:

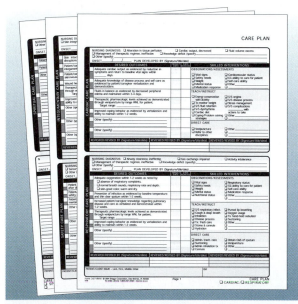

Fig. 2-5. A sample client care plan. (Reprinted with permission of Briggs Corporation, Des Moines, Iowa, 800-247-2343)

- range of motion exercises to be performed daily

- vital signs, such as temperature, pulse, and blood pressure to be taken at least once a day or more

- diet and fluid requirements

The care plan is a guide to help the client attain and maintain the best level of health possible. Activities not listed on the care plan should not be performed without permission from a supervisor. The HHA care plan is part of this overall plan of care. It must be followed very carefully.

Throughout this text you will read how important it is to make observations and report them to your supervisor. Sometimes even simple observations are very important. The information you collect, such as vital signs, and the changes you observe in the client, are both important in determining how that client's care plan needs to change.

3. Describe how each team member contributes to the care plan

Care planning should involve input from the client and/or the family, as well as healthcare professionals. Healthcare professionals will assess the client's physical, financial, social, and psychological needs. After the doctor prescribes treatment, the supervisor, nurses, and other care team members formulate the care plan.

Many factors are considered when formulating a care plan. These include the following:

- the client's health and physical condition

- the client's diagnosis and treatment

- whether additional services and resources, including transportation, equipment, or supplementary income, are needed

For example, a social worker may arrange transportation for the client to and from appointments with his or her physician.

The **psychological** (*sye-ka-LOJ-ik-ul*) and **socioeconomic** (*soh-shee-oh-ee-ka-NOM-ik*) status of the client and the family are other important factors. The agency will assess how the client and family are reacting to the medical problems. Family members may be absent or unavailable for some clients. For example, a client

may have only elderly and ailing relatives to help with care. Family members may have jobs to go to or children to care for. Some families may have relatives who are unwilling to assist in care. For some families, problems like alcoholism and substance abuse can make it difficult to provide care. Housing and financial resources may also be lacking. A medical social worker may be sent to the home to assess the situation and make referrals. The medical social worker can assist with long-term care planning.

Input from all members of the care team is needed to develop the client care plan. For instance, a 250-lb, elderly client requests a tub bath. The supervisor assigns it. The home health aide finds that the client has no adaptive equipment and is unable to move to the tub. The assignment puts the home health aide and the client at risk of injury. The home health aide must communicate this. The assignment needs to be changed to a sponge bath or shower, or the client needs to obtain adaptive equipment. The supervisor is responsible for reassessing the assignment and making necessary changes to the care plan.

Multiple care plans may be necessary for some clients. In these situations, the supervisor will coordinate the client's overall care. There will be one care plan for the home health aide to follow. There will be separate care plans for other providers, such as the physical therapist.

Care plans must be kept up-to-date as the client's condition changes. Reporting changes and problems to the supervisor is a very important role of the home health aide. That is how the care team revises care plans to meet the client's changing needs (Fig. 2-6).

4. Describe the role of the home health aide and explain typical tasks performed

The role of home health aides is to improve or maintain the health and well-being of clients. This is accomplished by providing or assisting

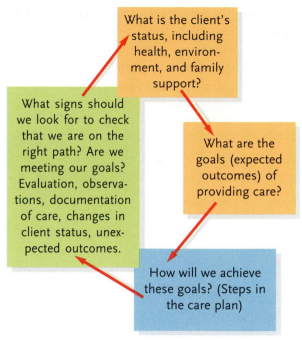

Fig. 2-6. The care planning process.

with personal care, assisting with ADLs (activities of daily living), and performing assigned healthcare tasks. Home health aides also fulfill goals indirectly by promoting self-care. HHAs can reinforce the teachings of other team members and promote behavior that improves health, such as diet and exercise.

Home health aides provide services directly to their clients in several ways:

HHAs provide care or assist with self-care, depending on the care plan. A care plan may include the following:

- bathing
- grooming
- feeding
- assisting with range of motion (ROM) exercises and ambulation
- reminding the client about medications
- measuring vital signs (temperature, pulse rate, respiratory rate, and blood pressure)

HHAs maintain a safe, secure, and comfortable home life for clients and their families. This may include light housekeeping, food shopping, meal preparation, and doing laundry.

Home health aides are also role models. They promote clients' independence by practicing good housekeeping, nutrition, and healthcare skills. For example, encouraging clients to do tasks for themselves helps ensure that health will be maintained between visits.

In addition, home health aides teach by example. By performing procedures and providing assistance efficiently and cheerfully, they provide the family with a model for caregiving.

5. Identify tasks outside the scope of practice for home health aides

Laws and regulations on what aides can and cannot do vary from state to state. A **scope of practice** defines the things you are allowed to do. However, some procedures are not performed by home health aides under any circumstances. These tasks are said to be outside the scope of practice of a home health aide.

HHAs do not administer medications unless trained and assigned to do so. Only a few states allow home health aides to do this. However, it **always** requires additional training. Home health aides may assist the clients with self-administered medications in certain situations.

HHAs do not insert or remove tubes or objects (other than a thermometer) in a client's body. These procedures are called "invasive," and are performed only by licensed professionals.

HHAs do not honor a request to do something outside the scope of practice, not listed in the job description, or not on the assignment sheet. In this situation an HHA should explain that he or she cannot do the task requested. The request should then be reported to a supervisor.

HHAs do not perform procedures that require sterile technique. For example, changing a sterile dressing on a deep, open wound requires sterile technique.

HHAs do not diagnose or prescribe treatments or medications.

HHAs do not tell the client or the family the diagnosis or the medical treatment plan. This is the responsibility of the doctor or nurse.

Your instructor or employer may provide a list of other tasks outside your scope of practice. In some cases, you may be trained to do a particular task that your employer does not want home health aides to perform. Know which tasks these are and do not perform them. Many of these specialized tasks require more training. It is important to learn how to refuse a task for which you have not been trained, or which is outside your scope of practice.

6. List the federal regulations that apply to home health aides

There are three basic federal regulations that apply to home health aides:

1. HHAs working in a Medicare-participating agency must complete 75 hours of training and/or they must pass a competency evaluation before they begin working. Training may be at a community college, high school, or home health agency (Fig. 2-7). State laws may require training in specific areas as well as certification through a standardized test. New rules also include passing a criminal background check prior to employment, and demonstrating the ability to read, write, and give oral reports.

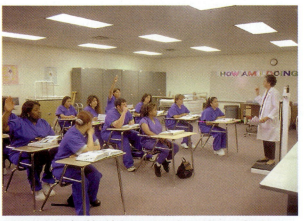

Fig. 2-7. Home health aides must complete 75 hours of training and/or pass a competency evaluation to work for a Medicare-participating agency.

2. HHAs must have at least twelve hours of education (in-service training) every year. Home health agencies are required to offer these courses for their employees. However, it is your responsibility to successfully complete twelve hours of courses each year. An agency will not allow you to work if you have not met the twelve-hour in-service training requirement. Many states require more than twelve hours.

3. HHAs must comply with Occupational Safety and Health Administration (OSHA) rules about bloodborne pathogens, Standard Precautions, and tuberculosis. OSHA is a federal government agency that makes rules to protect workers from hazards on the job. Information on following these rules is covered in chapter 5.

7. Describe the purpose of the chain of command

As a home health aide, you are carrying out instructions given to you by a nurse. The nurse is acting on the instructions of a physician or other member of the care team. This is called the **chain of command**. It guarantees that your clients get proper health care. It also protects you and your employer from **liability** (*lye-a-BIL-i-tee*). Liability is a legal term that means someone can be held responsible for harming someone else. For example, imagine that something you do for a client harms him. However, what you did was in the care plan and was done according to policy and procedure. In this case, you are not liable, or responsible, for hurting the client. However, if you do something not in the care plan that harms a client, you could be held responsible. That is why it is important to follow instructions in the care plan and for the agency to have a chain of command (Fig. 2-8).

Home health aides must understand what they can and cannot do. This is important so that you do not harm a client or involve yourself or your employer in a lawsuit. Some states certify that a home health aide is qualified to work. However, home health aides are not licensed

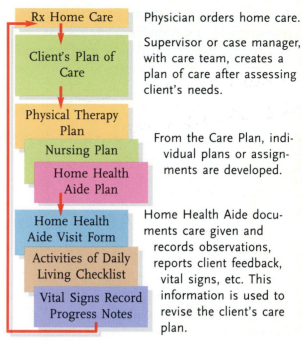

Fig. 2-8. The chain of command ensures that the client receives proper care.

healthcare providers. Everything you do in your job is assigned to you by a licensed healthcare professional. You do your job under the authority of another person's license. That is why these professionals will show great interest in what you do and how you do it.

Every state grants the right to practice various jobs in health care through licensure. Examples include granting a license to practice nursing, medicine or physical therapy. All members of the healthcare team work under each professional's scope of practice.

8. Define policies and procedures and explain why they are important

You will be told where to locate a list of policies and procedures that all staff members are expected to follow. A **policy** is a course of action that should be taken every time a certain situation occurs. For example, one policy at most agencies is that the care plan must be followed. That means that every time you visit a client, what you do will be determined by the care plan. A **procedure** (*proh-SEE-dyoor*) is a particular method, or way, of doing something. For example, your agency will have a procedure for

reporting information about your clients. The procedure tells you what form you fill out, when and how often to fill it out, and to whom it is given.

Common policies and procedures at home health agencies include the following:

- Keep all information confidential. Keeping information confidential means not telling anyone about it. This is not only an agency rule, it is also the law. See chapter 3 for more information on confidentiality, including the Health Insurance Portability and Accountability Act (HIPAA). The agency and all its employees must keep all information about clients and their families confidential. Be careful where you keep your notes and assignment sheets. Keeping your paperwork in the open where someone could read it, or losing your notes or assignments, is a breach of confidentiality. Confidentiality also extends to the agency's personnel files and clinical records. This means your employer cannot give out information about you from your job application or other records.

- Follow the client's care plan. Home health aides should perform all tasks assigned by the care plan. They should not do any tasks that are not included or approved by the case manager or supervisor. If the client or family requests changes, they should be told to speak to the supervisor.

- Report to the supervisor at regular arranged times, and more frequently if necessary. For example, home health aides must report the following to their supervisors: important events or changes in clients and their families, an accident on the job, and anything that delays or prevents them from going to or completing an assignment.

- Do not discuss personal problems with the client or the client's family. Discussing your personal problems is unprofessional. You must act in a professional manner. Clients should see you as someone whose job is to provide care, rather than as a friend.

- Be punctual and dependable. Employers expect this of all employees.

- Follow deadlines for documentation and paperwork. Timely and accurate documentation is very important. This topic is discussed in detail in chapter 4.

- Provide all client care in a pleasant, professional manner.

- Do not give or accept gifts. Gift giving and receiving is not allowed because it is unprofessional (Fig. 2-9). Gift giving can cause other problems as well. For example, a client may forget giving an object as a gift and report it as stolen. Some clients who give gifts may believe they deserve special treatment.

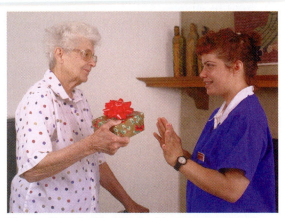

Fig. 2-9. Home health aides should not accept money or gifts because it is unprofessional and leads to conflict.

- Your employer will have policies and procedures for every client care situation. These have been developed to give quality care and protect client safety. You must always follow your employer's policies and procedures. Though written procedures may seem long and sometimes complicated, each step is important. This book includes general procedures for all the basic tasks you will do as a home health aide. Always follow your employer's procedures when caring for clients.

9. List examples of a professional relationship with a client and an employer

Professional means having to do with work or a job. The opposite of professional is **personal**,

which refers to your life outside your job, such as your family, friends, and home life. **Professionalism** is how you behave when you are on the job. It includes how you dress, the words you use, and the things you talk about. It also includes being on time, finishing assignments, and reporting to your supervisor. For an HHA, professionalism means participating in care planning, making important observations, and reporting accurately. Clients, coworkers, and supervisors respect employees who behave in a professional way. Professionalism will help you keep your job and may help you earn promotions and raises.

A professional relationship with a client includes the following:

- maintaining a positive attitude

- being cleanly and neatly dressed and groomed

- arriving on time, doing tasks efficiently, and leaving on time

- finishing an assignment

- doing only the tasks assigned

- speaking politely and cheerfully to the client, even if you are not in a good mood (Fig. 2-10)

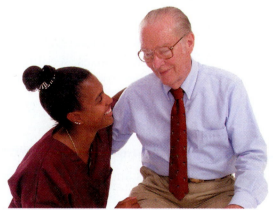

Fig. 2-10. Being polite and cheerful is something that will be expected of you.

- never cursing or using profanity, even if the client does

- never discussing your personal problems

- never giving or accepting gifts

- calling the client Mr., Mrs., Ms., or Miss, and his or her last name, or by the name he or she prefers

- listening to the client

- always explaining the care you will provide before providing it

- always following care practices, such as handwashing, to protect yourself and the client

A professional relationship with an employer includes the following:

- maintaining a positive attitude

- completing assignments efficiently

- consistently following policies and procedures

- documenting and reporting carefully and correctly

- communicating problems with clients or assignments

- reporting anything that keeps you from completing assignments

- asking questions when you do not know or understand something

- taking directions or criticism without getting upset

- being cleanly and neatly dressed and groomed

- always being on time

- participating in education programs offered

- being a positive role model for your agency at all times

10. Demonstrate how to organize care assignments

To finish all your assignments each day, you have to work efficiently. To be efficient, you need to decide the order in which to do your tasks. For example, you are assigned to work with an elderly client from 2:00 to 4:00 p.m. on Monday. Your supervisor has told you that this client needs some housekeeping, dinner preparation, and personal care. When you arrive at

The Home Health Aide and Care Team

2

the client's home, you see what tasks need to be done. It is a good idea to make a list of the tasks you will do and the order in which you will do them (Fig. 2-11).

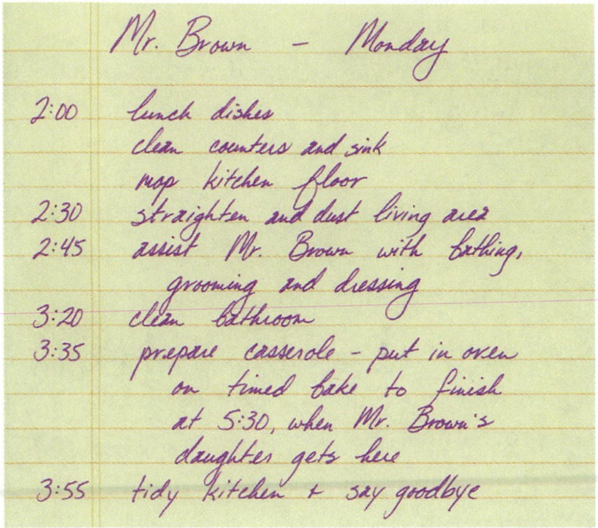

> Mr. Brown - Monday
>
> 2:00   lunch dishes
>   clean counters and sink
>   mop kitchen floor
> 2:30   straighten and dust living area
> 2:45   assist Mr. Brown with bathing,
>   grooming and dressing
> 3:20   clean bathroom
> 3:35   prepare casserole - put in oven
>   on timed bake to finish
>   at 5:30, when Mr. Brown's
>   daughter gets here
> 3:55   tidy kitchen + say goodbye

Fig. 2-11. Making a list of tasks to be done will help you organize to perform them efficiently.

Two hours is not a lot of time to do all those tasks. You will have to work quickly. You will not have any extra time to turn on the television or sit down and have coffee. If you had not planned the tasks before you started, you might have spent too long cleaning the kitchen and never have made dinner. Making a list of tasks helps you be most efficient. It is also helpful to include the client in your planning. A client may not cooperate with your schedule if he or she has different priorities. It takes good communication, and sometimes negotiation, to arrange a schedule that works.

If you run out of time with a client, you have to stay late to finish all your tasks. That makes you late to your next assignment. You then do not have enough time to do everything the next client needs. Completing assignments efficiently means you are not always running late. It means you will do a better job.

11. Demonstrate good personal grooming habits

Good grooming makes you feel great, and it makes others feel good about you (Fig. 2-12).

Grooming affects how confident clients feel about the care you give. Good employees have the following personal grooming habits:

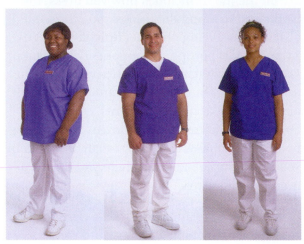

Fig. 2-12.

- bathing or showering daily and using deodorant or anti-perspirant (use little or no perfume, as some clients may be intolerant of some odors)

- brushing teeth frequently and using mouthwash when necessary

- keeping hair clean and neatly brushed or combed, tying long hair back in a bun or ponytail

- dressing neatly, in clothes that are washed and ironed

- not wearing clothes that are too tight or too baggy, torn or stained, or too revealing (short skirts, low-cut blouses, see-through fabrics)

- not wearing jewelry that is large or gets in the way

Your agency will have rules about your appearance. Know these rules and always follow them.

12. Identify personal qualities a home health aide must have

Home health aides must be:

- **Compassionate.** Being **compassionate** (*kum-PASH-on-et*) means being caring, concerned, considerate, **empathetic** (*em-pah-*

THEH-tik), and understanding. **Empathy** means being able to enter into the feelings of others. People who are compassionate understand other people's problems and care about them.

- **Honest**. A person who is honest tells the truth and can be trusted. Clients need to feel that they can trust the people who care for them. The care team will depend on your honesty in planning the care plan. Your employer counts on your truthful records of the care you provide, the hours you work, the time and mileage you spend traveling, and the observations you make.

- **Conscientious**. People who are **conscientious** (*kahn-shee-EN-shus*) always try to do their best. They are always alert, observant, accurate, and responsible. Conscientious care means making accurate observations, paying careful attention to the care plan, taking responsibility for actions, and reporting to other members of the care team (Fig. 2-13). For example, taking accurate measurements of vital signs, such as temperature, pulse, or respiration, is important. Other members of the care team will make treatment decisions based on the documented measurements. Without conscientious care, a client's health and well-being are in danger.

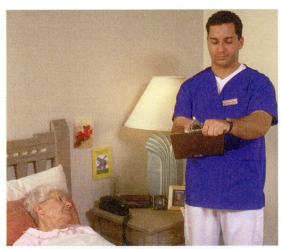

Fig. 2-13. Home health aides must be conscientious about documenting observations and procedures.

- **Dependable**. Healthcare providers must be able to make and keep commitments. You must report to work on time. You must skillfully perform the assigned tasks, avoid too many absences, and keep your promises. Dependability is especially important in home care, where the supervisor is not usually there to check on client care.

- **Respectful**. Being respectful means seeing value in other people's individuality, including age, religion, culture, feelings, and beliefs. People who are respectful treat others politely and considerately. You should care about people's self-esteem. Do not do or say anything that will damage it. You must not let people down by gossiping about them. Respect the various cultures and practices of your clients.

- **Unprejudiced**. You will work with many different people from different backgrounds. You must give every one of your clients the same quality care regardless of age, gender, sexual orientation, religion, race, or ethnic origin.

- **Non-judgmental**. You may not like or agree with things that your clients or their families do or have done. However, your job is to care for each client according to the care plan, not to judge him or her. Put aside your opinions and see each client as an individual who needs your care.

13. Identify an employer's responsibilities

Agencies should teach home health aides about their policies and procedures. Agencies must make sure that home health aides are educated and are able to perform all assigned tasks. Your employer's responsibilities include the following:

- Provide a written job description. The job description tells what you are expected to do during your working hours (Fig. 2-14).

- Provide competency testing and skills evaluation before you are sent to care for clients.

- Provide initial training and continuing in-service training. Initial training includes an

2

The Home Health Aide and Care Team

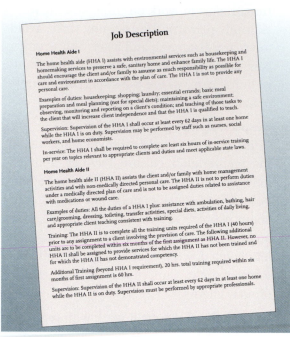

Job Description

Home Health Aide I

The home health aide (HHA I) assists with environmental services such as housekeeping and homemaking services to preserve a safe, sanitary home and enhance family life. The HHA I should encourage the client and/or family to assume as much responsibility as possible for care and environment in accordance with the plan of care. The HHA I is not to provide any personal care.

Examples of duties: housekeeping; shopping; laundry; essential errands; basic meal preparation and meal planning (not for special diets); maintaining a safe environment; observing, monitoring and reporting on a client's condition; and teaching of those tasks to the client that will increase client independence and that the HHA I is qualified to teach.

Supervision: Supervision of the HHA I shall occur at least every 62 days in at least one home while the HHA I is on duty. Supervision may be performed by staff such as nurses, social workers, and home economists.

In-service: The HHA I shall be required to complete are least six hours of in-service training per year on topics relevant to appropriate clients and duties and meet applicable state laws.

Home Health Aide II

The home health aide II (HHA II) assists the client and/or family with home management activities and with non-medically directed personal care. The HHA II is not to perform duties under a medically directed plan of care and is not to be assigned duties related to assistance with medications or wound care.

Examples of duties: All the duties of a HHA I plus: assistance with ambulation, bathing, hair care/grooming, dressing, toileting, transfer activities, special diets, activities of daily living, and appropriate client teaching consistent with training.

Training: The HHA II is to complete all the training units required of the HHA I (40 hours) prior to any assignment to a client involving the provision of care. The following additional units are to be completed within six months of the first assignment as HHA II. However, no HHA II shall be assigned to provide services for which the HHA II has not been trained and for which the HHA II has not demonstrated competency.

Additional Training (beyond HHA I requirement), 20 hrs. total training required within six months of first assignment is 60 hrs.

Supervision: Supervision of the HHA II shall occur at least every 62 days in at least one home while the HHA II is on duty. Supervision must be performed by appropriate professionals.

Fig. 2-14. Your employer should provide you with a job description.

orientation to the policies and procedures of the agency. You should also be trained in the agency's documentation system. In-service training is a federal requirement. It keeps your skills fresh and helps you do an even better job. OSHA regulations require employers to offer AIDS and Hepatitis B education as well.

- Provide appropriate preparation for each assignment. The agency should teach you to appropriately care for each client's special needs and conditions. You should be told why the client needs service and what the goals of care are. If other healthcare professionals are involved, their responsibilities should also be explained to you.

- Provide supervision. Supervisors support and teach you how to do new tasks. They help you find solutions to problems and adjust to new situations. Supervisors check with clients to assure the goals of the care plan are being met. They will also check to see that clients are satisfied with the care they are receiving.

- Provide information about supervision. Your employer should tell you when and where you will meet with your supervisor and what you will discuss in these meetings. You should also be told how the supervisor can be reached for assistance, and when and why the supervisor will visit your clients' homes.

- Provide adequate equipment and supplies for you to safely do your work. For example, your agency should provide the gloves you must sometimes wear to protect you and your client from infection.

Chapter Review

1. Choose three members of the care team and describe the roles they play.

2. Why are observing and reporting even simple observations about a client important?

3. What are the factors considered when forming a care plan?

4. How can home health aides be good role models for clients and their families?

5. Give an example of an "invasive" procedure. Give an example of sterile technique. Are HHAs supposed to perform these tasks?

6. Should an HHA tell a client about his or her diagnosis or medical treatment plan?

7. How many hours of training must HHAs complete to work for a Medicare-participating agency?

8. How many hours of in-service education are HHAs required to have per year?

9. Name one reason why the chain of command is important.

10. Why do home health agencies have written policies and procedures?

11. Describe professionalism and list five examples of professional behavior with a client.

12. List seven examples of professional behavior with an employer.

13. Write out a sample schedule for a two-hour morning visit to Mrs. Smith. Use tasks different from those listed in figure 2-11.

14. Why is it a good idea not to wear too much perfume when you are working in clients' homes?

15. What is one reason why you should keep your hair tied back if you have long hair?

16. What personal qualities will make you a good HHA?

17. Why should an employer provide competency testing and skills evaluation before sending you to care for clients?

The Home Health Aide and Care Team

2

3

Legal and Ethical Issues

1. List examples of legal and ethical behavior

Ethics and laws guide our behavior. **Ethics** are the knowledge of right and wrong. An ethical person has a sense of duty and responsibility toward others. He or she always tries to do what is right.

If ethics tell us what we *should* do, **laws** tell us what we *must* do. Laws are usually based on ethics. Governments establish laws to help people live peacefully together and to ensure order and safety. When someone breaks the law, he or she may be punished by having to pay a fine or spend time in prison.

Ethics and laws are extremely important in health care. They protect people receiving care and guide people giving care. Home health aides and other healthcare providers should be guided by a code of ethics. They must know the laws that apply to their jobs.

GUIDELINES
Legal and Ethical Behavior

- Be honest at all times. Stealing, and lying about what care you provided or how long it took are examples of dishonesty.

- Protect clients' privacy. Do not discuss their cases except with other members of the care team.

- Do not accept gifts or tips.

- Do not become personally or sexually involved with clients or family members.

- Report abuse or suspected abuse of a client.

- Follow the care plan/assignment.

- Do not perform any task outside your scope of practice.

- Report all client observations and incidents to your supervisor.

- Document accurately and on time.

- Follow OSHA rules about bloodborne pathogens, Standard Precautions, and tuberculosis.

2. List examples of clients' rights and explain why they are important

Clients' rights relate to how clients must be treated. They provide an ethical code of conduct for healthcare workers. Home health agencies give clients a list of these rights and review each right with them.

The first right listed in the box below states that clients have the right to receive considerate, dignified, and respectful care. This also means that clients have the right not to be neglected or abused by their caretakers. **Neglect** means failing to provide needed care. **Abuse** means purposely causing physical, mental, or emotional

pain or injury to someone. **Verbal abuse** is the use of words that do not show consideration and respect. **Physical abuse** refers to any treatment, intentional or unintentional, that causes harm to the client's body. **Sexual abuse** is forcing a client to perform or participate in sexual acts against his or her will. **Psychological or mental abuse** is any behavior that causes the client to feel threatened, fearful, or humiliated in any way. Many states require home health agencies to provide their clients with abuse hotline phone numbers.

Home health aides must never abuse clients in any way. They must also try to protect their clients from others who abuse them. If you ever see or suspect that another caregiver or a family member is abusing a client, report this immediately to your supervisor. Reporting abuse is not an option—**it's the law.**

Two other basic clients' rights are the right to be fully informed of the goals of care and of the care itself, and the right to participate in care planning. Your employer should develop an agreement with each client about the goals of care before service is provided. Your employer should also make every effort to involve clients and their families in care planning (Fig. 3-1). Each of us knows how our bodies work best and what makes us comfortable. People who feel in control of their bodies, lives, and health have greater self-esteem. They are more likely to continue a treatment plan and to cooperate with caregivers. Clients also have a right to know what the agency expects to happen as a result of

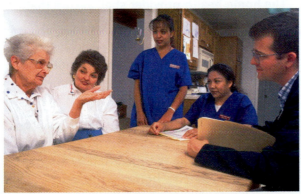

Fig. 3-1. Clients and their families should be involved in care planning.

their care. These expected outcomes are sometimes called the goals of the care plan. Clients should be informed of barriers to their care. For example, a client's consistent failure to eat enough healthy food can be an obstacle to getting well.

Client Bill of Rights

Home health clients and their formal caregivers have a right to not be discriminated against based on race, color, religion, national origin, age, gender, sexual orientation, or disability. Furthermore, clients and caregivers have a right to mutual respect and dignity, including respect for property. Caregivers are prohibited from accepting personal gifts and borrowing from clients.

Clients have the right:

* to have relationships with home health providers that are based on honesty and ethical standards of conduct;
* to be informed of the procedure they can follow to lodge complaints with the home health provider about the care that is, or fails to be, furnished and about a lack of respect for property. [The phone number to report this listed here].
* to know about the disposition of such complaints:
* to voice their grievances without fear of discrimination or reprisal for having done so; and
* to be advised of the telephone number and hours of operation of the state's home care hotline which receives questions and complaints about local home health agencies, including complaints about implementation of advance directive requirements. [Hours and the phone number listed here.]

Clients have the right:

* to be notified in advance about the care that is to be furnished, the types (disciplines) of the caregivers who will furnish

3

Legal and Ethical Issues

the care, and the frequency of the visits that are proposed to be furnished;

- to be advised of any change in the plan of care before the change is made;

- to participate in the planning of the care and in planning changes in the care, and to be advised that they have the right to do so;

- to be informed in writing of rights under state law to make decisions concerning medical care, including the right to accept or refuse treatment and the right to formulate advance directives;

- to be notified of the expected outcomes of care and any obstacles or barriers to treatment*

- to be informed in writing of policies and procedures for implementing advance directives, including any limitations if the provider cannot implement an advance directive on the basis of conscience;

- to have healthcare providers comply with advance directives in accordance with state law requirements;

- to receive care without condition or discrimination based on, the execution of advance directives; and

- to refuse services without fear of reprisal or discrimination.

* The home health provider or the client's physician may be forced to refer the client to another source of care if the client's refusal to comply with the plan of care threatens to compromise the provider's commitment to quality care.

Clients have the right:

- to confidentiality of the medical record as well as information about their health, social, and financial circumstances and about what takes place in the home; and

- to expect the home health provider to release information only as required by law or authorized by the client and to be informed of procedures for disclosure.

Clients have the right:

- to be informed of the extent to which payment may be expected from Medicare, Medicaid, or any other payer known to the home health provider;

- to be informed of the charges that will not be covered by Medicare;

- to be informed of the charges for which the client may be liable;

- to receive this information, orally and in writing, before care is initiated and within 30 calendar days of the date the home health provider becomes aware of any changes; and

- to have access, upon request, to all bills for service the client has received regardless of whether the bills are paid out-of-pocket or by another party.

Clients have the right:

- to receive care of the highest quality;

- in general, to be admitted by a home health provider only if it has the resources needed to provide the care safely and at the required level of intensity, as determined by a professional assessment; a provider with less than optimal resources may nevertheless admit the client if a more appropriate provider is not available, but only after fully informing the client of the provider's limitations and the lack of suitable alternative arrangements; and

- to be told what to do in the case of an emergency.

The home health provider shall assure that:

- all medically-related home care is provided in accordance with physicians' orders and that a plan of care specifies the services and their frequency and duration; and

- all medically-related personal care is provided by an appropriately trained home health aide who is supervised by a nurse or other qualified home health care professional.

3

Legal and Ethical Issues

Clients have the responsibility:

- to notify the provider of changes in their condition (e.g., hospitalization, changes in the plan of care, symptoms to be reported);
- to follow the plan of care;
- to notify the provider if the visit schedule needs to be changed;
- to inform providers of the existence of any changes made to advance directives;
- to advise the provider of any problems or dissatisfaction with the services provided;
- to provide a safe environment for care to be provided; and
- to carry out mutually-agreed-upon responsibilities.

To satisfy the Medicare certification requirements, the Centers for Medicare & Medicaid Services (CMS) requires that agencies:

1. Give a copy of the Bill of Rights to each client in the course of the admission process.
2. Explain the Bill of Rights to the client and document that this has been done. Agencies may have clients sign a copy of the client's Bill of Rights to acknowledge receipt.

3. List examples of behavior supporting and promoting clients' rights

You can help protect your clients' rights in the following ways:

- Watch for and report to your supervisor any signs of abuse or neglect.
- Involve clients in your planning.
- Always explain a procedure before performing it.
- Never abuse a client physically, psychologically, verbally, or sexually.
- Respect a client's refusal of care. Report the refusal to your supervisor immediately.

- Tell your supervisor if a client has questions about the goals of care or the care plan.
- Be truthful when documenting care.
- Do not talk or gossip about a client.
- Knock and ask permission before entering a client's room.
- Do not open a client's mail or look through his or her belongings (Fig. 3-2).

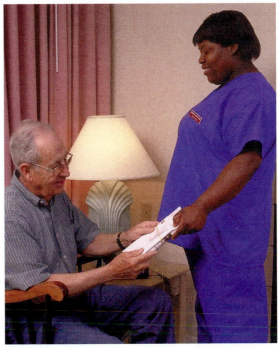

Fig. 3-2. Do not look through a client's mail or belongings.

- Do not accept gifts or money from a client.
- Respect your clients' property.
- Report observations regarding a client's condition or care.

4. Explain HIPAA and list ways to protect clients' confidentiality

To respect **confidentiality** means to keep private things private. You will learn confidential (private) information about your clients. You may learn about a client's state of health, finances, and personal relationships. Ethically and legally, you must protect the confidentiality of this information. This means you should not tell anyone other than members of the healthcare team anything about your clients.

Congress passed the Health Insurance Portability and Accountability Act (HIPAA) in 1996. It was further defined and revised in 2001 and 2002. One of the reasons this law was passed is to help keep health information private and secure. All healthcare organizations must take special steps to protect health information. They and their employees can be fined and/or imprisoned if they do not follow special rules to protect privacy. This applies to all healthcare providers, including doctors, nurses, home health aides, and any members of the care team.

Under this law a person's health information must be kept private. It is called protected health information (PHI). Examples of PHI include name, address, telephone number, social security number, e-mail address, and medical record number. Only people who must have information to provide care or to process records should know a person's private health information. They must make sure they protect the information so it does not become known or used by anyone else. It must be kept confidential.

HHAs cannot give any information about a client to anyone who is not directly involved in the client's care unless the client gives official consent or unless the law requires it. For example, if a neighbor asks you how your client is doing, you should reply, "I'm sorry but I cannot share that information. It's confidential." That is the correct response to anyone who does not have a legal reason to know about the client. Other ways HHAs can protect clients' privacy include the following guidelines:

GUIDELINES
Protecting Privacy

- Do not leave information for a client on an answering machine. Leave only your name and number when asking clients or family members to call you back.

- Make sure you are in a private area when you are listening to or reading your messages.

- Know with whom you are speaking on the phone. If you are not sure, get a name and number to call back after you find out it's okay to do so.

- Make or accept telephone calls about clients—even to or from the agency—in a private area.

- When calling another client to let him or her know you are running late, be aware that Caller ID can identify the client from whose house you are calling. Use another phone not in the home.

- When talking to a care team member on the phone, use regular phones, not cellular phones. Cell phones can be scanned.

- Do not talk about clients in public places. Public areas include elevators, the grocery store, lounges, waiting rooms, parking garages, schools, restaurants, etc.

- Use confidential rooms for reports to another care team member.

- If you see a client's family member or a former client in a public place, be careful in greeting him or her. He or she may not want others to know about the family member or that he or she has been a client.

- Do not bring family or friends to the client's home to meet the client. Do not leave family or friends in the car while you are visiting a client.

- Make sure nobody can see private and protected health or personal information on your computer screen while you are working. Log off when you are not working on your computer.

- Do not give confidential information in e-mails because you do not know who has access to your messages.

- Make sure fax numbers are correct before faxing any healthcare information. Use a cover sheet with a confidentiality statement.

- Do not leave papers or documents where others may see them.

- Store, file, or shred documents according to your agency's policy.

- If you find papers or documents with a client's information, give them to your supervisor.

All healthcare workers must comply with HIPAA regulations, no matter where they are or what they are doing. There are serious penalties for violating these regulations. Penalties differ depending upon the violation and can include:

- A fine of $100 per person per violation

- A fine of $50,000 and/or not more than one year imprisonment

- A fine of $100,000 and/or not more than five years imprisonment

- A fine of $250,000 and/or not more than ten years imprisonment

Maintaining confidentiality is a legal and ethical obligation. It is part of respecting your clients and their rights. Your clients have to trust you. Talking about them betrays this trust. Discussing a client's care or personal affairs with anyone other than your supervisor or another member of the healthcare team violates the law.

Chapter Review

1. List five examples of legal and ethical behavior for a home health aide.

2. If you see or suspect that a client is being abused, what is your responsibility?

3. What is the purpose of a client's Bill of Rights?

4. Pick three of the examples of behavior promoting clients' rights in learning objective 3. Describe how this behavior supports or promotes specific rights found in the client's Bill of Rights.

5. What are some examples of a person's protected health information (PHI)?

6. To whom is a HHA allowed to give information about a client?

7. To what members of the healthcare team is HIPAA applicable?

8. Do HIPAA's guidelines apply if you are shopping at the grocery store?

3

Legal and Ethical Issues

4

Communication and Cultural Diversity

1. Define communication

Communication is the process of exchanging information with others. It is a process of sending and receiving messages. People communicate by using signs and symbols, such as words, drawings, and pictures. They also communicate by their behavior.

The simplest form of communication takes place between two people (Fig. 4-1). The person who communicates first is the "sender" who sends a message. The person who receives the message is called the "receiver." Receiver and sender are constantly switching roles as they communicate.

The third step is providing feedback. The person who receives the message repeats it or responds to it in some way. This lets the sender know that the message was received and understood. All three steps must be taken before the communication process is complete. During a conversation, this three-step process is repeated over and over.

Effective communication is a critical part of your job. Home health aides must communicate with supervisors, members of the health care team, clients, and family members. A client's health depends on how well you communicate your observations and concerns to your supervisor. You will also need to be able to communicate clearly and respectfully in stressful or confusing situations. Some family members may need your help in communicating clearly with each other or with the care team.

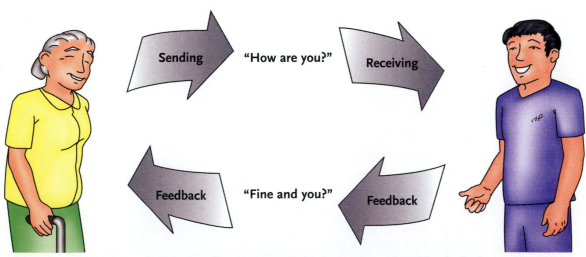

Sending — "How are you?" — Receiving

Feedback — "Fine and you?" — Feedback

Fig. 4-1. The communication process consists of sending a message, receiving a message, and providing feedback.

2. Explain verbal and nonverbal communication

Communication is either verbal or nonverbal. **Verbal communication** involves the use of words or sounds, spoken or written. Oral reports are an example of verbal communication. **Nonverbal communication** is the way we communicate without using words. Examples include shaking your head or shrugging your shoulders. Nonverbal communication also includes the way we say something using words. For example, you might say, "I'll be right there, Mr. Dodd." This communicates that you are ready and willing to help. But if you say the same phrase in a different tone or emphasizing different words, you communicate frustration and annoyance: "I'll *be* right *there*, Mr. Dodd!"

Body language is another form of nonverbal communication. Body movements, facial expressions, and posture can express different attitudes or emotions. Just as with speaking, you send messages with your body language. Other people receive them and interpret them. For example, slouching in a chair and sitting erect send two different messages (Fig. 4-2). Slouching sends the message that you are bored, tired, or hostile to the other person. Sitting up straight sends the message that you are interested and respectful.

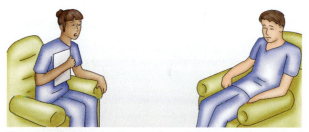

Fig. 4-2. Body language often speaks as plainly as words. Which of these people seems more interested in the conversation they are having?

Sometimes people send one message verbally and a very different message nonverbally. Nonverbal communication often tells us how someone is feeling. This message may be quite different from what he or she is saying. For example, a client who tells you "I'm feeling fine today," but stays in bed and winces in pain, is sending two very different messages. Paying attention to nonverbal communication helps you give better care. Communicate to your supervisor your observation that the client is staying in bed and appears to be wincing in pain despite what he or she says.

You must also be aware of your own verbal and nonverbal messages. If you say "It's nice to see you today, Mrs. Rodriguez," but you don't smile or look her in the eye, she will know that you aren't really all that happy to see her.

When communication is confusing, try to clarify it. Ask for an explanation of the message. Say something like "Mrs. Jones, you've just told me something that I don't understand. Would you explain it to me?" Or state what you have observed and ask if the observation is correct. For example, "Mrs. Jones, I see that you're smiling, but I hear by the sound of your voice that you may be depressed. Are you?" Take the time to clarify communication. It can help you know your clients better and avoid misunderstandings.

Cultural Sensitivity

Nonverbal communication may depend on personality or cultural background. Some people are more animated when they speak. They use lots of gestures and facial expressions. Other people speak quietly or calmly, regardless of their moods. Depending on their cultural background, people may make motions with their hands when they talk, stand close to the person they are talking to, or touch the other person.

People from some cultural groups stand further apart when talking than people from other groups. When one person shortens the distance, the other person may view it as a threat. Be sensitive to your clients' needs. Let them determine how close they want to be when talking to you.

The use of touch and eye contact also varies with cultural background and with personality (Fig. 4-3). For some people, touching is wel-

come. It expresses caring and warmth. For others, it seems intrusive, threatening, or even harassing. In the United States, we often talk about "looking someone straight in the eye" or speaking with each other "eye to eye." We regard eye contact as an indication of honesty. However, in some cultures, looking someone in the eye may seem overly bold or disrespectful.

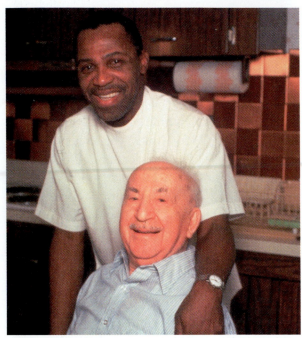

Fig. 4-3. How a person perceives your touch may depend on his or her cultural background.

Distinguishing what is nonverbal communication from what is culturally determined behavior can be a challenge. However, it is an important part of communication. It is especially important in a multicultural society (a society made up of many cultures), such as the United States. Be aware of all the messages you are sending and receiving. As you practice listening and observing carefully, you will learn to understand your clients' needs and feelings.

3. Identify barriers to communication

Communication can be blocked or disrupted in many ways (Fig. 4-4). Following are some barriers and ways to avoid them:

Client does not hear you, does not hear correctly, or does not understand. Stand directly facing the client. Speak more slowly than you

do with family and friends. Speak clearly. Speak in a low, pleasant voice. Do not whisper or mumble. If your client says he or she can't hear you, speak more loudly. However, use a pleasant, professional tone of voice. If your client wears a hearing aid, check to ensure it is on and is working properly.

Client is difficult to understand. Be patient and take time to listen. Ask client to repeat or explain. Rephrase the message in your own words to make sure you have understood.

Message uses words receiver does not understand. Do not use medical terminology with your client. Speak in simple, everyday words. Ask what a word means if you are not sure.

Using slang confuses the message. Avoid using slang words and expressions that are unprofessional or may not be understood.

Clichés make your message meaningless. **Clichés** (*klee-shays*) are phrases that are used over and over again and do not really mean anything. For example, "Everything will be fine" is a cliché. Instead, listen to what your client is really saying. Respond with a meaningful message. For example, if a client is afraid of having a bath, say "I understand that it seems scary to you. What can I do to make you more comfortable?" instead of saying, "Oh, it'll be over before you know it."

Asking "why" makes the client defensive. Avoid asking "why" when a client makes a statement. "Why" questions make people feel defensive. For example, a client may say she does not want to go for a walk today. If you ask "why not?" you may receive an angry response. Instead, ask, "Are you too tired to take a walk, or is there something else you want to do?" Your client may then be willing to discuss the issue.

Giving advice is inappropriate. Do not offer your personal opinion or give advice. Giving medical advice is not within the scope of your practice and could be dangerous. Giving advice about running the household can seem pushy and intrusive.

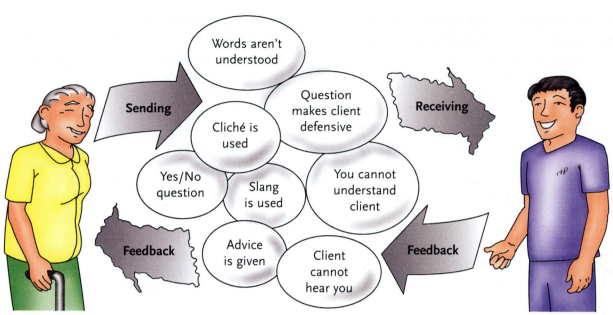

Fig. 4-4. Barriers to communication.

Yes/no answers end a conversation. Ask open-ended questions that need more than a yes or no answer. Yes and no answers bring any conversation to an end. For example, if you want to know what your client likes to eat, do not ask "Do you like vegetables?" Instead, try "Which vegetables do you like best?"

Nonverbal communication changes the message. Be aware of your body language and gestures when you are speaking. Be alert to nonverbal messages from your clients and clarify them. For example "Mr. Feldman, you say you're feeling fine but you seem to be in pain. Can I help?"

4. List ways to make communication accurate and complete

In addition to avoiding the barriers to communication listed above, the following techniques will help ensure that you send and receive clear, complete messages.

Be a good listener. Allow the other person to express his or her ideas completely. When he or she is finished, restate the message in your own words to make sure you have understood.

Provide feedback as you listen. Active listening means focusing on the person who is sending the message and providing feedback. Feedback might be an acknowledgment, a question, or a repetition of the sender's message. Offer general but leading responses, such as "Oh?" or "Go on," or "Hmm." By doing this you are actively listening, providing feedback, and encouraging the sender to expand the message.

Bring up topics of concern. If you know of a topic that might be of concern to your client, raise the issue in a general, nonthreatening way. This allows the client to decide whether or not to discuss it. For example, if you observe that your client is unusually quiet, you could say, "Mrs. Jones, you seem so quiet today." Or you may notice a certain emotion. You might say, "Mrs. Jones, you seemed upset earlier. Would you like to talk about it?"

Let some pauses happen. Use silence for a few moments at a time. This encourages the client to gather his or her thoughts and compose more messages.

Tune in to other cultures. Learn the words and expressions of your client's culture. This shows that you respect the culture and are interested in what the client has to say. It will help you understand your client's messages more fully. Be careful about using new words and terms yourself, however. Taken out of context, some words or expressions may have a different meaning than what you thought. The important thing is

to understand words and expressions when others use them. Never be judgmental; accept people who are different.

Ask for more. When clients report symptoms, events, or feelings, have them repeat what they have said and ask them for more information.

5. Describe the difference between facts and opinions

A fact is something that is definitely true. For example, "Mr. Ford has lost four pounds this month." You can back up this fact with evidence: weighing Mr. Ford and comparing his current weight to his weight last month. An opinion is something someone believes to be true, but is not definitely true. "I think Mr. Ford looks thinner," is an opinion. So is "Mr. Ford has lost weight because he won't eat what I cook." These statements might be true, but you cannot back them up with evidence. It is important to be able to separate facts from opinions.

Separating facts from opinions will make you a better communicator. When you give your opinion, you risk being wrong. If you say, "Mrs. Myers, drinking coffee is going to keep you awake tonight," you may make your client mad. Also, you might be wrong. Perhaps Mrs. Myers always drinks coffee, and it does not affect her sleep. Or maybe she does not sleep well because of medication, not because of the coffee.

Use facts to communicate more effectively. "Mrs. Myers, many people find that the caffeine (kaf-EEN) in coffee keeps them awake at night. Would you like to try skipping your coffee today to see if you might sleep better?" Now Mrs. Myers has no reason to get mad at you. You cannot be wrong, because it is a fact that caffeine keeps many people awake. Using facts instead of your opinion lets you communicate in a more professional way.

When communicating with members of the healthcare team, distinguish between facts and opinions. For example, "Mr. Morgan is acting like he had a stroke," is an opinion and could

very well be wrong. Instead, report the facts: "Mr. Morgan has lost strength on his right side and his speech is slurred." When you need to report your opinion, introduce it with "I think...." Then it is clear that you are offering your opinion and not a fact you have observed.

6. Explain how to develop effective interpersonal relationships

Developing good relationships with your clients, their family members, and other members of the care team will allow you to provide excellent care. You should not try to become friends with your clients. However, you should try to develop a warm professional relationship with them based on trust. Good communication skills will help you get to know your clients. It will also help them learn to trust you.

In addition to the strategies already discussed, the following suggestions can help you communicate effectively and develop good relationships.

Avoid changing the subject when your client is discussing something. This is true even if the subject makes you feel uncomfortable or helpless. For example, a client might say, "I'm having so much pain today." Do not try to avoid the topic by asking if he feels like watching television. This makes the client feel that you are not interested in him or what he is talking about.

Do not ignore a client's request. Ignoring a request is considered negligent behavior. Honor the request if you can. Otherwise, explain why the request cannot be fulfilled. Always report such requests to your supervisor.

Do not talk down to an elderly or disabled person or a child. Talk to your clients and their families as you would normally talk to any person. Make adjustments if someone is hearing-impaired or visually impaired.

Sit near the person who has started a conversation. Sitting near a person shows that you find what he or she is saying important and worth listening to.

Lean forward in your chair when someone is speaking to you. Leaning forward communicates interest. Pay attention to your nonverbal communication. If you fold your arms in front of you, you send the negative message that you are trying to distance yourself from the speaker.

Approach the person who is talking. Even if you are in another room, you should approach the person. This tells the person you are interested in him or her and what he or she has to say.

Put yourself in other people's shoes. Try to understand what they are going through. This is called **empathy** (*EM-pa-thee*). Ask yourself how you would feel if you were confined to bed, or needed help to go to the bathroom. Don't tell clients you know how they feel, because you don't know exactly how they feel. But do say things like, "I can imagine this must be difficult for you."

7. Describe basic medical terminology and approved abbreviations

Throughout your training, you will learn medical terms that describe specific conditions. For example, the medical term for a runny nose is nasal discharge; a client whose skin is pale or blue is called **cyanotic** (*sye-a-NOT-ik*). When communicating with your clients and their families, use simple, non-medical terms. But when you communicate with members of the health-care team, using medical terminology will help you give more complete information.

Abbreviations are another way to communicate more efficiently with other caregivers. Learn the standard medical abbreviations your agency uses. Use them to report information briefly and accurately. You may also need to know these abbreviations to read your client assignments or care plans. Not all agencies allow the use of abbreviations or use standard abbreviations.

Common Abbreviations

ā	before
abd	abdomen
ac, AC	before meals
ad lib	as desired
am	morning
amb	ambulate
AP	apical pulse
b.i.d., bid	twice daily
BM, B.M.	bowel movement
BP	blood pressure
c̄	with
C	Celsius degree
c/o	complains of
CHF	congestive heart failure
CPR	cardiopulmonary resuscitation
dc	discontinue
dx or DX	diagnosis
F	Fahrenheit degree
FBS	fasting blood sugar
ft	foot
FWB	full weight-bearing
GI	gastrointestinal
H_2O	water
hr.	hour
hs	hours sleep
I&O	intake and output
NKDA	no known drug allergies
NPO	nothing by mouth
NWB	absolutely no weight on leg
O_2	oxygen
OOB	out of bed
OD	right eye
OS	left eye
p	pulse
p̄	after
p.c., pc	after meals

po	by mouth
PRN	as necessary
PWB	partial weight-bearing
q	every
q.i.d., qid	four times a day
qod	every other day
qs	quantity sufficient
R	respirations
ROM	range of motion
s̄	without
SOB	shortness of breath
stat	at once
t.i.d., tid	three times a day
TPR	temperature, pulse, respiration
VS	vital signs
w/c	wheelchair

8. Explain how to give and receive an accurate oral report of a client's status

Home health aides must make brief and accurate oral and written presentations to clients and staff. Reports of a client's status are used in two ways. The first is to report something your supervisor needs to know about immediately. Signs and symptoms that should be reported will be discussed throughout this text. In addition, anything that endangers your client should be reported immediately. Examples include the following:

- falls
- chest pain
- severe headache
- difficulty breathing
- abnormal pulse, respiration, or blood pressure
- change in client's mental status
- sudden weakness or loss of mobility
- high fever
- loss of consciousness
- change in level of consciousness
- bleeding
- change in client's condition
- bruises, abrasions, or other signs of possible abuse

Use oral reports to discuss your experience with a client or family member and your observations of the client's condition and care. These reports should be facts, not opinions.

Even for oral reports, write notes so you do not forget to report any details. You will also have to make a written report later, so you'll need to recall all the facts accurately. Following an oral report, document when, why, about what, and to whom an oral report was given.

Sometimes your supervisor or another member of the healthcare team will give you a brief oral report on one of your clients. Listen carefully and take notes if you need to (Fig. 4-5). Ask about anything that you do not understand. At the end of the conversation, restate what you have been told to make sure you understand. An oral report from another home health aide who knows the client can be very helpful when you are new on a case.

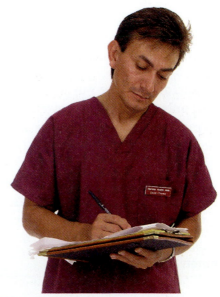

Fig. 4-5. Take notes on oral reports if you need to.

Be careful of misunderstandings when giving or receiving oral reports. If an oral report seems to require a change in your assignment sheet, request that the change be made.

9. Demonstrate how to report and document factual observations in written or oral form

When making any report, you must collect the right kind of information before documenting it. Facts, not opinions, are most useful to your supervisor and the care team. Two kinds of factual information are appropriate in your reporting. **Objective information** is based on what you see, hear, touch, or smell. **Subjective information** is something you cannot or did not observe, but that the client reported to you. An example of objective information is, "The client has lost two pounds." A subjective report of the same situation might be, "Client says he has no appetite." Your supervisor and care team need factual information in order to make decisions about care and treatment. Both objective and subjective reports are valuable.

The information you report should also be **pertinent** (*PER-ti-nent*). Pertinent means significant or useful. For example, "Mrs. Lee had rice for lunch" is factual information. However, it may not be pertinent unless carbohydrates are restricted in her diet. "Mrs. Lee refused to eat lunch" is objective and pertinent information.

In any report, make sure what you observe and what the client reports to you are clearly noted. You are not expected to make diagnoses based on signs and symptoms you observe. Your observations, however, can alert the care team to possible problems. In order to report accurately, observe your clients, their families, and their homes accurately. To observe accurately, use as many senses as possible to gather information (Fig. 4-6). Some examples follow.

Sight: Look for changes in client's appearance. These include rashes, redness, pale-

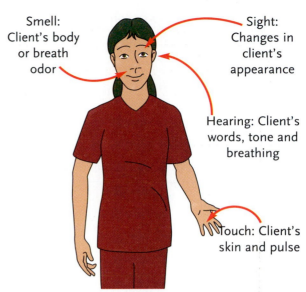

Fig. 4-6. Reporting what you observe means using more than one sense.

ness, swelling, discharge, weakness, sunken eyes, and posture or gait (walking) changes. Look for changes in the home. Does the home appear disorganized or dirty? Is food needed? Do safety hazards exist?

Hearing: Listen to what the client tells you about his or her condition, family, or needs. Is the client speaking clearly and making sense? Does the client show emotions such as anger, frustration, or sadness? Is breathing normal? Does the client wheeze, gasp, or cough? Is the area calm and quiet enough for your client to rest as needed?

Touch: Does your client's skin feel hot or cool, moist or dry? Is pulse rate normal? Use your sense of touch to test bath water and the home's heating or cooling system.

Smell: Do you notice odor from the client's body? Odors could suggest inadequate bathing, infections, or **incontinence** (*in-KON-ti-nens*). Incontinence is the inability to control the bladder or bowels. Breath odor could suggest use of alcohol or tobacco, indigestion, or poor oral care. Odors in the home may suggest housecleaning or repairs are needed. Food odors could indicate spoilage.

Using all your senses will allow you to make the most complete report of a client's situation.

10. Explain why documentation is important and describe how to document visit records and incident reports

Maintaining current documentation means keeping a record of everything you do and observe during a client visit. You and your agency must maintain current documentation for the following reasons:

1. It is the only way to guarantee clear and complete communication between all the members of the care team.

2. Documentation is a legal record of every part of a client's treatment. Medical charts can be used in court as legal evidence.

3. Documentation protects you and your employer from liability by proving what you did on every visit with your client.

Because you may see many clients in the course of a day, you cannot remember everything that each client ate, did, or said. Documentation gives you an up-to-date record of each of your clients' care. You must learn to document accurately. Always take the time to observe and record carefully. Always follow your agency's policies and procedures for documentation. Because documentation is so important, you should never put it off until later.

A medical chart is a legal document. What is written in the chart is considered in court to be what actually happened. If you worked in a client's home for four hours but never documented it, you could not necessarily prove that you actually visited the client. In general, if something does not appear in a client's chart, it did not legally happen. Failing to document your visits with clients could cause very serious legal problems for you and your employer. It could also cause harm to your client. Remember: if you didn't document it, you didn't do it.

Medical charts are confidential. As discussed in chapter 3, it is wrong and illegal to discuss information about your clients. It is important

that you are aware of the legal implications of documentation and that you record all your activities completely.

Employers have specific guidelines for completing written reports of your work. Always follow your employer's guidelines. Below are guidelines for completing two types of reports that most employers require: visit records or notes, and incident reports. **Visit records**, progress notes, or clinical notes, are the notes you make each time you visit a client. These notes serve as a record of your visit and the care you provided. Visit records also document observations of the client's condition, change, or progress (improvement).

GUIDELINES
Completing Visit Records and Incident Reports

- Write your notes immediately after the visit while everything is fresh in your mind. This helps you remember important details.

- Think about what you want to say before writing. Be as brief and as clear as possible.

- Write facts, not opinions. For example, "Client has lost 2 lb. Did not finish lunch," reports facts about the client's condition. It is more useful than "Client is thin and won't eat." When reporting something a client or family member told you, put the words in quotation marks (" "). Document the tasks that you performed, assisted with, or observed the client performing.

- Write as neatly as you can. Use black ink.

- If you make a mistake, draw one line through it and write the correct word or words. Above the crossed-out mistake, write "error" and put your initials and the date (Fig. 4-7). Never erase something you have written. Never use correction fluid.

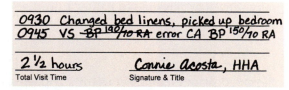

Fig. 4-7. Corrected visit notes.

Sign your full name, and write your title (Home Health Aide, Aide, or HHA). Write the date after each day's visit notes.

Document as specified in the care plan. Some agencies have a "check-off" sheet for documenting care. It is also called an ADL (activities of daily living) sheet (Fig. 4-8).

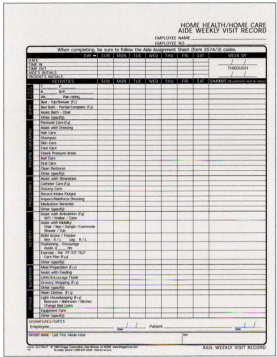

Fig. 4-8. Some agencies use check-off sheets to document care. (Reprinted with permission of Briggs Corporation, Des Moines, Iowa, 800-247-2343)

Incident reports must be completed when an accident or other significant event occurs during a visit. Report the incident as soon as possible. Report it before leaving the client's home. Always check with your supervisor before completing the report. Every agency has its own policies and procedures for incident reporting.

In general, file a report when any of the following incidents occur:

• your client falls

• you or a client break or damage something

• your client or a family member makes a request that is out of your scope of practice

• your client or a family member makes sexual advances or remarks

• anything happens that makes you feel uncomfortable, threatened, or unsafe

• you get injured on the job

• you are exposed to blood or body fluids

An incident report documents events that happen in the home and protects you. For example, if a client drops and breaks a vase and forgets what happened, you might be wrongly blamed. The report provides a written record of anything that happens and describes your part in it. Most agencies use incident reports in place of writing up the accident as a narrative on the visit form. You may be asked to document that you completed an incident report.

11. Demonstrate ability to use verbal and written information to assist with the care plan

You will spend much more time with each of your clients than other members of the care team will. Because of this, you may notice things about your clients that the nurses or doctor cannot know. You will not diagnose or recommend treatment. However, you will have a lot of valuable information about your clients that will help in care planning.

When you attend care planning meetings, do not be afraid to speak up. Share your observations of your clients. If you are not sure what is important to mention, talk to your supervisor before the meeting to find out.

Writing accurate records of your visits is an important contribution to care planning. A thorough written record shows your observations to others and helps you remember details about each client.

12. Demonstrate effective communication on the telephone

You will use the telephone to communicate with your supervisor. Always ask permission before using a client's phone. You may also need

to answer the phone for your clients, and know how to take messages.

When making a call, follow these steps:

1. Always identify yourself before asking to speak to someone. Never ask "Who is this?" when someone answers your call.

2. After you have identified yourself, ask for the person with whom you need to speak.

3. If the person you are calling is available, identify yourself again. State why you are calling. Planning your call before you pick up the phone will help you be as efficient as possible.

4. If the person is not available, ask if you can leave a message. Always leave a brief message, even if it is only to say you called. The message shows that you were trying to reach someone.

5. Leave a brief and clear message. Do not give more information than necessary. A basic message includes your name, the phone number you are calling from, how long you will be at that number, and a brief description of the reason for your call.

6. Thank the person who takes the message for you. Always be polite over the telephone, as you would be in person.

When answering calls for clients, be sensitive to their privacy. Do not ask for more information than the client needs to return the call: a name and phone number is enough. Do not give out any information about your client. Simply say "Mr. Schmidt is not available right now. May I take a message?" Write down the name and phone number of the caller. Tell your client about the call.

Your side of a phone conversation with your supervisor might sound like this:

—*This is Ella Ferguson. I am calling from Mrs. Lee's house. She has a question about her medication and I need to know what to tell her.*

—*Her question is this: She forgot to take her pill this morning when she had breakfast. She wants to know if she should take two now with lunch.*

—*She should take one now and one with a snack around 3:00 p.m.? Okay, I'll tell her. I'll write in my visit notes that you told me to tell her to take one now, and one again with a snack at 3:00. I'll still be here then so I can help her remember.*

—*Thank you for your help, Ms. Crier. Goodbye.*

If you could not reach Ms. Crier, your side of the conversation might go like this:

—*Hello, this is Ella Ferguson calling. Is Ms. Crier there, please?*

—*Could you take a message for me, please?*

—*My name is Ella Ferguson. I'm an aide, and I am at Mrs. Lee's house. The number is 873-9042. I will be here until 4:30 this afternoon. I'm calling because Mrs. Lee has a question about her medication and I need to know how to answer it.*

—*Thank you very much. Goodbye.*

13. Describe cultural diversity and religious differences

Imagine if there were only one restaurant, one place to worship, or one style of clothing or house. It would be very boring. Luckily, in most developed countries, people have many different cultural backgrounds and religious traditions. You will take care of clients with different backgrounds and traditions than your own. Respect and value each person as an individual. Sometimes it is easier to accept different practices or beliefs if you understand a little about them.

There are so many different cultures that they cannot all be listed here. A **culture** is a system of behaviors people learn from the people they grow up and live with. One might talk about American culture being different from Japanese culture. But within American culture there are

thousands of different groups with their own cultures: Japanese-Americans, African-Americans, and Native Americans, to name just a few. Even people from a particular region, state, or city can be said to have a different culture (Fig. 4-9). The culture of the South is not the same as the culture of New York City.

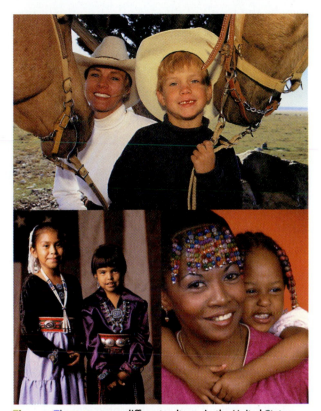

Fig. 4-9. There are many different cultures in the United States.

Cultural background affects how friendly people are to strangers. It can affect how they feel about having you in their houses, or how close they want you to stand to them when talking. Be sensitive to your clients' backgrounds. You cannot expect to be treated the same way by all of your clients. You may have to adjust your behavior around some of your clients. Regardless of their background, you must treat all clients with respect and professionalism. Expect them to treat you respectfully as well.

A resident's primary language may be different from yours. If he or she speaks a different language, an interpreter may be necessary. Take time to learn a few common phrases in a client's native language. Picture cards and flash cards can assist with communication.

Religious differences also influence the way people behave. Religion can be very important in people's lives, particularly when they are ill or dying. You must respect the religious beliefs and practices of your clients, even if they are different from your own. Never question your clients' religious beliefs. Do not discuss your own beliefs with them. Understanding a little bit about common religious groups in America may be useful.

Christianity: Christians believe Jesus Christ was the son of God and that he died so their sins would be forgiven. Christians may be Catholic or Protestant. There are many subgroups or denominations (such as Baptists, Episcopalians, Evangelicals, Lutherans, Methodists, Mormons, or Presbyterians). Christians may go to church on Saturdays or Sundays; read the Bible, including the Old and New Testaments; take communion as a symbol of Christ's sacrifice; and be baptized. Some Christians may try to share their beliefs and convert others to their faith. Religious leaders may be called priests, ministers, pastors, or deacons.

Judaism: Divided into Reform, Conservative and Orthodox movements, Jews believe that God gave them laws through Moses and in the Bible, and that these laws should order their lives. Jewish services are held on Friday evenings and sometimes on Saturdays, in synagogues or temples. Some Jewish men wear a **yarmulke** (*YAR-mul-ke*), or small skullcap, as a sign of their faith. Some Jews observe special dietary restrictions. Jewish people may not do certain things, such as work or drive, on the Sabbath, which lasts from Friday sundown to Saturday sundown. Religious leaders are called **rabbis** (*RAB-eyes*).

Islam (*IS-lahm*): Muslims, or followers of Mohammed, believe that Allah (God) wants people to follow the teachings of the prophet Mohammed in the Koran (*koh-RAN*). Many Muslims pray five times a day facing Mecca, the holy city for their religion. Muslims worship at mosques (*mosks*) and generally do not drink alcohol. There are other dietary restrictions, too.

Other major world religions include Hinduism (*HIN-doo-ism*), practiced in India and elsewhere. Confucianism (*kon-FYOO-shan-ism*) is practiced in China and Japan. Buddhism (*BOO-dism*) started in Asia but has followers in other parts of the world. Native Americans follow many spiritual traditions throughout North America.

14. List examples of cultural and religious differences

In addition to showing respect for different cultural and religious traditions, be aware of specific practices that affect your work. Many religious beliefs include **dietary restrictions**. These are rules about what and when followers can eat. Some examples are listed below.

Many Jewish people eat kosher foods, do not eat pork, and do not eat meat products at the same meal with dairy products. Kosher food is food prepared in accordance with Jewish dietary laws. When you work in a Jewish client's home, you may be asked to separate meat and dairy products. This can include using separate basins to wash dishes, separate pans for cooking, and separate utensils for eating. Respect and follow the client's practices.

Many Muslims do not eat pork or shellfish. They may not drink alcohol. Muslims may have regular periods of fasting. **Fasting** means not eating food or eating very little food. Some Catholics do not eat meat on Fridays. Some people are vegetarians and do not eat any meat for religious or moral reasons. Some people are vegans. **Vegans** do not eat any animals or animal products, such as eggs or dairy products. Be aware of any dietary restrictions. Honor them.

Some people's backgrounds may make them less comfortable being touched by others. Be sensitive to your clients' feelings. You must touch clients to do your job. However, recognize that some clients feel more comfortable when there is little physical contact. Learn about your clients. Adjust your care to their needs.

15. List ways of coping with combative behavior

Clients may sometimes display **combative** (*kom-BA-tiv*), meaning violent or hostile, behavior. Such behavior may include hitting, pushing, kicking, or verbal attacks. Such behavior may be the result of disease affecting the brain. It may also be an expression of frustration. Or it may just be part of someone's personality. In general, combative behavior is not a reaction to you. Do not take it personally.

Always report combative behavior to your supervisor. Document it. Even if you do not find the behavior upsetting, the healthcare team needs to be aware of it.

GUIDELINES
Combative Behavior

g Block physical blows or step out of the way, but never hit back (Fig. 4-10). No matter how much a client hurts you, or how angry or afraid you are, never hit or threaten a client.

g Leave the client alone if you can safely do so. Sometimes getting out of the room for a moment or two will calm everyone down. Call for help if you need to physically restrain someone. If you are afraid, leave the home. Call your supervisor immediately.

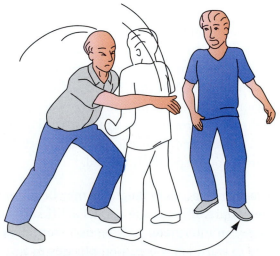

Fig. 4-10. Step out of the way but never hit back.

🄖 Try not respond to verbal attacks. If you must respond, say something like, "I understand that you're angry and frustrated. How can we make things better?"

🄖 Consider what provoked the client. Did you do or say something that upset him or her? Sometimes something as simple as a change in caregiver or routine can be very upsetting to a client. Do not blame yourself. Try to learn from the situation and avoid it in the future.

16. List ways of coping with inappropriate behavior

Inappropriate behavior from a client includes trying to establish a personal, rather than a professional, relationship. Examples include asking personal questions or revealing personal information, requesting visits on personal time, asking for or doing favors, giving tips or gifts, and loaning or borrowing money. It is also inappropriate for a client to ask a home health aide to perform tasks that would not be in the care plan, like scrubbing floors or cleaning the garage. Inappropriate behavior includes making sexual advances and comments. Sexual advances include any sexual words, comments, or behavior that makes you feel uncomfortable.

When clients or family behave inappropriately, report the behavior to your supervisor, even if you think the behavior was harmless. Reporting is the only way to protect yourself. It does not violate the client's privacy.

GUIDELINES
Inappropriate Behavior

🄖 If you think a light approach will work, say something like "I'm sorry, I'm not allowed to do that."

🄖 Address the behavior directly, saying something like, "That makes me very uncomfortable." If the client persists, tell him or her that you will have to leave if the behavior continues.

🄖 Respond to personal questions by saying, "I really can't talk about my personal life on the job." If the client is sharing thoughts or feelings that make you uncomfortable, say "That's not something I can help you with. If you'd like to speak with a social worker I can let the nurse/doctor know."

🄖 Firmly refuse gifts, tips, and favors. Say, "I really can't accept that. It's against the agency's rules."

🄖 Report inappropriate behavior to your supervisor.

While working in people's homes, you may see family interactions that make you feel uncomfortable. This may include fighting or verbal abuse. Report this behavior to your supervisor.

Chapter Review

1. Write out a short sample conversation you might have with a client. Use the three basic steps of communication.

2. Which of the following is an example of nonverbal communication?

   a. telling a joke
   b. laughing at a joke

3. How can you show a client that you are listening and encourage him or her to provide more information?

4. One example of nonverbal communication that may be affected by cultural background is:

   a. making hand motions while talking
   b. use of eye contact
   c. standing far away from the other person
   d. all of the above

5. For each statement, decide whether it is an example of a fact or an opinion. Write "F" for fact and "O" for opinion.

   ____ Mrs. Connelly doesn't eat enough.

   ____ Mr. Moore looked terrible today.

_____ Mr. Gaston had a fever of 100.7.

_____ Ms. Martino needs to make some friends.

_____ Ms. Martino hasn't had a visitor since last week.

_____ The doctor says you have to walk once a day.

6. Why should you sit near a person who has started a conversation with you?

7. What does the abbreviation "ROM" stand for?

8. What does the abbreviation "NPO" stand for?

9. What should you do before giving an oral report to your supervisor?

10. For each of the following, decide whether it is an objective observation or a subjective observation. Write "O" for objective and "S" for subjective.

_____ Client says he is depressed.

_____ Red skin on client's hip.

_____ Client is running a fever.

_____ Client has noisy breathing.

_____ Client complains of chest pain.

_____ Client says she has a toothache.

11. Is it okay to document a client's care a few hours after your visit? Why or why not?

12. If you forget to document an entire visit, did the visit legally happen?

13. Should you use facts or opinions when writing visit notes?

14. Name three situations in which you would file an incident report.

15. What person generally spends more time with the client than other members of the care team?

16. What should you do before using a client's phone?

17. What does the word "culture" mean?

18. You prepared a cheeseburger for Mr. Klein. He tells you that it is not kosher and he won't eat it. How should you respond?

19. How should you respond if a combative client makes you fear for your safety?

20. How would you respond to a client who asks about your personal life?

21. What should you always do after a client behaves inappropriately?

5

Infection Control and Standard Precautions

1. Define asepsis and explain the chain of infection

Asepsis (*ay-SEP-sis*) means sterility, or that no infection is present. It refers to the clean conditions you want to create in your clients' homes. In this chapter you will learn about the importance of preventing infection and how to protect yourself and your clients from disease.

Infections occur when harmful microorganisms (*my-kro-OR-gan-izms*), called **pathogens** (*PATH-oh-gens*), enter the body. To understand how to prevent disease you must first understand how it is spread.

The **chain of infection** is a way of describing how disease is transmitted from one living being to another (Fig. 5-1). Definitions and examples of each of the six links in the chain of infection follow.

Link 1: The **causative agent** is a pathogen or microorganism that causes disease. Examples include bacteria, viruses, fungi, and protozoa.

Link 2: A **reservoir** is a place where the pathogen lives and grows. Examples include the lungs, blood, and large intestine.

Link 3: The **portal of exit** is any body opening on an infected person that allows pathogens to leave, such as the nose, mouth, eyes, or a cut in skin (Fig. 5-2).

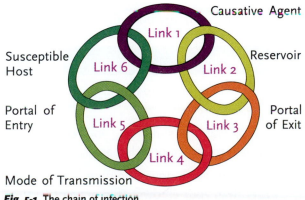

Fig. 5-1. The chain of infection.

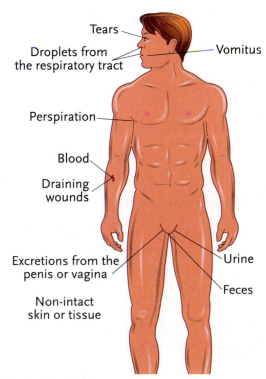

Fig. 5-2. Portals of exit.

Link 4: The **mode of transmission** describes how the pathogen travels from one person to the next person. Transmission can happen through the air or through direct contact or indirect contact.

Link 5: The **portal of entry** is any body opening on an uninfected person that allows pathogens to enter. This can occur through the nose, mouth, eyes, other mucous membranes, a cut in the skin, or dry/cracked skin (Fig. 5-3).

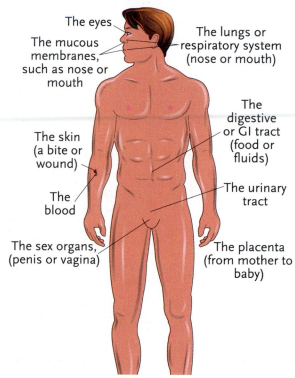

The eyes
The mucous membranes, such as nose or mouth
The lungs or respiratory system (nose or mouth)
The digestive or GI tract (food or fluids)
The skin (a bite or wound)
The blood
The urinary tract
The sex organs, (penis or vagina)
The placenta (from mother to baby)

Fig. 5-3. Portals of entry.

Link 6: A **susceptible host** is an uninfected person who could get sick. Examples include all healthcare workers and anyone in their care who is not already infected with that particular disease.

If one of the links in the chain of infection is broken, then the spread of infection is stopped. By using infection control practices, you can help stop the pathogens from traveling (Link 4), and getting on your hands, nose, eyes, mouth, skin, etc. (Link 5). You can also reduce your own chances of getting sick by having immunizations (Link 6) for diseases such as hepatitis B and influenza.

Transmission of most **infectious** (*in-FEKT-shus*) or contagious diseases can be prevented by always taking a few simple precautions. Washing your hands is an important and easy way to greatly reduce the spread of infection. All caregivers should wash their hands frequently. Practicing what you learn when caring for clients offers the best protection from infection—for everyone.

2. Identify when to wash hands

Washing your hands is the single most important thing you can do to prevent the spread of disease to yourself and others.

You should wash your hands

- when arriving at a client's home
- before and after touching a client
- before and after making meals or working in the kitchen
- before and after you eat
- before feeding a client
- after using the restroom
- after touching any item used by or for a client
- before leaving a client's home
- before reaching into the clean area of your supply bag
- before putting on gloves
- after removing your gloves or any type of personal protection equipment (PPE)
- after touching a surface that may be contaminated with any body fluid

Washing hands

Equipment: bar or liquid soap provided by your employer, paper towels

1. Turn on water at sink. Keep your clothes dry, because moisture breeds bacteria.

2. Angle your arms down, holding your hands lower than your elbows. This prevents water

from running up your arm. Wet hands and wrists thoroughly (Fig. 5-4).

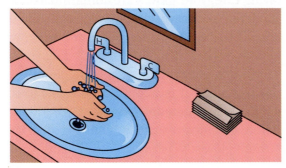

Fig. 5-4.

3. Use a generous amount of soap. Rub hands together and fingers between each other to create a lather. Lather all surfaces of fingers and hands, including above the wrists, producing friction, for at least 10 seconds. Friction helps clean (Fig. 5-5).

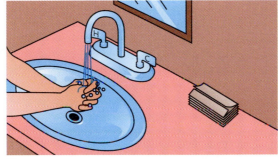

Fig. 5-5.

4. Clean your nails by pushing soap under your fingernails and cuticles with a brush or by rubbing them in the palm of your hand (Fig. 5-6).

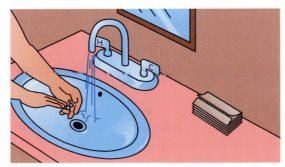

Fig. 5-6.

5. Being careful not to touch the sink, rinse thoroughly under running water. Rinse from just above the wrists down to fingertips. Do not run water over unwashed arms down to clean hands (Fig. 5-7).

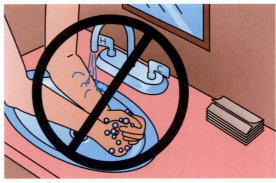

Fig. 5-7.

6. Use a clean, dry paper towel to dry from tips of fingers up to clean wrists. Do not wipe towel on unwashed forearms and then wipe clean hands. Dispose of towel without touching waste container. If your hands touch the sink or waste container, start over.

7. Use a clean, dry paper towel to turn off the faucet without contaminating your hands (Fig. 5-8). Properly discard towel.

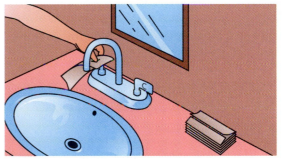

Fig. 5-8.

3. Identify when to wear gloves

You must wear gloves when there is a chance you might come into contact with body fluids, open wounds, or **mucous** (*MYOO-kus*) **membranes**. Mucous membranes are the membranes that line body cavities such as the mouth or nose. Your agency will have specific policies and procedures on when to wear gloves. Learn and follow these rules. Always wear gloves for the following tasks:

*   anytime you might touch blood or any body fluid, including vomitus, urine, feces, or saliva

*   performing or assisting with mouth care or care of any mucous membrane

5

Infection Control and Standard Precautions

- performing or assisting with care of the **perineal** (payr-i-NEE-al) area (the area between the anus and the genitals)

- performing personal care on a client whose skin is broken by abrasions, cuts, rash, acne, pimples, or boils

- assisting with a client's personal care when you have open sores or cuts on your hands

- shaving a client

- disposing of soiled bed linens, gowns, dressings, and pads

If you have cuts or sores on your hands, first cover these areas with bandages or gauze and then put on gloves. Disposable gloves are to be worn only once. They may not be washed or disinfected for reuse. Replace disposable gloves as soon as they are torn. Wash hands before putting on fresh gloves. Some people develop allergies to latex gloves. If you notice a reaction, contact your supervisor immediately. Your employer will provide you with a kind of glove you can wear.

Putting on gloves

1. Wash your hands.

2. If you are right-handed, slide one glove on your left hand (reverse if left-handed).

3. With gloved hand, take second glove and slide the other hand into the glove.

4. Interlace fingers to smooth out folds and create a comfortable fit.

5. Carefully look for tears, holes, or discolored spots. Replace the glove if necessary.

6. If wearing a gown, pull the cuff of the gloves over the sleeve of the gown (Fig. 5-9).

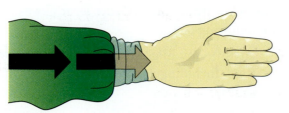

Fig. 5-9.

Remember you are wearing gloves to protect your skin from becoming contaminated. After giving care, your gloves are contaminated. If you open a door with the gloved hand, the doorknob becomes contaminated. Later, when you open the door with an ungloved hand, you will be infected even though you wore gloves during the procedure. It is a common mistake to contaminate the room around you. Do not do it. Before touching a surface, such as a doorknob, remove gloves. Wash your hands. Afterward, put on new gloves if necessary.

Taking off gloves

1. Touching only the outside of one glove, pull the first glove off by pulling down from the cuff (Fig. 5-10).

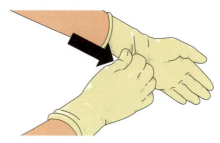

Fig. 5-10.

2. As the glove comes off your hand, it should be turned inside out.

3. With the fingertips of your gloved hand, hold the glove you just removed. With your ungloved hand, reach two fingers inside the remaining glove, being careful not to touch any part of the outside of glove (Fig. 5-11).

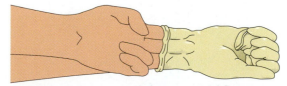

Fig. 5-11.

4. Pull down, turning this glove inside out and over the first glove as you remove it.

5. You should now be holding one glove from its clean inner side and the other glove should be inside it.

6. Drop both gloves into the proper container.

7. Wash your hands.

4. Identify when to use personal protective equipment (PPE)

Personal protective equipment (PPE) includes gowns, masks, and eye shields (goggles), as well as gloves. Your employer will provide you with PPE as necessary for your client assignments. The guidelines for wearing PPE are the same as for gloves. You should wear PPE if there is a chance you could come into contact with body fluids, mucous membranes, or open wounds. Masks and eye shields are worn when splashing of body fluids or blood could occur. Masks should also be worn when caring for clients with respiratory illnesses. With some of your clients or for some types of care, this might mean you wear PPE all the time. If you are unsure of the risk, don't take any chances: wear PPE (Fig. 5-12).

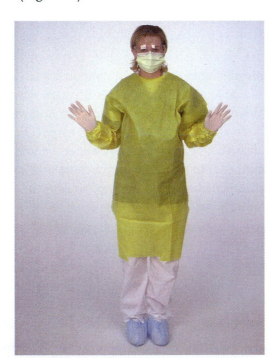

Fig. 5-12. Dress for the occasion!

Putting on a gown

1. Wash your hands.
2. Open gown. Hold out in front of you and allow gown to open (Fig. 5-13). Do not shake it. Slip your arms into the sleeves and pull the gown on.

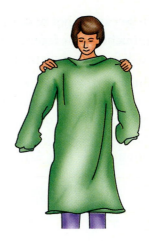

Fig. 5-13.

3. Tie the neck ties into a bow so they can be easily untied later.
4. Reaching behind you, pull the gown until it completely covers your clothes. Tie the back ties (Fig. 5-14).

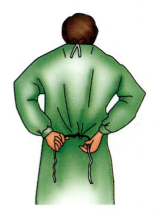

Fig. 5-14.

5. Remember, use a gown only once and then remove and discard it. When removing a gown, roll the dirty side in and away from the body. If your gown ever becomes wet or soiled, remove it. Check your clothing, and put on a new gown. The Occupational Safety and Health Administration (OSHA) requires non-permeable gowns—gowns that liquids cannot penetrate—when working in a bloody situation.
6. Put on gloves after putting on gown.

Putting on mask and eye shield

1. Wash your hands.
2. Pick up mask by the top strings or the elas-

5

Infection Control and Standard Precautions

tic strap. Be careful not to touch the mask where it touches your face. Do not wear the same mask from one client to another.

3. Adjust the mask over your nose and mouth. Tie top strings first, then bottom strings. Masks must always be dry or they must be replaced. Never wear a mask hanging from only the bottom tie (Fig. 5-15).

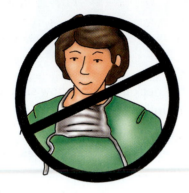

Fig. 5-15.

4. Put on eye shield.

5. Put on gloves after mask and eye shield.

When applying PPE, remember this order:

1. Apply mask and eye shield.

2. Apply gown.

3. Apply gloves last.

When removing PPE, remember this order:

1. Remove gloves.

2. Remove gown.

3. Remove mask and eye shield.

5. Explain how to handle spills

Spills, especially those involving blood, body fluids, or glass, can pose a serious risk of infection. Clean spills using proper equipment and procedure.

GUIDELINES
Cleaning Spills Involving Blood, Body Fluids, or Glass

🄶 When blood or body fluids are spilled, put on gloves before starting to clean up the spill. In some cases, industrial-strength

gloves are best because they won't tear if you are handling glass.

🄶 When glass has been broken, do not pick up any pieces, no matter how large, with your hands. Use a dustpan and broom or other tools.

🄶 If blood or body fluids are spilled on a hard surface such as a linoleum floor or countertop, clean immediately using a solution of one part household bleach to ten parts water. You can mix the solution in a bucket and, with gloves on, wipe up the spill with rags or paper towels dipped in the solution. Or, mix the solution in a plastic spray bottle and spray the spill before wiping. Be careful not to spill bleach or bleach solution on clothes, carpets, or bedding. It can discolor and damage fabrics. Your employer may provide commercial sprays for cleaning spills.

🄶 If blood or body fluids are spilled on fabrics such as carpets, bedding, or clothes, do not use bleach to clean the spill. Commercial disinfectants that do not contain bleach are available. If you have no disinfectant, wear gloves and wipe spills using soap and water. Then clean carpet with regular carpet cleaner. Use gloves to load soiled bedding or clothes into the washing machine and add color-safe bleach to the washer with the laundry detergent.

🄶 Waste containing broken glass, blood, or body fluids should be properly bagged. Put the waste in one trash bag and close it properly. Then put the first bag inside a second, clean trash bag and close it. This is called **double-bagging**. Waste containing blood or body fluids may need to be placed in a special biohazard waste bag and disposed of separately from household trash. Follow your agency's policy.

6. Explain and follow Standard Precautions

State and federal government agencies have guidelines and laws concerning infection control. The **Occupational Safety and Health**

Administration (OSHA) is a federal government agency that makes rules to protect workers from hazards on the job. The **Centers for Disease Control and Prevention** (CDC) issues guidelines on protecting and improving our health.

In 1996, the CDC recommended a comprehensive new infection control system for reducing the risk of contracting infectious diseases. There are two tiers of precautions within this system: Standard Precautions and Transmission-Based Precautions.

Following **Standard Precautions** means treating all blood, body fluids, non-intact skin (like abrasions, pimples, or open sores), and mucous membranes (openings of eyes, mouth, nose, rectum, or genitals) as if they were infected with an infectious disease. Following Standard Precautions is the only safe way of performing your job. You cannot tell by looking at your clients or their charts whether they are infected with a contagious disease such as HIV, hepatitis, or influenza.

Under Standard Precautions, "body fluids" include saliva, sputum (fluid coughed up), urine, feces, semen, vaginal secretions, and pus or other wound drainage. It does not include sweat.

Standard Precautions and Transmission-Based Precautions provide a way to stop the spread of infection by interrupting the mode of transmission. In other words, these guidelines do not stop an infected person from giving off pathogens (germs). However, by following these guidelines you help prevent those pathogens from infecting you or other persons in your care.

1. **Always** practice Standard Precautions with every single person in your care.

2. Transmission-Based Precautions vary based on how an infection is transmitted. These precautions are used **in addition** to the Standard Precautions. You will learn more about these precautions later in this chapter.

Standard precautions include the measures listed below.

- **Wear gloves** if you may come into contact with the following: blood; any body fluids or secretions; broken skin (including abrasions, acne, cuts, stitches or staples, and pinpricks); or mucous membranes (such as the linings of the mouth, nose, eyes, vagina, rectum, and penis). In the home, such situations may include mouth care, bathroom assistance, perineal care, assistance with a bedpan or urinal, ostomy care, cleaning up spills, cleansing basins, urinals, bedpans, and other containers that have held body fluids; and disposing of wastes.

- **Wash your hands** before putting on gloves. Wash your hands immediately after removing your gloves.

- **Remove gloves** immediately when finished with a procedure.

- **Immediately wash all skin surfaces that have been contaminated** with blood and body fluids.

- **Wear a disposable gown** if you may come into contact with blood or body fluids. If your client has a contagious illness, you should wear a gown even if it is not likely you will come into contact with blood or body fluids.

- **Wear a mask and protective goggles** if the possibility exists that you will come into contact with splashing blood or body fluids (for example, emptying a bed pan).

- **Wear gloves and use caution when handling razor blades and other sharp objects**. Discard these objects carefully in a puncture-resistant biohazard container.

- **Avoid nicks and cuts** when shaving clients.

- **Carefully bag all contaminated supplies.** Dispose of them according to your agency's policy.

- **Clearly label body fluids that are being saved for a specimen** with the client's name and a biohazard label. Keep in a container with a lid.

- **Never handle a client's needles or syringes**. Never attempt to put a cap on a needle or syringe. Request that the client dispose of them in a hard, plastic biohazardous waste container. (Fig. 5-16).

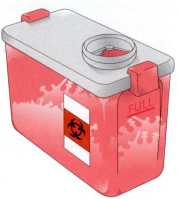

Fig. 5-16. One type of biohazardous waste container.

- **Contaminated wastes should be disposed of** according to your agency's procedure.

- **Waste containing blood or body fluids** is considered biohazardous waste. It should be disposed of separately from household garbage. Your agency will have a policy on how to dispose of biohazardous waste.

7. Explain guidelines of care for clients with infectious diseases

Caring for persons who are infected or suspected of being infected with a disease requires **additional** precautions beyond the Standard Precautions. These precautions are called Transmission-Based or isolation precautions. To **isolate** means to keep something separate, or by itself.

These precautions will always be listed in the client's care plan and on your assignment sheet. It is for your safety and the safety of family members that these precautions must be followed.

The three categories of Transmission-Based Precautions are

- Airborne Precautions

- Droplet Precautions

- Contact Precautions

The category used depends on the disease and how it spreads to other people. They may also be used in combination for diseases that have multiple routes of transmission.

Airborne precautions are used for diseases that can be transmitted or spread through the air after being expelled by the client (Fig. 5-17). The pathogens are so small that they can attach to moisture in the air and remain floating for some time. For certain care procedures you may be required to wear a special mask, such as N95 or HEPA masks, to avoid being infected. Airborne diseases include tuberculosis, measles, and chicken pox. More information on tuberculosis is found later in this chapter.

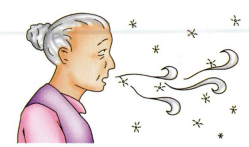

Fig. 5-17. Airborne diseases stay suspended in the air.

Droplet precautions are used when the disease-causing microorganism does not stay suspended in the air and usually travels only short distances after being expelled. Droplets can be generated by coughing, sneezing, laughing, or talking (Fig. 5-18). Droplet precautions can include wearing a face mask during care procedures and restricting visits from uninfected people. Cover your nose and mouth with a tissue when you sneeze or cough and ask clients, family, and others to do the same. If you sneeze on your hands, wash them promptly. Always follow your agency's procedures and the client's care plan.

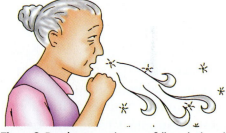

Fig. 5-18. Droplet precautions are followed when the disease-causing microorganism does not stay suspended in the air.

Contact precautions are used when the client is at risk of transmitting or contracting a microorganism from touching an infected object or person (Fig. 5-19). For example, bacteria could infect an open skin wound. Lice, scabies (a skin disease that causes itching), and conjunctivitis (pink eye) are other examples. Transmission can occur with skin-to-skin contact during transfers or bathing.

Precautions include personal protective equipment and client isolation. Contact precautions require washing hands with antimicrobial soap, and not touching infected surfaces with ungloved hands or uninfected surfaces with contaminated gloves.

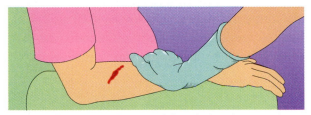

Fig. 5-19. Contact precautions are followed when the person is at risk of transmitting or getting a microorganism from touching an infected object or person.

Two important points to remember about isolation precautions are

1. Isolation precautions are always used **in addition** to Standard Precautions.

2. The client must be reassured that it is the disease, not the person with the disease, that is being isolated. Communicate with your client. Explain why these special steps are being taken.

GUIDELINES
Isolation Procedures

- Serve food using disposable dishes and utensils that are discarded in specially marked bags and stored in covered garbage containers. When items cannot be discarded, they must be washed thoroughly in very hot water with detergent and bleach. Family members should use separate dishes and utensils.

- Wear disposable gloves when handling soiled laundry. Bag laundry in the client's

room and carry it to the laundry area in the bag. Wash the client's laundry separately. Use hot water and detergent.

- A solution of bleach and water (1:10) should be mixed in a clearly labeled, plastic spray bottle and stored in a safe place. The bleach solution can be used to clean up spills of blood or body fluids and to disinfect surfaces that may have been contaminated.

- A client in contact or airborne isolation should use a separate bathroom if possible. If the client uses the same bathroom as others, disinfect it after each use by the client.

8. Explain sterilization and disinfection

Measures like sterilization and disinfection are used to decrease the spread of pathogens and disease. **Sterilization** means all microorganisms are destroyed, not just pathogens. **Disinfection** means that only pathogens are destroyed. However, disinfection does not destroy all pathogens.

In home care, you may disinfect items used by the client. You will also disinfect some areas while doing housekeeping tasks. The care plan and your assignments will specify what disinfection you need to do. General methods of disinfection are by wet and dry heat and by chemicals. Wet heat disinfection uses boiling water to disinfect. Dry heat disinfection means baking in the oven. See chapter 21 for information on household chemical disinfecting solutions. The method used depends on the type of item that needs to be disinfected. Your agency will have policies and procedures for disinfection in the home.

Disinfecting using wet heat

Equipment: items to be disinfected, clean pot with enough room to hold items, clean lid for pot, cold water, timer or clock, stove, potholders

1. Wash your hands.

2. Place items in the pot and fill it with water. Make sure water covers all items, leaving

enough room at the top for steam to escape.

3. Place lid on pot and place covered pot on burner on stove.

4. Turn on heat and bring water to a boil. Do not open the lid at any time during boiling.

5. Boil for 20 minutes. You should see steam escaping from the sides of the pot.

6. Turn off heat. Allow items and water to cool.

7. After items have cooled, remove the cover with the potholders.

8. Remove the items. Place on a rack or a clean towel to air dry.

9. Wash and dry the disinfecting equipment. Return to proper storage.

10. Wash your hands.

11. Document the procedure.

Disinfecting using dry heat

Equipment: items to be disinfected, clean metal pan (cookie sheet, cake pan, etc.), timer or clock, oven, potholders

1. Wash your hands.

2. Place items in the pan.

3. Place sheet or cake pan in the oven.

4. Turn on oven to 350° F. Bake for one hour. Keep oven door closed while items are baking.

5. Turn off heat. Allow items to cool.

6. After items have cooled, remove with the potholders.

7. Store the items.

8. Wash and dry the disinfecting equipment. Return to proper storage.

9. Wash your hands.

10. Document the procedure.

9. Explain how bloodborne diseases are transmitted

Microorganisms carried in blood transmit bloodborne diseases. These microorganisms may also be present in body fluids, non-intact skin (such as open sores or acne), and mucous membranes.

Bloodborne diseases can be transmitted by infected blood entering your bloodstream, or if infected semen or vaginal secretions contact your mucous membranes. Mucous membranes include the linings of the vagina, penis, rectum, nose, and mouth. You can become infected with a bloodborne disease by having sexual contact with someone carrying that disease. It is not necessary to have sexual intercourse to transmit disease. Other kinds of sexual activity can just as easily cause infection. Using a needle to inject drugs and sharing needles with others can also transmit bloodborne diseases. In addition, infected mothers may transmit bloodborne diseases to their babies in the womb or during birth.

In healthcare, contact with infected blood or body fluids is the most common way to be infected with a bloodborne disease. Standard Precautions, handwashing, isolation, and using PPE are all methods of preventing transmission of bloodborne diseases. Employers are required by law to help prevent exposure to bloodborne pathogens. Understand and follow Standard Precautions and other procedures to protect yourself from bloodborne diseases.

Remember that you can safely touch, hug, and spend time talking with clients who have a bloodborne disease. They need the same thoughtful, personal attention you give to all your clients. Follow Standard Precautions but never isolate a client emotionally because he or she has a bloodborne disease.

10. Explain the basic facts regarding HIV and hepatitis infection

The major bloodborne diseases in the United States are HIV/AIDS and **hepatitis** (*hep-a-TYE-tis*). HIV stands for **human immunodeficiency** (*im-yoo-no-de-FISH-en-see*) **virus**. HIV weakens the immune system so that people cannot effec-

tively fight infections. After a number of years, a person with HIV usually develops acquired immune deficiency syndrome (AIDS). People with AIDS lose all ability to fight infection and can die from illnesses that a healthy body could handle.

Hepatitis refers to swelling (-itis) of the liver (hepa-) caused by infection. Liver function can be permanently damaged by hepatitis, which can lead to other chronic, life-long illnesses. Several different viruses can cause hepatitis. The most common types of hepatitis are A, B, and C. Hepatitis B and C are bloodborne diseases that can cause death. Many more people have hepatitis B (HBV) than HIV. The risk of acquiring hepatitis is greater than the risk of acquiring HIV. HBV poses a serious threat to healthcare workers. Your employer must offer you a free vaccine to protect you from hepatitis B. There is no vaccine for hepatitis C.

11. Identify high risk behaviors that allow the spread of HIV/AIDS and HBV

Behaviors that put people at high risk for HIV/AIDS or HBV infection include

- Sharing drug needles
- Having unprotected sex (not using latex condoms during sexual contact)
- Having sexual contact with many partners
- Engaging in any sexual activity that involves exchange of body fluids with a partner who has not tested negative for HIV or who has had many sexual partners. Be aware that it may take six months after coming into contact with the virus for an HIV test to show positive results.

Ways to protect against the spread of HIV and AIDS include

- Never share needles for injections of any type of drug.
- Practice safer sex by using latex condoms during sexual contact.

- Stay in a monogamous relationship with a partner who has tested negative for HIV. Being monogamous means having only one sexual partner.

- Practice abstinence. Abstinence means not having sexual contact with anyone.

- Get tested if you think you may have been infected with HIV. It can take up to six months from the time you become infected with HIV for the antibodies to be detected in your blood. Get re-tested periodically if necessary. It is especially important that pregnant women get tested.

- Follow Standard Precautions at work to protect yourself.

12. Demonstrate knowledge of the legal aspects of AIDS, including testing

The right to confidentiality is especially important to people with HIV/AIDS because others may pass judgment on people with this disease. A person with HIV/AIDS cannot be fired from a job because of the disease. However, a healthcare worker with HIV/AIDS may be reassigned to job duties with a lower risk of transmitting the disease.

HIV testing requires consent. That means no one can test you for HIV unless you agree. HIV test results are confidential and cannot be shared with a person's family, friends, or employer without his or her consent. If you are HIV-positive, you might want to confide in your supervisor so your assignments can be adjusted to avoid putting you at high risk for exposure to other infections. Everyone has a right to privacy regarding their health status. Never discuss a client's status with anyone.

13. Identify community resources and services available to clients with HIV/AIDS

Depending on the community, many resources

and services may be available for people with HIV/AIDS. These may include counseling, meal services, access to experimental drugs and any number of other services. Look in the phone book or on the Internet for resources available in your area. Speak to your supervisor if you feel a client with HIV/AIDS needs more help. A social worker or another member of the care team may be able to coordinate services for clients with HIV/AIDS.

14. Explain tuberculosis and list infection control guidelines

Tuberculosis (*too-ber-kyoo-LOH-sis*), or TB, is an airborne disease carried on mucous droplets suspended in the air. When a person infected with TB talks, coughs, breathes, or sings, he or she may release mucous droplets carrying the disease. TB usually infects the lungs, causing coughing, difficulty breathing, fever, and fatigue. If left untreated, TB may cause death.

There are two types of TB. **TB infection**, also called **latent TB**, and **TB disease**, also called **active TB**. Someone with TB infection carries the disease but does not show symptoms and cannot infect others. A person with active TB, or TB disease, shows symptoms of the disease and can spread TB to others. TB infection can progress to TB disease. The signs and symptoms of TB include the following:

- fatigue
- loss of appetite
- weight loss
- slight fever and chills
- night sweats
- prolonged coughing
- coughing up blood
- chest pain
- shortness of breath
- difficulty breathing

Tuberculosis is more likely to be spread in small, confined, or poorly ventilated places. TB disease is more likely to develop in people whose immune systems are weakened by illness, malnutrition, alcoholism or drug abuse. People with cancer and people with HIV/AIDS are especially susceptible to developing TB disease when exposed. This is due to their weakened immune systems.

GUIDELINES

Infection Control for Clients with Known or Suspected TB

g Follow Standard Precautions and airborne precautions.

g Wear a mask and gown during client care. Special masks, such as N95 or high efficiency particulate air (HEPA) masks, may be needed (Fig. 5-20). These masks filter out very small particles, such as the germs that cause TB.

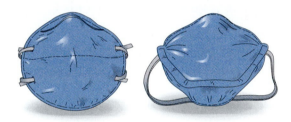

Fig. 5-20. a. N-95 respirator mask and b. PFR-95 respirator mask.

g Use special care when handling sputum or phlegm.

g Ensure proper ventilation in the client's room. Open windows when possible.

g Follow isolation procedures for airborne diseases if indicated in the care plan.

g Help the client remember to take all medication prescribed. Failure to take all medication is a major factor in the spread of TB.

15. Explain the importance of reporting a possible exposure to an airborne or bloodborne disease

If you think you may have been exposed to TB, HIV/AIDS, or hepatitis at work, report this to your supervisor immediately. Fill out an incident report or a special exposure report form.

Your employer will help you find out if you have been infected and take steps to prevent you from becoming sick. In order to protect your health and the health of your family members and other clients, report any potential exposures right away. Steps will also be taken to help prevent similar incidents from occurring again. Depending on the exposure, your agency may require tests and other measures to keep you healthy.

16. Explain the terms MRSA and VRE

MRSA is **methicillin** (*meth-i-SILL-in*)-**resistant Staphylococcus** (*staff-il-oh-KAH-kus*) **aureus**. In the past, the most serious bacterial infections were treated with a certain type of antibiotic related to penicillin. Treatment of these infections has become more difficult because bacteria have become resistant to various antibiotics. This includes the commonly used penicillin-related antibiotics and cephalosporins. These resistant bacteria are called MRSA.

MRSA can spread among people having close contact with infected people. MRSA is almost always spread by direct physical contact, and not through the air. This means that if a person has MRSA on his skin, especially on the hands, and touches another person, he may spread MRSA. Spread also occurs through indirect contact by touching objects (for example, towels, sheets, wound dressings, clothes) contaminated by the infected skin of a person with MRSA.

You can prevent MRSA by practicing good hygiene. Handwashing, using soap and warm water, is the single most important measure to control the spread of MRSA. Keep cuts and abrasions clean and covered with a proper dressing (e.g., bandage) until healed. Avoid contact with other people's wounds or material contaminated from wounds.

VRE is **vancomycin** (*van-co-MY-a-sin*)-**resistant enterococcus** (*en-ter-oh-KAH-kus*). Enterococcus are bacteria that live in the digestive and genital tracts. They normally do not cause any problems in healthy people. Vancomycin is a powerful antibiotic that is often the antibiotic of last resort. It is generally limited to use against bacteria that are already resistant to penicillin and other antibiotics. Vancomycin-resistant enterococcus is a mutant strain of enterococcus that originally developed in individuals who were exposed to the antibiotic.

VRE is dangerous because it cannot be controlled with antibiotics. It causes life-threatening infections in people with compromised immune systems—the very young, the very old, and the very ill.

VRE is spread through direct and indirect contact. Once VRE establishes itself, it is very difficult to get rid of. Preventing VRE is much easier. You can help prevent its spread by washing your hands often. Handwashing is very important in stopping the spread of VRE. Wear PPE as directed. Disinfect items according to the care plan.

17. List employer and employee responsibilities for infection control

Several state and federal government agencies have guidelines and laws concerning infection control. OSHA requires employers to provide for the safety of their employees through rules and suggested guidelines. The Centers for Disease Control and Prevention issues guidelines for healthcare workers to follow on the job. Some states have additional requirements. Home health agencies consider these rules very carefully when writing their policies and procedures. It is very important that you learn these and follow them. They exist to protect you. Some of the infection control requirements for you and your employer are listed below.

Employer's responsibilities for infection control include the following:

1. Establish infection control procedures and an exposure control plan to protect workers.

2. Provide continuing in-service education on infection control, including education on bloodborne and airborne pathogens.

3. Have written procedures to follow should an exposure occur, including medical treatment and plans to prevent any similar exposures.

4. Provide personal protective equipment for employees to use and teach them when and how to properly use it.

5. Provide free hepatitis B vaccinations for all "at-risk employees." (As a home health aide, you are considered at risk.)

Employee's responsibilities for infection control include the following:

1. Follow Standard Precautions.

2. Follow all agency policies and procedures.

3. Follow client care plans and assignments.

4. Use provided personal protective equipment as indicated or appropriate.

5. Take advantage of the free hepatitis B vaccination.

6. Immediately report any exposure you have to infection, blood, or body fluids.

7. Participate in annual education programs covering the control of infection.

Chapter Review

1. What does "asepsis" mean?

2. Wearing gloves breaks which link(s) in the chain of infection and why?

3. What is the single most important thing you can do to prevent the spread of disease?

4. How many times can disposable gloves be worn?

5. List two situations in which you should wear a mask.

6. In what order should PPE be applied? In what order should it be removed?

7. Kelley, a home health aide, is helping her client, Mrs. McClain, prepare dinner. Mrs. McClain wants to use her large glass bowl for the salad she is making. As she takes it down from the cabinet, she loses her grip and the bowl crashes to the floor. Kelley calmly and gently leads a visibly upset Mrs. McClain to the living room. Kelley returns to clean up the mess before continuing with dinner. She stoops to pick up the large broken pieces. She notices a trickle of blood and thinks that Mrs. McClain probably cut her hand. She wipes it up with a sponge. When finished, she takes the large pile of glass and throws it into the nearest trash can. She then goes back to cooking dinner.

Did Kelley follow the proper procedure? If not, what should Kelley have done?

8. Under Standard Precautions what does the phrase "body fluids" include?

9. On whom should Standard Precautions be practiced?

10. What are Transmission-Based or isolation precautions?

11. How should you handle a client's needles?

12. When should you wear gloves?

13. Which precautions are used when a disease can be transmitted or spread through the air after being expelled by the client?

14. Which precautions are used when the disease-causing microorganism does not stay suspended in the air and usually travels only short distances after being expelled?

15. Which precautions are used when the client is at risk of transmitting or contracting a microorganism from touching an infected object or person?

16. When serving food to an infectious client using dishes and utensils that cannot be discarded, what should you do?

17. How would you disinfect using wet heat? How would you disinfect using dry heat?

18. How are bloodborne diseases transmitted? What is the most common way to be infected with a bloodborne disease in the healthcare setting?

19. Name three ways of preventing transmission of a bloodborne disease.

20. What is hepatitis?

21. What does HIV do to a person's immune system?

22. List four ways to protect against the spread of HIV/AIDS.

23. Why is confidentiality especially important to people with HIV/AIDS?

24. What types of resources may be available to clients with HIV/AIDS?

25. What is the difference between TB infection and TB disease?

26. TB is more likely to develop in which people?

27. In what kind of setting is TB most likely to spread?

28. List four guidelines you should follow when caring for clients with known or suspected TB.

29. What is the first thing you should do if you suspect you have been exposed to TB, HIV/AIDS or hepatitis at work?

30. What is one of the best ways you can prevent the spread of MRSA and VRE?

31. List three employer's responsibilities for infection control.

32. List three employee's responsibilities for infection control.

6

Safety and Body Mechanics

1. Explain the principles of body mechanics

Body mechanics is the way the parts of the body work together whenever you move. Good body mechanics help save energy and prevent injury. Good body mechanics helps you push, pull, and lift objects or people who are not able to fully support or move their own bodies. Understanding some basic principles of body mechanics will help you.

Alignment: Alignment is based on the word "line." When you stand up straight, a vertical line could be drawn right through the center of your body and your center of gravity (Fig. 6-1). When the line is straight, the body is in alignment. Whether standing, sitting or lying down, you should try to have your body in alignment. This means that the two sides of the body are mirror images of each other, with body parts lined up naturally. Maintain correct body alignment when lifting or carrying an object by keeping the object close to your body. Point your feet and body in the direction you are moving. Avoid twisting at the waist.

Base of support: The base of support is the foundation that supports an object. The feet are the body's base of support. The wider your support, the more stable you are. Standing with legs apart allows for a greater base of support.

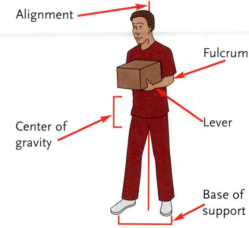

Fig. 6-1. Proper body alignment is important when standing and sitting.

Fulcrum and lever: A **lever** moves an object by resting on a base of support, called a fulcrum. Think of a seesaw on the playground. The flat board you sit on is the lever. The triangular base the board rests on is the fulcrum. When two children sit on opposite sides of the seesaw, they easily move each other up and down. They can do this because the fulcrum and lever of the seesaw are actually doing the work.

If you think of your body as a set of fulcrums and levers, you can find smart ways to lift without working as hard. Think of your arm as a lever with the elbow as the fulcrum. When you lift something, resting it against your forearm will shorten the lever and make it easier to lift than holding it in your hands (Fig. 6-2).

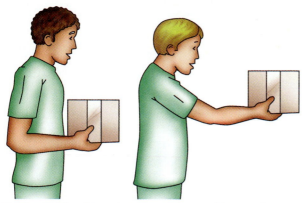

Fig. 6-2. Holding things close to you moves weight toward your center of gravity. In this illustration, whose arms will tire first?

Center of gravity: The center of gravity in your body is the point where the most weight is concentrated. This point will depend on the position the body is in. When you stand, your weight is centered in your pelvis. A low center of gravity gives a more stable base of support (Fig 6-3). Bending your knees when lifting an object lowers your pelvis and, therefore, lowers your center of gravity. This gives you more stability and makes you less likely to fall or strain the working muscles.

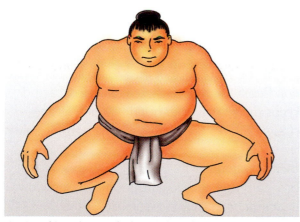

Fig. 6-3. This sumo wrestler knows that taking a wide stance and lowering his center of gravity make him much harder to knock over.

2. Apply principles of body mechanics to your daily activities

By applying the principles of body mechanics to your daily activities, you can avoid injury and use less energy. Some examples of applying good body mechanics include the following:

Lifting a heavy object from the floor. Spread your feet shoulder-width apart and bend your knees. Using the strong, large muscles in your thighs, upper arms, and shoulders, lift the object. Pull it close to your body, to a point level with your pelvis. By doing this you are keeping the object close to your center of gravity and base of support. When you stand up, push with your strong hip and thigh muscles to raise your body and the object together (Fig. 6-4).

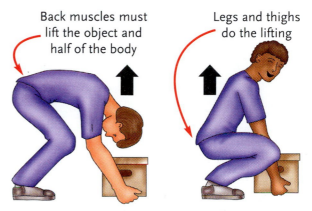

Back muscles must lift the object and half of the body

Legs and thighs do the lifting

Fig. 6-4. In this illustration, which person is lifting correctly?

Do not twist when you are moving an object. Always face the object or person you are moving. Pivot your feet instead of twisting at the waist.

Helping a client sit up, stand up, or walk. Whenever you support a client's weight, protect yourself by assuming a good stance. Place your feet twelve inches, or hip-width apart, one foot in front of the other, and knees bent. Your upper body should stay upright and in alignment. If the client starts to fall, you will be in a good position to help support him or her. Never try to "catch" a falling client. If a client falls, assist him or her to the floor. If you try to reverse a fall in progress, you will probably injure yourself and/or the client (Fig. 6-5).

Bend your knees to lower yourself, rather than bending from the waist. Any time a task requires bending, use a good stance. This allows you to use the big muscles in your legs and hips rather than straining the smaller muscles in your back.

6

Safety and Body Mechanics

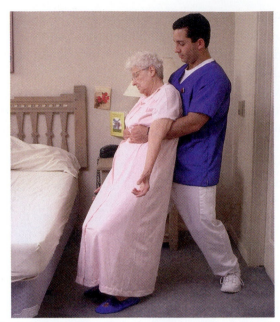

Fig. 6-5. Maintaining a wide base of support and low center of gravity will enable you to assist a falling client.

If you are making an adjustable bed, adjust the height to a safe working level, usually waist high. If you are making a regular bed, put one knee on the bed, lean, or even kneel to support yourself at working level. Avoid bending at the waist.

Back strain or injury is one of the greatest risks home health aides face. Prevention is very important. Throughout this text you will learn correct procedures for assisting with client transfers, positioning, and ambulation. These procedures will include instructions for maintaining proper body mechanics. In addition, always keep the following tips in mind:

- Use both arms and hands when lifting, pulling, pushing, or carrying objects.

- Hold objects close to you when you are lifting or carrying them.

- Push, slide, or pull objects rather than lifting them.

- Avoid bending and reaching as much as possible. Move or position furniture so that you do not have to bend or reach.

- Avoid twisting at the waist. Instead, turn your whole body. Your feet should point toward what you are lifting.

- Get help whenever possible for lifting or assisting clients.

- When moving a client, let him know what you will do so he can help if possible. Count to three and lift or move on three so everyone moves together.

Report to your supervisor if your assignments include tasks that you feel you cannot safely perform. Never attempt to lift an object or a client that you feel you cannot handle.

3. List ways to adapt the home to principles of good body mechanics

Following are several strategies that can help you apply good body mechanics in the home:

Have the right tools for a job. For example, if you cannot reach an object on a high shelf, use a step stool rather than climbing on a counter or straining to reach.

Have footrests and pillows available. You can make any position safer and more comfortable by using footrests and pillows to keep the body in alignment. For example, tasks that require standing for long periods can be more comfortable if you rest one foot on a footrest. This position flexes the muscles in the lower back and keeps the spine in alignment. When sitting, using a footrest allows for a more comfortable leg position. Crossing the legs disrupts alignment. It should be avoided. Using pillows can make any chair more comfortable. Use pillows behind the back to keep the back straight.

Keep tools, supplies, and clutter off the floor. Keep frequently-used items on shelves or counters where they can be easily reached without lifting. Keeping things organized will also help you find what you need without straining.

Sit when you can. Whenever you can sit to do a job, do so. Chopping vegetables, folding clothes, and other tasks can be done easily while sitting. For jobs like scouring the bathtub, kneel or use a low stool. Avoid bending at the waist.

Use gait or transfer belts when assisting clients with ambulation or transfers. In chapter 12 you will learn correct procedures for safely assisting clients with ambulation and transfers.

Make sure the homes you work in are safe for your clients, their family members, and yourself. Working in a home that is neglected puts you at risk of injury. Do remember, however, that you are a visitor in the client's home. Unless an immediate danger exists, check with your supervisor and the client before making any significant changes.

A nurse or case manager will assess the safety of the homes in which you work. However, you will spend more time in the home than any other member of the care team. Look for safety hazards. Immediately report to your supervisor any hazards you observe.

4. Identify five common types of accidents in the home

Common types of accidents that occur in the home include the following:

Falls: Falls can be caused by an unsafe environment or by loss of abilities. Falls are particularly common among the elderly. Older people are often more seriously injured by falls because their bones are more fragile. Be especially alert to the risk of falls with your elderly clients.

Factors that raise the risk of falls include the following:

- clutter
- throw rugs
- exposed electrical cords
- slippery floors
- uneven floors or stairs
- poor lighting

Personal conditions that raise the risk of falls include medications, loss of vision, gait or balance problems, weakness, paralysis, and disorientation. **Disorientation** means confusion about time or place.

Follow these tips to guard against falls:

- Clear all walkways of clutter, throw rugs, and cords (Figs. 6-6 and 6-7).

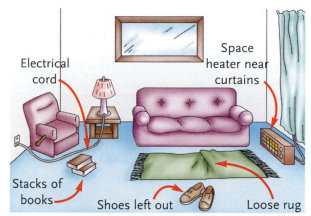

Fig. 6-6. Be aware of unsafe conditions in your clients' homes. This living room contains many tripping and fire hazards.

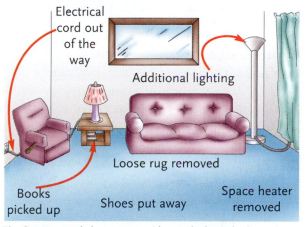

Fig. 6-7. You can help prevent accidents. The hazards shown in Fig. 6-6 have been removed. Talk with your client about changes that need to be made to avoid hazards.

- Avoid waxing floors, and use non-skid mats or carpeting where appropriate.
- Keep frequently used personal items close to client.
- Immediately clean up spills on the floor.
- Mark uneven flooring or stairs with red tape to indicate a hazard.
- Improve lighting where necessary.

The HHA needs to be able to identify hazards and take action to remove them. This will include working with the client, the client's family, and/or other members of the care team.

Burns: Burns can be caused by stoves and by

electrical appliances, hot water or liquids, or heating devices. Small children, older adults, or people with loss of sensation due to paralysis are at the greatest risk of burns. Follow these tips to guard against burns:

- Roll up sleeves and avoid loose clothing

when working at or near the stove (Figs. 6-8 and 6-9).

- Check that the stove and appliances are off when you leave.

- Suggest that the hot water heater be set lower than normal. It should be set at 120°F

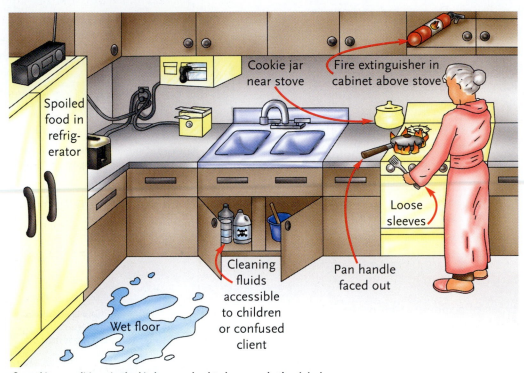

Fig. 6-8. Unsafe working conditions in the kitchen can lead to burns and other injuries.

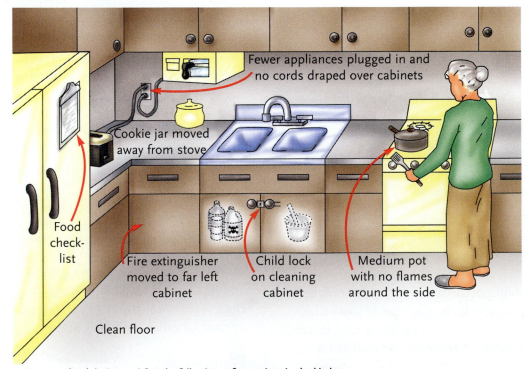

Fig. 6-9. Prevent burns, other injuries, and fires by following safe practices in the kitchen.

to 130°F to avoid burns from scalding tap water.

- Always check water temperature with water thermometer or on wrist before using.

- Check temperatures of liquids on your wrist before serving.

- Keep space heaters away from clients' beds, chairs, and draperies. Never allow space heaters to be used in the bathroom.

- Report frayed electrical cords or unsafe-looking appliances immediately. Do not use these appliances.

Poisoning: Homes contain many harmful substances that should not be swallowed. These include cleaning products, paints, medicines, toiletries, and glues. Lock these products away from confused clients, clients with limited vision, and children. Have the number for the Poison Control Center posted by the telephone.

Clients who have a diminished sense of taste or smell due to stroke or head injury might eat spoiled food. Check the refrigerator and cabinets frequently for foods that are moldy, sour or otherwise spoiled. Investigate any odors you notice. Clients with dementia may hide food and let it spoil in closets, drawers or other places.

Cuts: Cuts typically occur in the kitchen or bathroom. Keep any sharp objects, including knives, peelers, graters, food processor blades, scissors, nail clippers, or razors out of reach of children. Lock sharp objects away if there is a confused client in the home. If you are preparing food, cut away from yourself, use a cutting board, and keep your fingers out of the way. Know proper first aid for cuts (see chapter 7).

Choking: Choking can occur when eating, drinking or swallowing medication. Babies and young children who put objects in their mouths are at great risk of choking. People who are weak, ill, or unconscious may choke on their own saliva. A person's tongue can also become swollen and obstruct the airway.

To guard against choking, keep small objects out of the reach of babies and small children.

Cut food into bite-sized pieces for clients who have trouble with utensils and for children. Position infants on their backs for sleeping after feeding. Infants should sleep on their backs to prevent sudden infant death syndrome (SIDS). Never put pillows, small toys, or other objects in a crib. Clients should eat in as upright a position as possible to avoid choking. Elderly clients with swallowing difficulties may have a special diet with liquids thickened to the consistency of honey. Thickened liquids are easier to swallow.

Household Tips for Preventing Accidents

Bathroom

Falls: Use nonskid bathmats in tubs and showers. Request grab bars for the tub, shower, and toilet if the client is weak and unsteady (Figs. 6-10 and 6-11).

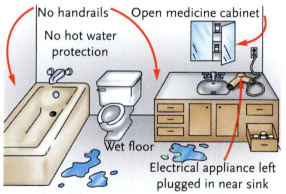

Fig. 6-10. The bathroom is full of safety hazards if it is not properly maintained.

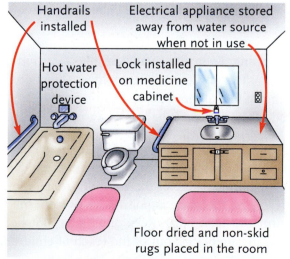

Fig. 6-11. This bathroom has been made safer by using special devices and by cleaning and straightening.

Burns: Check water temperature with a bath thermometer or on your wrist. Put away electrical appliances when they are not in use. Do not use electrical appliances near a water source.

Drowning: Do not leave young children unattended near any water. This includes bathtubs, swimming pools, buckets or basins of water, puddles, ponds, drainage ditches, toilets, or sinks. Do not leave anyone who is ill and weak alone in a tub. Do not leave clients who are dizzy or confused alone in the tub or shower.

Poisoning: Suggest that all medications be stored in containers with childproof caps and in locked cabinets. Never tell children that medication is candy. Be sure all medicines are labeled and your client reads medicine labels with his or her eyeglasses if reading glasses are necessary. Store client's medications separately from medications taken by other members of the family. Discard old and unused medications.

Cuts: Put away razors and other sharp objects (such as nail scissors) when they are not in use.

Kitchen

Falls: Fasten high chair safety belt.

Burns: Turn pot handles out of sight and toward the back of the stove. Stir food, especially if cooked in a microwave. This ensures that it is uniformly warm and not too hot before serving. Cool hot liquids with an ice cube before serving, as appropriate.

Poisoning: Keep emergency numbers, including the Poison Control Center, near the phone. Suggest that all household cleaning products and other chemicals be locked away.

Cuts: Keep cutlery put away. If you are using a knife and put it down for a moment, place it away from the edge of the counter or table. Make sure the blade is pointed away from the counter or table edge. Keep other sharp kitchen tools in safe places, out of the reach of children.

Choking: Do not give infants and toddlers popcorn, peanuts, hard candy, gum, or foods such as hot dogs or grapes. These items are easily inhaled, causing choking. Cut all foods into small, bite-size pieces suitable for the age of the child. For elderly clients who have difficulty swallowing, serve softer foods and foods cut into small pieces. Encourage clients to take small bites of food, chew thoroughly, and eat slowly. Keep plastic storage bags out of reach. Discard plastic bags from dry cleaners or other vendors.

Bedroom

Falls: If available, keep a nightlight on to illuminate pathways. Do not leave children unattended on high surfaces. This includes cribs, beds, changing tables, high chairs or play pens. Do not turn your back when you are changing a child on a high surface. Be sure the crib side rails are raised before you leave the room.

Burns: Do not allow clients to smoke in bed or when unattended. Especially do not allow smoking around oxygen tanks or equipment. When a client is unattended, place a call signal nearby.

Poisoning: Some window blinds have been found to collect lead-contaminated dust, which can cause lead poisoning if ingested.

Cuts: Be sure sharp objects are put away.

Choking: Report any cribs that have wide spaces between the slats. The infant's head could become wedged between them. Keep crib away from drapes and blinds. Infants and toddlers can strangle on the cords. Do not prop up bottles for infants and toddlers. Keep pillows out of cribs to avoid suffocation. Examine all toys for loose or removable parts.

Living area

Falls: Request walkers or canes for clients who need support when walking. Talk to your supervisor about having handrails installed where necessary. Keep the floors clear. Keep electrical and extension cords out of the way. Be sure shoes are sturdy and shoelaces are tied. For

small children, place safety gates, if available, at the tops and bottoms of stairs. Be certain the gates are secure and closed. Use hardware-mounted gates at the top of stairs.

Burns: Suggest that electrical outlets be covered with baby-proof plugs. Keep lighters and matches out of reach and out of sight. Never smoke around children.

Poisoning: Keep plants out of children's reach. Many common plants are poisonous.

Cuts: Keep sharp objects out of children's reach. Do not allow children to run, jump, or play roughly with any toy or object that could stab.

Choking: Do not permit young children to play with balloons or rubber bands. These objects are easily inhaled. Do not allow children to run and jump with food in their mouths.

Garage and outdoors

Never leave children at home alone or alone in a vehicle.

Make sure all children are fastened into an approved car seat. Child car seats should be placed in the back seat of the automobile. Children should never sit in the front seat of a car equipped with dual airbags.

Supervise children at play.

Keep walkways clear of toys and other obstructions, as well as snow and ice.

5. List home fire safety guidelines and describe what to do in case of fire

Recognize and report fire hazards. Any of the following can be a fire hazard:

- wood stoves, kerosene, gas or electric heaters that appear old, damaged, or faulty
- unvented heaters used in small, enclosed areas or sleeping areas
- space heaters used near fabrics such as

draperies, bedspreads, or towels, or used to dry clothing or towels

- flammable materials such as gasoline, kerosene, or paint thinner stored near stoves, heaters, furnaces, hot water heaters, or other appliances
- frayed or exposed electrical wires
- matches or lighters left within reach of children or incapacitated adults
- careless smoking, smoking in bed, cigarettes left burning, or confused clients smoking

GUIDELINES
Reducing Fire Hazards

- Never work wearing loose or flowing clothing, especially around the stove. Roll up clients' sleeves and avoid loose clothing when client may be cooking or around the stove.
- Store potholders, dish towels, and other flammable kitchen items away from the stove.
- Never store cookies, candy, or other items that may attract children above or near the stove.
- Discourage careless smoking and smoking in bed. If clients must smoke, check to be sure that cigarettes are extinguished. Empty ashtrays frequently.
- Stay in or near the kitchen when anything is cooking or baking.
- Do not leave the dryer on when you leave the house. Lint can catch fire.
- Turn off space heaters when no one is home or everyone is asleep.
- Be sure there are working smoke alarms. Check monthly to see that alarms are working. Replace batteries when needed.
- Have fire extinguishers on hand. Every home should have a fire extinguisher in the kitchen. Do not store the kitchen fire extinguisher near or above the stove, because you need to be able to get to it if the stove is on fire. Check that the homes you work in have fire extinguishers that have not expired.

Know where the extinguisher is stored and how to operate it (Fig. 6-12):

Pull the pin.

Aim at the base of the fire when spraying.

Squeeze the handle.

Sweep back and forth at the base of the fire.

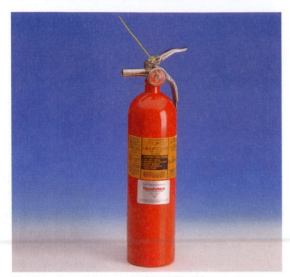

Fig. 6-12. Know how to use a fire extinguisher.

In case of fire, RACE is a good rule to follow:

Remove clients from danger.

Activate 911.

Contain fire if possible.

Extinguish, or call fire department to extinguish.

In addition, follow these guidelines for helping clients and family members exit the building safely:

- Remain calm.

- Be sure all family members know how to exit in case of fire, and have a designated meeting place outside the home.

- If windows or doors have locking bars, keep keys in the lock or close by. Mark windows of children's rooms outside with stickers that indicate a child sleeps in the room.

- Remove anything blocking a window or door that could be used as a fire exit.

- If clothing catches fire, do not run. Stop, drop to the ground, and roll to extinguish flames.

- Do not try to put out a large fire. Get out of the house and call for emergency help. Fires can quickly get out of control.

6. Discuss the use of restraints and related problems

A **restraint** is a physical or chemical way to limit a person's movement. Examples of physical restraints are leg and arm ties, vests and jacket restraints, and chair or wheelchair bars. Side rails on a bed and special chairs that restrict movement are also considered physical restraints. Chemical restraints are medications given to control a person's behavior.

Certain kinds of physical restraints can be used to protect clients' safety. For example, side rails keep clients from rolling out of bed. In the past some restraints have been abused by caregivers. This led to new restrictions and laws on the use of restraints. Check with your supervisor for laws and policies on the use of restraints.

There are many problems associated with restraints. Some of the negative effects of restraint use include the following:

- loss of dignity

- loss of independence

- reduced blood circulation

- stress on the heart

- incontinence

- weakened muscles and bones

- pressure sores

- increased agitation or depression

- poor self-esteem

- less activity, leading to poor appetite

- risk of suffocation

- pneumonia

Some restraints designed to safeguard clients have caused injury and even death. Due to serious problems caused by restraints, they are only used when ordered by a physician. There are several types of pads, belts, special chairs, and alarms that can be used instead of restraints.

Never use a restraint unless your supervisor has told you to do so, and you have been instructed in the proper use of the restraint. Follow the care plan. Instructions should always include frequent monitoring and repositioning.

7. Identify ways to reduce the risk of automobile accidents

Since you may be driving to and from clients' homes, you will need to protect your safety.

Plan your route. Trying to read a map or directions while driving can be very dangerous. When you must drive to a new location, study the map or directions before you start your car. Plan the route you will take.

Minimize distractions. Paying attention to the road can help you avoid accidents. Keep your eyes on the road and your hands on the wheel. If music is distracting, don't listen in the car.

Use turn signals. Using your turn signals lets other drivers know what you are planning to do. Always use turn signals when preparing to turn or change lanes.

Use caution when backing up. Many accidents occur when drivers back up. When you back up, look around you carefully. Turn your head to both sides and look behind your car. It is safest to turn your head and look behind you while backing up rather than relying on your rear view mirror.

Drive at a safe speed. Follow speed limits to be sure you are not driving too fast. Road conditions such as ice or heavy rain may mean you have to drive at a slower speed.

Always wear your seat belt. Although it may not help you avoid an accident, it will certainly help protect you if an accident occurs. Always buckle up, no matter how short the distance you must drive. Require your passengers to wear their seat belts as well.

8. Identify guidelines for using your car on the job

Keep the following in mind when using your car on the job:

* Park in safe, well-lit areas.
* Lock doors, both when driving and when you leave your car.
* Don't leave valuables in the car. If you must leave something in the car, put it out of sight.
* Have valid car insurance and carry the insurance card with you.
* Keep your proof of registration or registration card with you, not in the car. If your car is stolen, you do not want the thief to have this important document.
* Keep track of the miles you drive for work. Document them accurately. Lying about your mileage is the same as stealing from your employer.
* Keep your car in good working order. Get your car serviced at the appropriate times. Make sure you have good tires. Keep the gas tank full.

9. Identify guidelines for working in high-crime areas

If an assignment takes you to an area where crime is a problem, use caution. If you are using public transportation, be alert at all times.

The following tips can help you avoid trouble:

* Park in well-lit areas as close as possible to the home you are visiting.
* Try to leave valuables at home when you must work in a dangerous area.
* If possible, do not take your purse with you. If you must take it, hold your purse or bag tightly, close to your body.
* Lock your car and don't leave any valuables in it.

6

Safety and Body Mechanics

- Walk confidently. Look as though you know where you are going (Fig. 6-13).

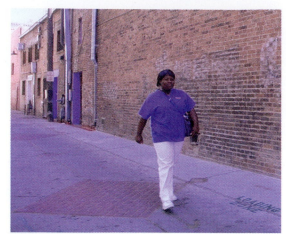

Fig. 6-13. Be cautious but look confident if you enter a high-crime area.

- Carry a whistle so you can make a loud noise to startle an attacker and get help.
- Carry your keys in your hand to unlock your car as soon as you arrive. If necessary, you can also use them as a weapon.
- Do not sit in your car, even with the doors locked. Drive away as soon as you reach your car.
- Try to avoid unsafe areas after dark.
- If you are concerned about your safety in a particular area, leave the area immediately. Contact your supervisor.
- Do not approach a home where strangers are hanging around. Go to the nearest phone in a safe area. Call your supervisor.
- Call your client before you visit so they know approximately when to expect you.
- Never enter a vacant home.
- If necessary, ask your supervisor to arrange for an escort or another care provider to go with you.
- Be sure someone knows your schedule. Call the office at the end of your work day.

Chapter Review

1. _____ is the way the parts of the body work together whenever you move.

2. The foundation that supports an object is called the _____.

3. The point where most weight is concentrated is called the

   _____.

4. When the two sides of the body are mirror images of each other, the body is in

   _____.

True or False. Mark each statement with either a "T" for true or an "F" for false.

5. ___ By applying the principles of good body mechanics to your work, you can avoid injury and save energy.

6. ___ To lift a heavy object from the floor, you must first place your feet together and keep your knees straight.

7. ___ The muscles of the thighs, upper arms, and shoulders are not as strong as the muscles in the back.

8. ___ A wide base of support and a low center of gravity means the feet are apart and the knees are bent.

9. ___ When moving an object, pivot your feet instead of twisting at the waist.

10. ___ It is a good idea to hold an object away from your body, because this helps you balance the weight more evenly.

11. ___ Never try to catch a falling client, as you could seriously injure yourself and/or the client.

12. ___ Bending from the waist allows you to use the big muscles in your legs and hips rather than smaller muscles in your back.

13. Name three things you can do as you work in a client's home that will help you use good body mechanics.

14. List five factors that increase the risk of falls.

6

Safety and Body Mechanics

15. Describe five ways to guard against burns.

16. In what position should clients eat to avoid choking?

17. List seven guidelines to reduce fire hazards while you work.

18. Why are restraints no longer used very often?

19. Why might you need to drive at a speed lower than the speed limit?

20. Why is not a good idea to leave your car registration document in your car?

21. Is it okay to guess the number of miles you drove to a client's house and back? Why or why not?

22. You are riding the city bus on your way to a client's home. As the bus approaches your stop, you notice a person near the bus stop who is swearing loudly and appears to be drunk. What should you do?

    a. Get off the bus and ignore the person.

    b. Get off the bus and tell the person to stop swearing in public.

    c. Stay on the bus and get off at the next stop.

    d. None of the above

6

Safety and Body Mechanics

7

Emergency Care and Disaster Preparation

1. Demonstrate how to recognize and respond to medical emergencies

Medical emergencies may be the result of accidents or sudden illnesses. This chapter discusses how to respond appropriately to medical emergencies. Heart attacks, strokes, diabetic emergencies, choking, automobile accidents, and gunshot wounds are all medical emergencies. Falls, burns, and cuts can also be emergencies when they are severe.

In an emergency situation, it is important to remain calm, act quickly, and communicate clearly. Memorizing the following steps will help you respond calmly and quickly in an emergency:

Assess the situation. Try to determine what has happened. Make sure you are not in danger. Notice the time.

Assess the victim. Ask the injured or ill person what has happened. If the person is unable to respond, he may be unconscious. To determine whether a person is conscious, tap the person and ask if he is all right. Speak loudly. Use the person's name if you know it. If there is no response, assume the person is unconscious and that you have an emergency situation. Call for help right away or send someone else to call.

Reporting Emergencies

When in doubt about calling for help, call! If you need to call emergency medical services, call 911 or dial 0 for the operator to get emergency medical services. If you are alone, make the call yourself. If you are not alone, shout for help and have someone make the call for you and then return to you.

When calling emergency services, be prepared to give the following information:

- the phone number and address of the emergency, including exact directions or landmarks if necessary
- the person's condition, including any medical background you know
- your name and position
- details of any first aid being given

The dispatcher you speak with may need other information or may want to give you other instructions. Do not hang up the phone until the dispatcher hangs up or tells you to hang up. If you are in a home, unlock the front door so emergency personnel can get in when they arrive.

If a person is conscious and able to speak, then he is breathing and has a pulse. Talk with the client about what happened, and check the person for injury. Check for the following:

- severe bleeding
- changes in consciousness
- irregular breathing
- unusual color or feel to the skin
- swollen places on the body
- medical alert tags
- anything the clients says is painful

If one of these conditions exists, you may need professional medical help. Follow your agency's policies about whom to call in different types of situations.

If the injured or ill person is conscious, he may feel panic about his condition. Listen to the person. Tell him what actions are being taken to help him. Be calm and confident to reassure him that he is being taken care of.

Once the emergency is over, you will need to document the emergency in your notes and complete an incident or an accident report. Try to remember as many details as possible. Remember, report the facts only. If a client had a heart attack, your notes should record the signs and symptoms you observed and the actions you took. Knowing the kind of information you will have to document will help you remember the important facts during the emergency. For instance, it is especially important to remember the time at which a client becomes unconscious.

2. Demonstrate knowledge of first aid procedures

Cardiopulmonary resuscitation (CPR) refers to medical procedures used when a person's heart or lungs have stopped working. CPR is used until medical help arrives.

Quick action is necessary. CPR must be started immediately. Brain damage may occur within four to six minutes after the heart stops beating and the lungs stop breathing. The person can die within ten minutes.

Only properly trained people should administer CPR. Your agency will probably arrange for you to be trained in CPR. If your agency does not schedule you for training, ask about Heart Association or Red Cross CPR training or contact one of these agencies yourself. CPR is an important skill to learn. **If you are not trained, do not attempt to perform CPR.** Performing CPR incorrectly can further injure a person. This textbook is not a CPR course. **The following is intended as a brief review for people who have had CPR training:**

1. Check whether the person is responsive. Gently shake the person and shout, "Are you okay?"

2. If there is no response, call 911 immediately or send someone to call 911. Remain calm.

3. After calling 911, kneel at the person's side near his or her head to start CPR.

4. Open the airway. Tilt the head back slightly by lifting the chin with one hand while pushing down on the forehead with the other hand. (head tilt-chin lift method) (Fig. 7-1).

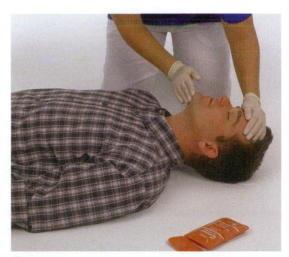

Fig. 7-1.

5. Hold the airway open and check for breathing:

   - Look for the chest to rise and fall.

   - Listen for sounds of breathing. Put your ear near the person's nose and mouth.

- Feel for the person's breath on your cheek.

6. If the person is not breathing, you will have to breathe for the person. Give two rescue breaths. To give rescue breaths:

   - Pinch the nose to keep air from escaping from the nostrils. Cover the person's mouth completely with your mouth.

   - Blow into the person's mouth slowly, watching for the chest to rise (Fig. 7-2). Blow two full breaths, approximately two seconds each. (Rescue breaths for an infant or a child should last 1 to 1 1/2 seconds for each breath.) Turn your head to the side to listen for air. If the chest does not rise when you give a rescue breath, reopen the airway using the head tilt-chin lift method. Try to give rescue breaths again.

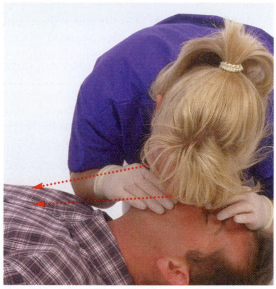

Fig. 7-2.

   - If a barrier device, such as a special face mask, is available, use the barrier device to give rescue breathing (Fig. 7-3).

7. After giving rescue breaths, look for signs of circulation. The person may start moving, breathing normally, or coughing. If you do not see signs of circulation, give 15 chest compressions only if you have been trained to do so. Be sure the person is lying flat on a hard surface. To give chest compressions:

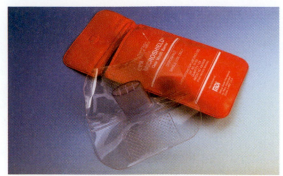

Fig. 7-3. A barrier device protects you and the person you are helping from contacting body fluids.

   - Find the lower end of the person's sternum. Do this by following the rib cage up to the center of the chest.

   - Place your index finger next to your middle finger where the ribs meet the sternum. Place the heel of your other hand next to the upper finger over the lower half of the sternum (Fig. 7-4).

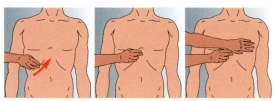

Fig. 7-4.

   - Place the heel of your other hand on top of the positioned hand. Interlace your fingers. Position your body directly over your hands. Keep your elbows straight. Look down on your hands.

   - Use the heels of your hands to give 15 chest compressions. Push in 1 1/2 to 2 inches with each compression. Allow the chest to relax between compressions. Do not take your hands off the chest between compressions.

8. Continue giving two breaths followed by 15 compressions. After about a minute of CPR, check for signs of circulation. If you see signs of circulation, stop compressions and continue to provide rescue breathing as necessary.

When medical help arrives, follow their directions. Assist them as necessary. Report details of the incident.

7

Emergency Care and Disaster Preparation

Choking

When something is blocking the tube through which air enters the lungs, the person has an **obstructed airway**. When people are choking, they usually put their hands to their throats and cough (Fig. 7-5). As long as a person can speak, breathe, or cough, do nothing. Encourage him to cough as forcefully as possible to get the object out. Stay with the person at all times, until he stops choking or can no longer speak, breathe, or cough.

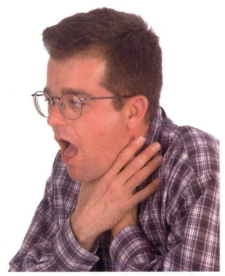

Fig. 7-5. People who are choking usually put their hands to their throats and cough.

If a person can no longer speak, breathe, or cough, call 911 immediately. After calling 911 return to the person.

The Heimlich maneuver is a procedure used for choking. It uses abdominal thrusts to move the blockage upward, out of the throat. Make sure the person needs help before starting the Heimlich maneuver. If the person cannot speak or cough, or if his response is weak, start the Heimlich maneuver.

Heimlich maneuver for the conscious person

1. Stand behind the person and bring your arms under his arms. Wrap your arms around the person's waist.

2. Make a fist with one hand. Place the flat, thumb side of the fist against the person's abdomen, above the navel but below the breastbone.

3. Grasp the fist with your other hand. Pull both hands toward you and up, quickly and forcefully (Fig. 7-6).

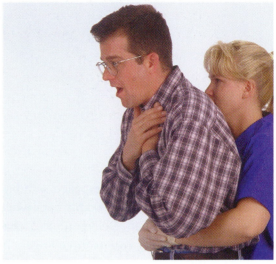

Fig. 7-6.

4. Repeat until the object is pushed out or the person loses consciousness.

5. Report and document the incident properly.

If the person becomes unconscious while choking, help him to the floor gently so he is lying on his back with his face up. He probably has a completely blocked airway and needs professional medical help immediately. Call 911, then attempt CPR if you are trained to do so. If someone else is present, send that person to call 911 while you begin CPR.

For an infant who is choking, you will need to give back blows and chest thrusts.

Clearing an obstructed airway in a conscious infant

1. Lie the infant face down on your forearm; if you are sitting, rest the arm holding the infant's torso on your lap or thigh. Support his jaw and head with your hand.

2. Using the heel of your free hand, deliver up to 5 back blows. **Back blows** are performed by striking the infant between the shoulder blades (Fig. 7-7).

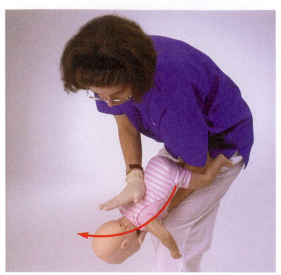

Fig. 7-7.

3. If the obstruction is not expelled with back blows, turn the infant onto his back while supporting the head. Deliver up to 5 **chest thrusts** by placing two or three fingers in the center of the breastbone (Fig. 7-8). This is the same position used for chest compression during CPR.

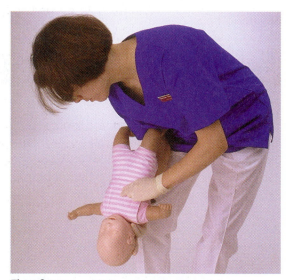

Fig. 7-8.

4. Repeat alternating 5 back blows and 5 chest compressions until the object is pushed out or the infant loses consciousness.

5. Report and document the incident properly.

Shock

Shock occurs when organs and tissues in the body do not receive an adequate blood supply.

Bleeding, heart attack, severe infection, and conditions that cause the blood pressure to fall can lead to shock. Shock can become worse when the person is extremely frightened or in severe pain.

Shock is a dangerous, life-threatening situation. Signs of shock include pale or bluish skin, staring, increased pulse and respiration rates, decreased blood pressure, and extreme thirst. Always call for help if you suspect a person is experiencing shock. To prevent or treat shock, do the following:

Shock

1. Have the person lie down on her back. If the person is bleeding from the mouth or vomiting, place her on her side (unless you suspect that the neck, back, or spinal cord is injured).

2. Control bleeding. This procedure is described later in the chapter.

3. Check pulse and respirations if possible. (See chapter 14.)

4. Keep the person as calm and comfortable as possible.

5. Maintain normal body temperature. If the weather is cold, place a blanket around the person. If the weather is hot, provide shade.

6. Elevate the feet unless the person has a head or abdominal injury, breathing difficulties, or a fractured bone or back (Fig. 7-9). Elevate the head and shoulders if a head wound or breathing difficulties are present. Never elevate a body part if a broken bone exists.

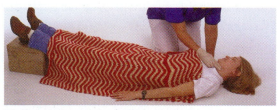

Fig. 7-9.

7. Do not give the person anything to eat or drink.

8. Call for help immediately. Victims of shock

should always receive medical care as soon as possible.

9. Report and document the incident properly.

Myocardial Infarction or Heart Attack

Myocardial infarction (MI) (*mye-oh-KAR-dee-al in-FARK-shun*), or heart attack, occurs when the heart muscle itself does not receive enough oxygen because blood vessels are blocked. The following are signs and symptoms of MI:

- sudden, severe pain in the chest, usually on the left side or in the center behind the sternum
- a feeling of indigestion or heartburn
- nausea and vomiting
- **dyspnea** (*DISP-nee-a*) or difficulty breathing
- dizziness
- skin color may be pale, gray, or bluish (**cyanotic**) (*sye-a-NOT-ik*), indicating lack of oxygen
- perspiration
- cold and clammy skin
- weak and irregular pulse rate
- low blood pressure
- anxiety and a sense of impending doom

You must take immediate action if a client experiences any of these symptoms. Follow these steps:

Heart attack

1. Call or have someone call emergency services. Call your supervisor.
2. Place the person in a comfortable position. Encourage him to rest, and reassure him that you will not leave him alone.
3. Loosen clothing around the neck (Fig. 7-10).
4. Do not give the person liquids.
5. If the person takes heart medication, such as nitroglycerin, find the medication and

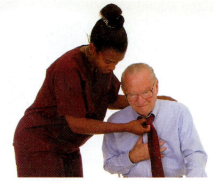

Fig. 7-10.

offer it to him. Never place medication in someone's mouth.

6. Monitor the person's breathing and pulse. If the person stops breathing or has no pulse, perform CPR if you are trained to do so.
7. Stay with the person until help arrives.
8. Report and document the incident properly.

Bleeding

Severe bleeding can cause death quickly and must be controlled. Call for help immediately, then follow these steps to control bleeding.

Bleeding

1. Put on gloves.
2. Hold a thick sterile pad, a clean pad, or a clean cloth such as a handkerchief or towel against the wound. Have the injured person use his bare hand until you can get a clean pad. Also have the client hold the pad if he is able until you can put on gloves.
3. Press down hard, directly on the bleeding wound, until help arrives. Do not decrease pressure (Fig. 7-11). Put additional pads over the first pad if blood seeps through. Do not remove the first pad.

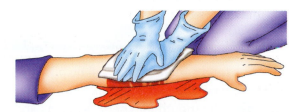

Fig. 7-11. Hold pad over wound and press down hard. Do not decrease pressure.

4. Raise the wound above the heart to slow down the bleeding. If the wound is on an arm, leg, hand, or foot, and there are no broken bones, prop up the limb on towels, blankets, coats, or other absorbent material.

5. When bleeding is under control, secure the dressing to keep it in place. Check the person for symptoms of shock (pale skin, increased pulse and respiration rates, decreased blood pressure, and extreme thirst). Stay with the person until medical help arrives.

6. Wash hands thoroughly when finished.

7. Report and document the incident properly.

Poisoning

First aid kits in the home should contain syrup of ipecac (*IH-pi-kak*), activated charcoal, and Epsom salts for the treatment of accidental poisoning (Fig. 7-12). Always have the poison control center phone number available and know if the client has syrup of ipecac in the house. Suspect poisoning when a client suddenly collapses, vomits, and has heavy, labored breathing. If you suspect poisoning, take the following steps:

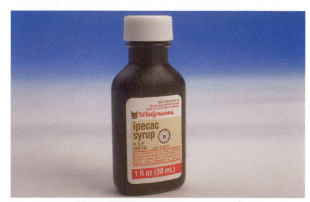

Fig. 7-12. Ipecac syrup causes vomiting. It should only be used when directed by a doctor or by a poison control center.

Poisoning

1. Look for a container that will help you determine what the client has taken or eaten. Check the mouth for chemical burns and note the breath odor.

2. Call the local or state poison control center immediately. Follow instructions from poison control.

3. Notify your supervisor.

4. Report and document the incident properly.

Burns

Care of a burn depends on its depth, size, and location. There are three types of burns: first degree, second degree, and third degree burns (Fig. 7-13).

First degree burns involve just the outer layer of skin. The skin becomes red, painful, and swollen, but no blisters occur. Second degree burns extend from the outer layer of skin to the next deeper layer of skin. The skin is red, painful, swollen, and blisters occur. Third degree burns involve all three layers of the skin and may extend to the bone. If the nerves are destroyed, no pain occurs. The skin is shiny and appears hard. It may be white in color.

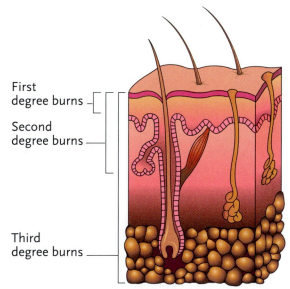

First degree burns

Second degree burns

Third degree burns

Fig. 7-13.

You should call for emergency help in any of the following situations:

- An infant or child, or an elderly, ill or weak person has been burned, unless burn is very minor.

- The burn occurs on the head, neck, hands,

7

Emergency Care and Disaster Preparation

feet, face, or genitals, or burns cover more than one body part.

- Person who has been burned is having trouble breathing.

- The burn was caused by chemicals, electricity, or explosion.

Burns

To treat a minor burn:

1. Use cool, clean water (not ice) to decrease the skin temperature and prevent further injury (Fig. 7-14). Ice will cause further skin damage. Dampen a clean cloth and place it over the burn.

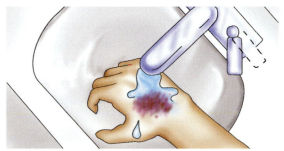

Fig. 7-14.

2. Once the pain has eased, you may cover the area with a dry, sterile gauze.

3. Never use any kind of ointment, salve, or grease on a burn.

For more serious burns:

1. Remove the person from the source of the burn. If clothing has caught fire, smother it with a blanket or towel to extinguish flames. Protect yourself from the source of the burn.

2. Check for breathing, pulse, and severe bleeding.

3. Call for emergency help.

4. Do not apply water. It may cause infection.

5. Remove as much of the person's clothing around the burned area as possible, but do not try to pull away clothing that sticks to the burn. Cover the burn with thick, dry, sterile gauze if available, or a clean cloth. A dry, insulated cool pack may be used over the dressing (Fig. 7-15). Again, never use any kind of ointment, salve, or grease on a burn.

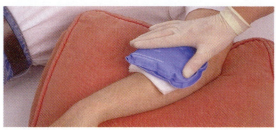

Fig. 7-15.

6. Ask the person to lie down and elevate the affected part if this does not cause greater pain.

7. If the burn covers a larger area, wrap the person or the extremity in several thicknesses of a dry, clean sheet and apply an ice pack if possible. Take care not to rub the skin.

8. Wait for emergency medical help.

9. Report and document the incident properly.

Seizures

Seizures are involuntary, often violent, contractions of muscles. They can involve a small area or the entire body. Seizures are caused by an abnormality in the brain. They can occur in young children who have a high fever. Older children and adults who have a serious illness, fever, head injury, or a seizure disorder such as **epilepsy** may also have seizures.

The main goal during a seizure is to make sure the client is safe. During a seizure, a person may shake severely and thrust arms and legs uncontrollably (Fig. 7-16). He may clench his jaw, drool, and be unable to swallow. The following emergency measures should be taken if a client has a seizure:

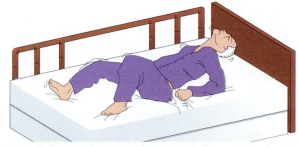

Fig. 7-16. A person having a seizure may shake severely and thrust his arms and legs uncontrollably.

Seizures

1. Lower the person to the floor.

2. Have someone call for emergency medical help if needed. Do not leave the person during the seizure unless you must do so to get medical help.

3. Move furniture away to prevent injury. If a pillow is nearby, place it under his or her head.

4. Do not try to restrain the person.

5. Do not force anything between the person's teeth. Do not place your hands in the person's mouth for any reason. You could be bitten.

6. Do not give liquids.

7. When the seizure is over, check breathing.

8. Report and document the incident properly.

Fainting

Fainting, called **syncope** (*SING-ke-pee*), occurs when the blood supply drops, causing a loss of consciousness. Fainting may be the result of hunger, fear, pain, fatigue, standing for a long time, poor ventilation, or overheating.

Signs and symptoms of fainting include dizziness, perspiration, pale skin, weak pulse, shallow respirations, and blackness in the visual field. If someone appears likely to faint, follow these steps:

Fainting

1. Have the person lie down or sit down before fainting occurs.

2. If the person is in a sitting position, have her bend forward and place her head between her knees (Fig. 7-17). If the person is lying flat on her back, elevate the legs.

3. Loosen any tight clothing.

4. Have the person stay in position for at least five minutes after symptoms disappear.

5. Help the person get up slowly. Continue to observe him for symptoms of fainting.

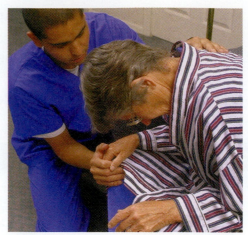

Fig. 7-17.

6. Report and document the incident properly.

If a person does faint, lower him to the floor or other flat surface. Position him on his back. Elevate his legs eight to twelve inches. Loosen any tight clothing. Check to make sure the person is breathing. He should recover quickly, but keep him lying down for several minutes. Report the incident to the nurse immediately. Fainting may be a sign of a more serious medical condition.

Nosebleed

A nosebleed can occur spontaneously, when the air is dry, or when injury has occurred. The medical term for a nosebleed is **epistaxis** (*ep-i-STAK-sis*). If a client has a nosebleed, take the following steps:

Nosebleed

1. Elevate the head of the bed or tell the client to remain in a sitting position. Offer tissues or a clean cloth to catch the blood. Do not touch blood or bloody clothes, tissues or cloths without gloves.

2. Put on gloves. Apply firm pressure over the bridge of the nose. Squeeze the bridge of the nose with your thumb and forefinger (Fig. 7-18). Have the client do this until you are able to get gloves on.

3. Apply the pressure consistently until the bleeding stops.

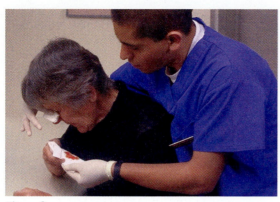

Fig. 7-18.

4. Use a cool cloth or ice wrapped in a cloth on the back of the neck, the forehead, or the upper lip to slow the flow of blood. Never apply ice directly to skin.

5. Report and document the incident properly.

Falls

Falls can be minor or severe. All falls should be reported to your supervisor, and incident reports should be completed. In the case of a severe fall, call emergency medical services immediately. Take the following steps to help a client who has fallen:

Helping a client who has fallen

1. Assess client's condition. Determine if client is unconscious, not breathing, has no pulse, or is bleeding severely. Get emergency medical help if any of these conditions exist.

2. Look for broken bones. Pain and body parts lying in an unnatural position or bones protruding through the skin are indications.

3. If client seems unhurt, encourage her to stay down until you can check her thoroughly.

4. Ask client to move each body part separately to be sure there are no strains, sprains, or fractures.

5. If you find no evidence of injury, make the client as comfortable as possible.

6. Call your supervisor and report the fall immediately. Do not move the client until you have spoken with your supervisor.

3. Identify emergency evacuation procedures

During a fire or other disaster, you may need to get yourself, the client, and the client's family out of the home immediately. Leaving in an emergency is called **evacuation** (*ee-vac-yoo-AY-shun*). Because you may not have time to think or plan in an emergency, know how to evacuate each client's home.

Plan for evacuation by doing the following:

- Locate all the doors and windows that could serve as exits in an emergency.

- In an apartment building, know where fire stairs are located. Elevators may be unsafe in an emergency.

- Know the location of disaster supplies if they are available in the home. These include fire extinguishers, ladders for escape from upper floors, first aid kits or supplies, and utility shut-off points.

- Discuss a plan for evacuation with your clients and their family members. Emphasize that everyone should keep calm in an emergency.

- Know who will be responsible for helping the disabled and children in emergencies.

- Agree on a place outside the home for everyone to meet after evacuation.

Chapter 6 includes fire safety information.

4. Demonstrate knowledge of disaster procedures

Disasters can include fire, flood, earthquake, hurricane, tornado, or severe weather. The disasters you may experience will depend on where you live. Know the appropriate action to take to protect yourself and your client. During natural disasters, most agencies rely on local or state management groups to assume overall responsibility for the ill and disabled. Each agency has a local and area-specific disaster plan. Know your agency's disaster plan.

The following guidelines apply in any disaster situation:

- Remain calm.

- Listen to radio or television bulletins to keep informed. A battery-powered radio will help you to stay informed if power goes out.

- If a disaster is forecast (for example, a tornado or hurricane), be ready. Wear appropriate clothing and shoes. Have family members dressed and ready in case evacuation is necessary.

- Stay in contact with your supervisor or others if possible. Let someone know where you are, what conditions are, and where you will go if you must evacuate.

- Locate disaster supplies. Ideally, a disaster supply kit should be assembled before disaster strikes. See below.

Emergency Supplies

Keep enough supplies in your home to meet your needs for at least three days. Assemble a disaster supply kit with items you may need in an evacuation. Store kit in sturdy, easy-to-carry containers such as backpacks, duffel bags or covered trash containers.

Include

- A three-day supply of water (one gallon per person per day) and food that won't spoil.

- One change of clothing and footwear per person, and one blanket or sleeping bag per person.

- A first aid kit that includes your family's prescription medications.

- Emergency tools, including a battery-powered radio, flashlight, and plenty of extra batteries.

- An extra set of car keys and a credit card, cash, or traveler's checks.

- Sanitation supplies.

- Special items for infant, elderly, or disabled family members.

- An extra pair of glasses.

- Important family documents in a water-proof container.

Chapter Review

1. List two steps to follow when you come upon an emergency situation.

2. What information should you be prepared to give when calling emergency services?

3. Why would remaining calm and confident help in an emergency situation?

4. Why should you not perform CPR if you are not trained to do so?

5. How is the Heimlich maneuver used to help someone who is choking?

6. If the person becomes unconscious while choking, what should you do first?

7. Why should you not use ice on a burn?

8. List seven signs of a heart attack.

9. What does ipecac syrup do?

10. What can be done to a wound to slow the bleeding?

11. List the signs of shock.

12. Why should you not force anything into the mouth of a person who is having a seizure?

13. If a person feels like he is going to faint, in what position should he be placed?

14. Why should you put on gloves if a client has a nosebleed?

15. If a client falls, but it is only a minor fall, do you need to report it to your supervisor?

16. Why is it important to know in advance of an emergency how best to evacuate a home?

17. Describe how you can prepare for disasters that are common in your area.

8

Physical, Psychological, and Social Health

1. Identify basic human needs

People have different genes, physical appearances, cultural backgrounds, ages, and social or financial positions. But all human beings have the same basic physical needs:

- food and water
- protection and shelter
- activity
- sleep and rest
- safety
- comfort, especially freedom from pain

You will be helping your clients meet these basic physical needs. Activities of daily living (ADLs), such as eating, toileting, bathing, and grooming, are the ways we meet our most basic physical needs. By assisting with ADLs or helping clients learn to perform them independently, you help clients meet their basic needs.

We also have **psychosocial** needs, which involve social interaction, emotions, intellect, and spirituality. Psychosocial needs are not as easy to define as physical needs. However, all human beings have the following psychosocial needs:

- love and affection
- acceptance by others
- security
- self-reliance and independence in daily living

- interaction with other people (Fig. 8-1)
- accomplishments and self-esteem

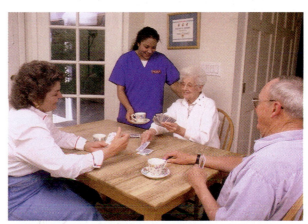

Fig. 8-1. Interaction with other people is a basic psychosocial need. Encourage your clients to be with friends or relatives. Social contact is important. Accommodate visitors, even if doing so throws off your schedule.

Our health and well-being are affected by how well our psychosocial needs are met. Stress and frustration occur when basic needs are not met. This can lead to fear, anxiety, anger, aggression, withdrawal, indifference, and depression. Stress can also cause physical problems that may eventually lead to illness.

Abraham Maslow, a researcher of human behavior, wrote about human physical and psychosocial needs. He arranged these needs into an order of importance. He thought that physical needs must be met before we can work on meeting our psychosocial needs. His theory is called "Maslow's Hierarchy of Needs" (Fig. 8-2).

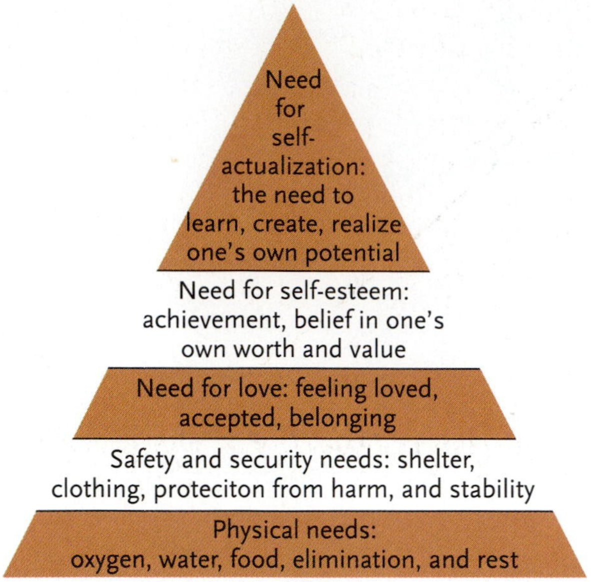
Need for self-actualization: the need to learn, create, realize one's own potential
Need for self-esteem: achievement, belief in one's own worth and value
Need for love: feeling loved, accepted, belonging
Safety and security needs: shelter, clothing, proteciton from harm, and stability
Physical needs: oxygen, water, food, elimination, and rest

Fig. 8-2. **Maslow's Hierarchy of Needs.**

People also have sexual needs. These needs continue throughout their lives. The ability to engage in sexual activity, such as intercourse and masturbation, continues unless a disease or injury occurs. Always knock and wait for permission before entering a client's bedroom. If you encounter a sexual situation, provide privacy and leave the room.

Clients have the right to choose how they express their sexuality. In all age groups, there is a variety of sexual behavior. This is true of your clients also. Do not judge any sexual behavior you see. An attitude that any expression of sexuality by the elderly is "disgusting" or "cute" deprives your clients of their right to dignity and respect.

2. Define holistic care

Holistic (*hole-IS-tik*) means considering a whole system, such as a whole person, rather than dividing the system up into parts. Holistic care means caring for the whole person—the mind as well as the body (Fig. 8-3). A simple example of holistic care is taking time to talk with your clients while helping them bathe. You are meeting the physical need with the bath and meeting the psychosocial need for interaction with others at the same time.

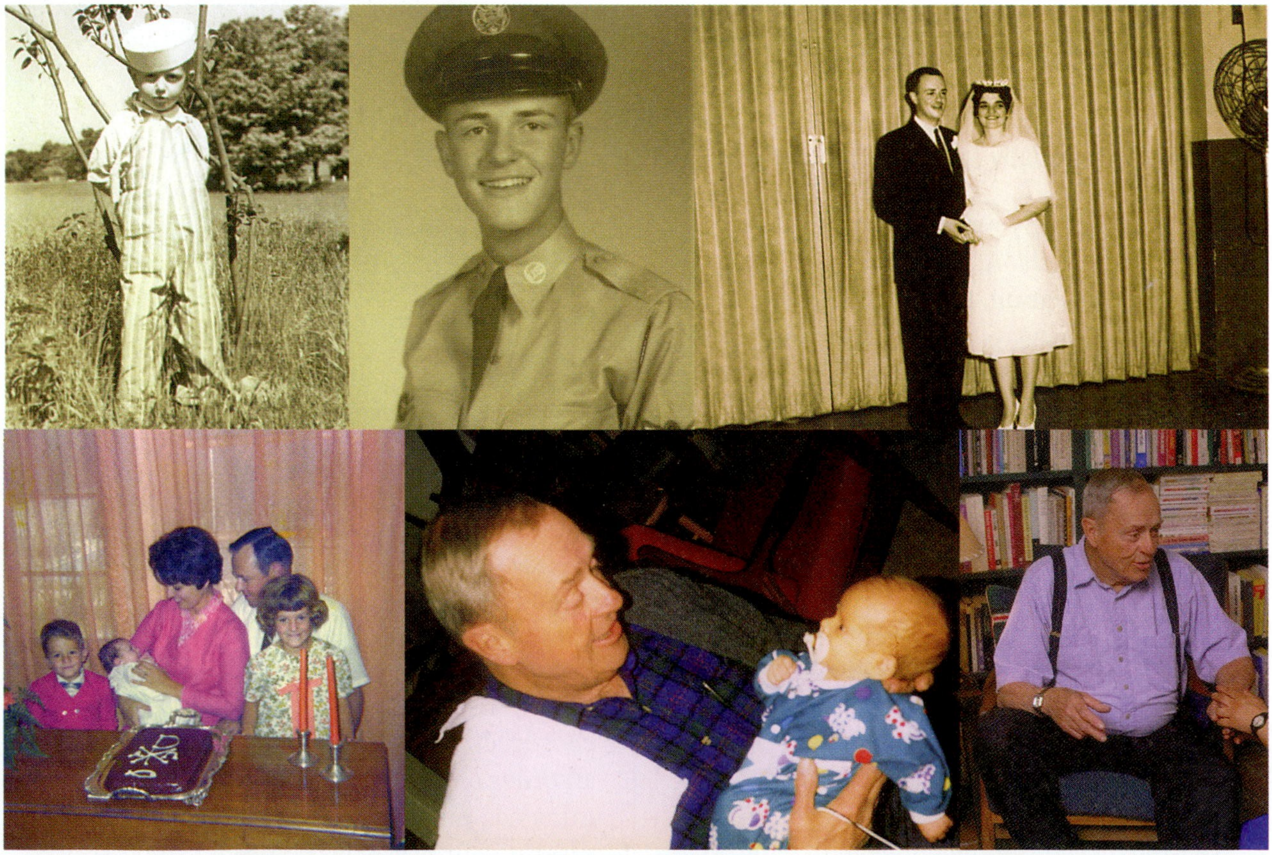

Fig. 8-3. **Remember that clients are people, not just lists of illnesses and disabilities. They have many needs, like you. Many have had rich lives with wonderful experiences. Take time to experience and care for your clients as whole people.**

Another way of practicing holistic care is considering psychosocial factors in illness, as well as physical factors. For example, Mr. Bollinger looks thin and tired. The cause might be depression rather than an infection. You do not need to determine the cause of his condition. However, by talking with him you might learn something that would help the rest of the care team. For example, you might learn that last year at this time his wife died, and he is still coping with that loss. You can and should share this information with the care team and document it.

3. Identify ways to help clients meet their spiritual needs

Clients have spiritual needs. You can assist with these needs, too. Helping clients meet their spiritual needs can help them cope with illness or disability. Remember that spirituality is a sensitive area. Do not offend your clients by making judgments or imposing your beliefs.

Following are some ways you can help clients meet their spiritual needs:

- Learn a little bit about your client's religion or beliefs (Fig. 8-4).
- Accommodate practices such as dietary restrictions. Never make judgments about them. Also, respect your client's decision to refrain from food-related rituals.
- Respect all religious items.
- Get to know the priest, rabbi, or minister who visits or calls your client.
- Allow privacy for clergy visits.
- If a client asks you, help find spiritual resources available in the area. The yellow pages usually list churches, synagogues, and other houses of worship.

You should never do the following:
- try to change someone's religion
- tell clients their belief or religion is wrong
- express judgments about a religious group
- insist clients join religious activities
- interfere with religious practices

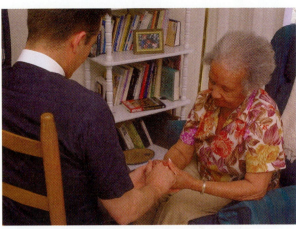

Fig. 8-4. Be open to your clients' spiritual needs. Be welcoming when they receive visits from a spiritual leader.

4. Discuss family roles and their significance in health care

Families are the most important unit within our social system (Fig. 8-5). Families play a huge role in many people's lives. Some examples of family types are listed below.

- Single-parent families include one parent with a child or children.
- Nuclear families include two parents with a child or children.
- Blended families include widowed or divorced parents who have remarried, with children from previous marriages as well as from this marriage.
- Multigenerational families include parents, children, and grandparents.
- Extended families may include aunts, uncles, cousins, or even friends.
- Families may also be made up of unmarried couples of the same sex or opposite sexes, with or without children.

Today a family is defined more by supporting each other than by the particular people involved. Your clients' families may not look like the kind of family you are used to. Clients with no living relatives may have friends or neighbors who function as a family. Whatever kinds of families your clients have, recognize the important role they can play. Family members help in many ways:

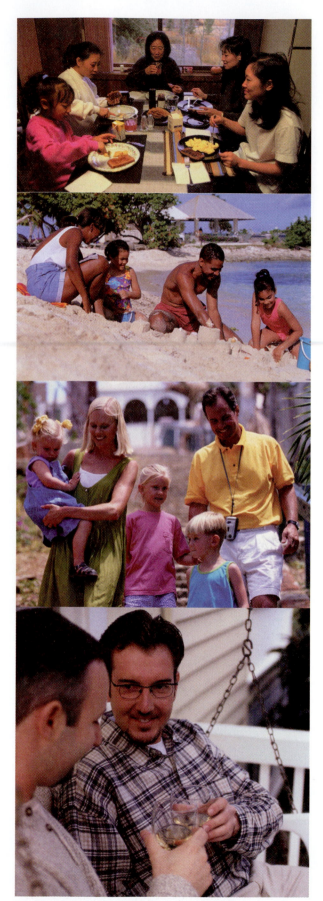

- helping clients make care decisions
- communicating with the care team
- providing daily care when home health aide is not present
- giving support and encouragement
- connecting the client to the outside world
- giving assurance to dying clients that family memories and traditions will be valued and carried on

5. Describe personal adjustments of the individual and family to illness and disability

Illness or disability requires clients and families to make adjustments. Making these adjustments may be difficult (Fig. 8-6). It depends on the family's emotional, spiritual, and financial resources. Some personal adjustments include the following:

- accepting the illness or disability and its long-term consequences or results
- finding money needed to pay expenses of hospitalization or home care
- dealing with paperwork involved in insurance, Medicaid, or Medicare benefits
- taking care of tasks the client can no longer handle
- understanding medical information and making difficult care decisions
- providing daily care when the aide cannot be there

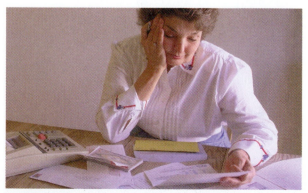

Fig. 8-6. Family members may have a hard time adjusting to the additional responsibilities when a loved one becomes ill or disabled.

Fig. 8-5. Families come in all shapes and sizes.

Be sensitive to the big adjustments your clients and their families may be making. Help them by doing your job well. Refer them to your supervisor if more help is needed.

6. Identify community resources for individual and family health

The larger community—the local government or social service agencies, church or synagogue—can provide families with resources. These resources can help them through difficult times and help solve problems. Such resources include meal or transportation services, **hospice care** (*HA-spis*, or care for the dying), counseling, and support groups (Fig. 8-7). Be familiar with resources available in your community. If clients ask you for more help, refer them to these resources. If no one asks but you think help is needed, speak to your supervisor.

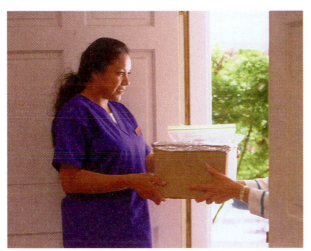

Fig. 8-7. "Meals on Wheels" and similar services provide nutritious meals to people unable to cook for themselves.

7. List ways to respond to emotional needs of your clients and their families

Clients or family members may come to you with problems or needs. Your response will depend on many factors. These include how comfortable you feel with emotions in general, how well you know the person, and what need or problem is brought up. Try to **empathize** (*EM-pa-thyze*), or understand how the person feels.

The following are three good ways to respond in this situation:

Listen. Often just talking about a problem or concern can make it easier to handle. Sitting quietly and letting someone talk or cry may be the best help you can give (Fig. 8-8).

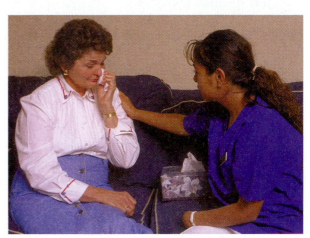

Fig. 8-8. Sometimes listening to someone is the best way to provide emotional support.

Offer support and encouragement. Saying things like "You have really been under a lot of stress, haven't you?" or "I can imagine that really is scary," can provide a lot of comfort. Avoid using **clichés** (*kli-SHAYS*, or common phrases that really don't mean anything), like "It'll all work out." Things may not all work out. It is more comforting to the client if you acknowledge how hard the situation is rather than simply dismissing her feelings with a cliché.

Refer the problem to a social worker or your supervisor. When you feel that you cannot help the client, or when someone is asking you for help outside your scope of practice, get someone else on the care team to handle the situation. Say something like, "Mrs. Pfeiffer, I need to get you the help you need. Can I have my supervisor call you?"

Chapter Review

1. How do you feel when you are hungry, tired, or cold?

2. How can you help clients meet their needs for love, acceptance, and independence?

3. According to Maslow, which needs must be met first, physical or emotional?

4. How can you help the care team provide holistic care to your clients?

5. List four ways you can help clients meet their spiritual needs.

6. List four ways that families can help the client.

True or False. Mark each statement with a "T" for true or an "F" for false.

7. ___ Emotional, spiritual, and financial resources can affect how well the family adjusts to the client's illness or disability.

8. ___ If you think your client's family needs help adjusting, you should refer them to your supervisor.

9. ___ You should only report on your client's condition, never on the family's condition.

10. List three types of community resources available to clients and families in need.

11. When should you refer a client's or family member's problem to a social worker or your supervisor?

9
The Human Body in Health and Disease

Our bodies are organized into body systems. Each system in the body has a condition under which it works best. **Homeostasis** (*hoh-mee-oh-STAY-sis*) is the name for the condition in which all of the body's systems are working their best. To be in homeostasis, the body's **metabolism** (*me-TAB-oh-lism*), or physical and chemical processes, must be operating at a steady level. When disease or injury occur, the body's metabolism is disturbed. Homeostasis is lost. Changes in metabolic (*me-tah-BOL-ic*) processes are called **signs and symptoms**. For instance, changes in body temperature could indicate that the body is fighting an infection. Noticing and reporting changes in your clients is a very important part of your job. The changes you notice could be signs of significant problems.

Each system in the body has its own unique structure and function. The body's systems can be broken down in different ways. In this book we divide the human body into ten body systems.

1. Integumentary (*in-teg-you-MEN-tar-ee*), or skin
2. Musculoskeletal (*mus-kyoo-lo-SKEL-e-tal*)
3. Nervous (*NERV-us*)
4. Circulatory (*SER-kyoo-la-tor-ee*) or cardiovascular (*kar-dee-oh-VAS-kyoo-lar*)
5. Respiratory (*RES-spir-a-tor-ee*)
6. Urinary (*YOOR-i-nayr-ee*)
7. Gastrointestinal or digestive (*di-JEST-iv*)
8. Endocrine (*EN-doh-krin*)
9. Reproductive (*ree-pro-DUK-tiv*)
10. Immune (*i-MYOON*) and Lymphatic (*lim-FAT-ik*)

Body systems are made up of **organs**. Organs are made up of **tissues**. Tissues are made up of groups of cells that perform a similar function. For example, in the circulatory system, the heart is one of the organs. It is made up of tissues and cells. **Cells** are the building blocks of our bodies. Living cells divide, develop, and die, renewing the tissues and organs of our body systems.

1. Describe the integumentary system

The largest organ and system in the body is the skin, a natural protective covering, or **integument** (*in-TEG-you-ment*). Skin prevents injury to internal organs. It also protects the body against entry of bacteria or germs. Skin also prevents the loss of too much water, which is essential to life. Skin is made up of tissues and **glands** (structures that secrete fluids) (Fig. 9-1).

The skin is also a *sense organ* that feels heat, cold, pain, touch, and pressure. Body temperature is regulated in the skin, which has blood vessels that **dilate** (*DYE-late*), or widen, when the outside temperature is too high. This brings

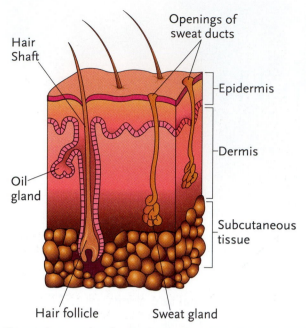

Fig. 9-1. Cross-section showing details of the integumentary system.

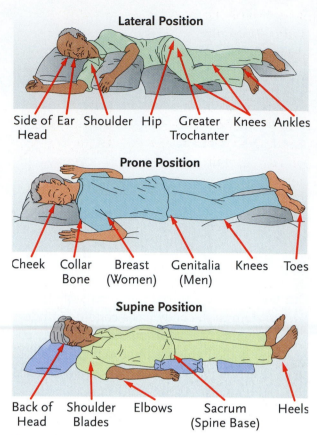

Fig. 9-2. Pressure sore danger zones.

more blood to the body surface to cool it off. The same blood vessels **constrict**, or close, when the outside temperature is too cold. By restricting the amount of blood reaching the skin, the blood vessels help the body retain heat.

COMMON DISORDERS
Integumentary System

Pressure sores occur when the skin deteriorates (breaks up) from pressure and shearing (pressure from sliding skin across another surface). Eventually blood does not circulate properly and sores or ulcers form, swell, and may become infected. **Decubitus ulcer** is another name for pressure sore.

Pressure sores usually occur on **bony prominences**, which are areas of the body where bone is close to the skin. The skin here is at a much higher risk for skin breakdown. These areas include elbows, shoulder blades, tailbone, hip bones, ankles, heels, and the back of the neck and head. Other areas at risk are the ears, the area under the breasts, and the scrotum (Fig. 9-2).

Pressure sores are painful and difficult to heal. They can lead to life-threatening infection. Prevention is very important. See chapter 15 for more information.

OBSERVING AND REPORTING
Integumentary System

Report to a supervisor the following signs and symptoms:

- rashes or scales
- bruising
- cuts, boils, sores, wounds, abrasions
- changes in color or moistness/dryness
- swelling
- scalp or hair changes
- skin that appears different from normal or that has changed

2. Describe the musculoskeletal system

Muscles, bones, ligaments, tendons, and cartilage (*KAR-ti-lidj*) give the body shape and structure. They work together to allow the body to move (Fig. 9-3). Besides allowing the body to

move, **bones** also protect organs. Two bones meet at a **joint**. Some joints make movement possible in all directions. Other joints permit movement in one direction only. **Muscles** provide movement of body parts to maintain posture and to produce body heat.

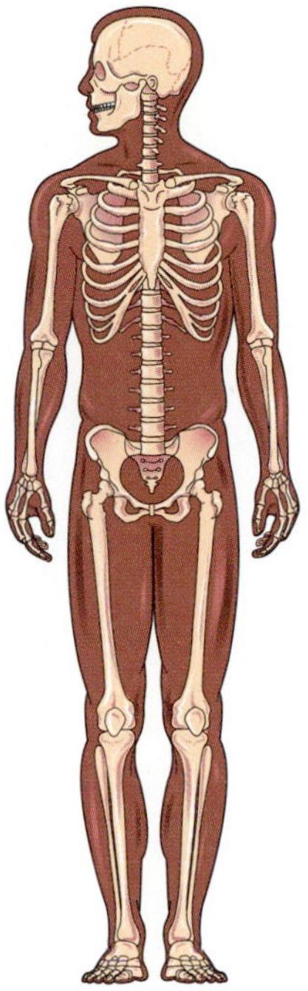

Exercise is important for improving and maintaining physical and mental health. Inactivity and immobility can result in loss of self-esteem, depression, pneumonia, urinary tract infection, constipation, blood clots, and dulling of the senses. Clients who are ill or elderly can develop **muscle atrophy** (*AT-roh-fee*) or **contractures** (*kon-TRAK-churz*). When atrophy occurs, the muscle wastes away, decreases in size, and becomes weak. When a contracture develops, the muscle shortens, becomes inflexible, and "freezes" in position. This causes permanent disability of the limb.

Range of motion (ROM) exercises can help prevent these conditions. With ROM exercises, the joints are extended and flexed in the measured degrees of a circle (Fig. 9-4). Exercise increases circulation of blood, oxygen, and nutrients and improves muscle tone. See chapter 15 for more information on ROM exercises.

Fig. 9-3. The skeleton is composed of 206 bones that help movement and protect organs.

COMMON DISORDERS
Musculoskeletal System

- A **fracture** (*FRAKT-chur*) is a broken bone. To treat fractures, bones are held immobile (by a cast if possible) until the bone can fuse itself back together. This process can take longer in elderly clients than in younger people.

- **Osteoporosis** (*os-tee-oh-poh-ROH-sis*) is a disease that causes bones to become

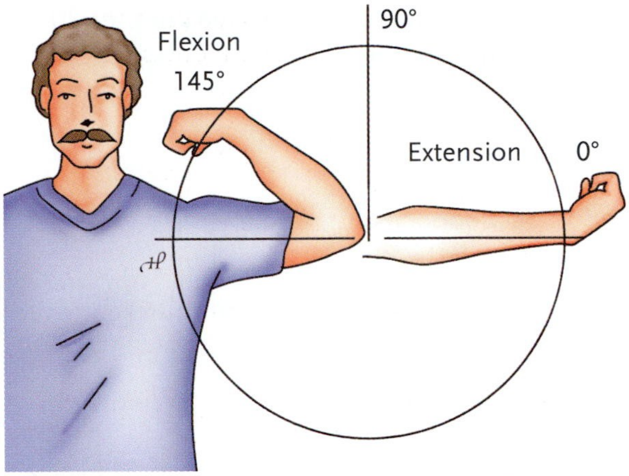

Fig. 9-4. A complete circle is 360 degrees. Degrees of a circle are used to determine how far the client's joints flex or extend during ROM exercises.

porous and brittle. Brittle bones can fracture easily. Weakness in bones may be due to age, lack of hormones, not enough calcium in bones, alcohol consumption, or lack of exercise. It occurs more commonly in women after **menopause** (*MEN-oh-paws*). Menopause is the stopping of menstrual periods. Extra calcium and regular exercise can help prevent osteoporosis. Signs and symptoms of osteoporosis include low back pain, stooped posture, and becoming shorter over time (Fig. 9-5).

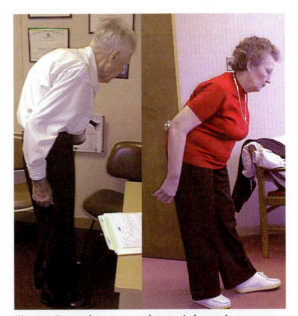

Fig. 9-5. Stooped posture, or dowager's hump, is a common sign of osteoporosis. (Photos courtesy of Jeffrey T. Behr, MD)

- **Arthritis** (*ar-THRYE-tis*) is inflammation, or swelling, of a joint. It can result in pain and

The Human Body in Health and Disease

9

difficulty with movement. See chapter 20 for more information.

OBSERVING AND REPORTING
Musculoskeletal System

Report to a supervisor the following signs and symptoms:

- changes in ability to perform routine movements and activities
- any changes in clients' ability to perform ROM exercises
- pain during movement
- any new or increased swelling of joints
- white, shiny, red, or warm areas over a joint
- bruising
- aches and pains clients report to you

3. Describe the nervous system

The nervous system is the control center and message center of the body. It controls and co-ordinates all body functions. The nervous system also senses and interprets information from the environment outside the human body.

The nervous system has two main parts: the **central nervous system** (CNS) and the **peripheral** (*per-IF-er-al*) **nervous system** (Fig. 9-6). The central nervous system is composed of the brain and spinal cord. The peripheral nervous system deals with the periphery, or outer part of the body, via the nerves that extend throughout the body.

COMMON DISORDERS
Central Nervous System

- **Dementia** refers to changes in the brain that alter personality and impair the ability to think and remember. **Alzheimer's disease** (AD) is an example of a dementia with an unknown cause. It cannot be cured, is irreversible, and gets worse over time. See chapter 20 for more information on AD.

- A **cerebrovascular** (*se-ree-broh-VAS-kyoo-lar*) **accident** (CVA), or stroke, occurs when blood supply to a part of the brain is cut off

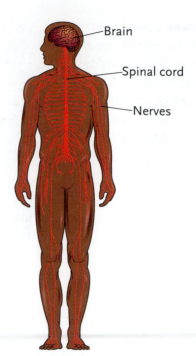

Fig. 9-6. The nervous system includes the brain, spinal cord, and nerves throughout the body.

suddenly by a clot or a ruptured blood vessel. A CVA can cause sudden paresis (weakness) or paralysis (immobility) of certain parts of the body. Paresis and paralysis usually affect one side of the body. Other functions of the body may be impaired, including the ability to speak and swallow. See chapter 20 for more information.

- **Parkinson's disease** causes a section of the brain to degenerate slowly and progressively. See chapter 17 for more information.

- When a person has **multiple sclerosis** (MS), the **myelin** (*MYE-e-lin*) **sheath** that covers the nerves, spinal cord, and white matter of the brain breaks down over time. Without the myelin sheath, the nerves cannot conduct impulses to and from the brain in a normal way. See chapter 17 for more information.

- **Epilepsy** is an illness of the brain that produces seizures. Epileptic seizures can range from mild tremors or brief blackouts to violent convulsions lasting several minutes. The cause of most cases of epilepsy is unknown. However, excessive alcohol intake, substance abuse, brain tumors, or injuries can sometimes cause it.

Cerebral palsy is the result of an injury to the cerebrum that occurs during pregnancy or the birth process. The resulting brain damage causes a loss of muscle control, poor coordination, problems with balance, and difficulty in speaking. See chapter 17 for more information.

Head injuries can cause permanent brain damage. The extent of **spinal cord injuries** depends on the force of the impact and where on the spinal cord the injury is located. See chapter 17 for more information.

OBSERVING AND REPORTING
Central Nervous System

Report to a supervisor the following signs and symptoms:

- fatigue or pain with movement or exercise
- shaking or trembling
- inability to speak clearly
- inability to move one side of body
- disturbance or change in vision or hearing
- changes in eating patterns or fluid intake
- difficulty swallowing
- bowel and bladder changes
- depression or mood changes
- memory loss or confusion
- violent behavior
- any unusual or unexplained change in behavior
- decreased ability to perform ADLs

The Nervous System: Sense Organs

The eyes, ears, nose, tongue, and skin are the body's major sense organs. They are considered part of the central nervous system because they contain receptors that receive impulses from the environment. They relay these impulses to nerves (Figs. 9-7 and 9-8).

COMMON DISORDERS
Eyes and Ears

Cataracts (*KAT-a-rakts*) are milky or cloudy

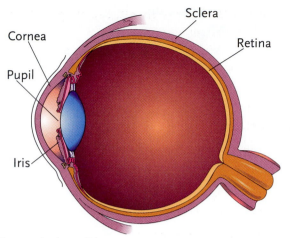

Fig. 9-7. The parts of the eye.

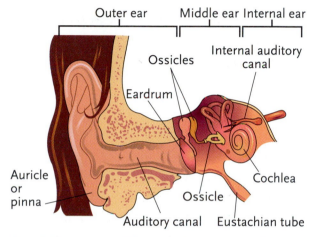

Fig. 9-8. The outer ear, middle ear, and inner ear are the three main divisions of the ear.

spots that develop in the eye. Cataracts eventually impair vision and can affect one or both eyes. **Glaucoma** (*glaw-KOH-ma*) is a condition in which the fluid inside the eyeball is unable to drain. Pressure inside the eye increases and causes damage that often leads to blindness. See chapter 17 for more information.

Otitis media (*oh-TYE-tis MEE-dee-a*) is an infection of the middle ear that can be caused by a variety of microorganisms.

Deafness is partial or complete loss of hearing. It can occur as the result of heredity, disease, or injury. In the elderly, aging commonly causes loss of hearing, as well as impaired vision, smell, and taste.

Vertigo (*VER-ti-goh*), or dizziness, is usually the result of an inner ear disturbance. Diseases of the brain can also cause it.

9

The Human Body in Health and Disease

Eyes and Ears

Report to a supervisor the following signs and symptoms:

- changes in vision or hearing
- signs of infection
- dizziness
- client complaints of pain in eyes or ears

4. Describe the circulatory or cardio-vascular system

The circulatory system is made up of the heart, blood vessels, and blood. The heart pumps blood through the blood vessels to the cells. The interior of the heart is divided into four chambers (Fig. 9-9). The two upper chambers are called the left atrium and right atrium. They receive blood. The two lower chambers or **ventricles** (*VEN-tri-kuls*) pump blood. The blood carries food, oxygen, and other substances that cells need to function properly (Fig. 9-10).

The heart functions in two phases: the contracting phase or **systole** (*SIS-toh-lee*), when the ventricles pump blood through the blood vessels and the resting phase or **diastole** (*dye-AS-toh-lee*), when the chambers fill with blood.

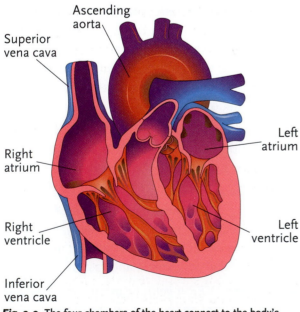

Fig. 9-9. The four chambers of the heart connect to the body's largest blood vessels.

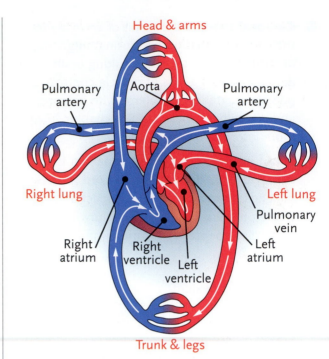

Fig. 9-10. The flow of blood through the heart.

When a person's blood pressure is taken, the numbers measure these two phases.

The circulatory system performs the following major functions:

- supplying food, oxygen, and hormones to cells
- producing and supplying antibodies and other infection-fighting blood cells
- removing waste products from cells
- controlling body temperature

Circulatory System

- **Atherosclerosis** (*ath-er-oh-skle-ROH-sis*) is a hardening and narrowing of the blood vessels.

- **Myocardial infarction** (MI) (*mye-oh-KAR-dee-al in-FARK-shun*), or heart attack, occurs when the heart muscle itself does not receive enough oxygen because blood vessels are blocked. See chapters 7 and 20 for more information.

- **Angina pectoris** (*an-JYE-na PEK-tor-is*) is a condition that causes temporary constriction of a coronary artery. Angina is a squeezing

pain or feeling of pressure in the chest, left arm, or jaw. See chapter 20 for more information.

Hypertension (*high-per-TEN-shun*) is high blood pressure. If untreated, hypertension can cause injury to the heart, brain, and kidneys. See chapter 20 for more information.

Congestive heart failure (CHF) can result from untreated hypertension, MI, infection, and other illnesses. Congestive heart failure occurs when the heart is no longer able to pump effectively. Blood backs up into the heart instead of circulating. See chapter 20 for more information.

Peripheral vascular disease (PVD) is a disease in which the legs, feet, arms, or hands do not have enough blood circulation. This is due to fatty deposits in the blood vessels that harden over time. The legs, feet, arms, and hands feel cool or cold. Nail beds become ashen or blue. Swelling occurs in the hands and feet. Clients may develop ulcers of the legs and feet that can become infected.

OBSERVING AND REPORTING
Circulatory System

Report to a supervisor the following signs and symptoms:

- changes in pulse rate
- weakness, fatigue
- loss of ability to perform activities of daily living (ADLs)
- swelling of hands and feet
- pale or blue appearance of hands, feet, or lips
- chest pain
- weight gain
- shortness of breath, changes in breathing patterns, inability to catch breath
- severe headache
- inactivity (which can lead to circulatory problems)

5. Describe the respiratory system

Respiration (*res-pir-AY-shun*), the body taking in oxygen and removing carbon dioxide, involves breathing in, **inspiration** (*in-spir-AY-shun*), and breathing out, **expiration** (*ex-pir-AY-shun*). The lungs accomplish this process (Fig. 9-11).

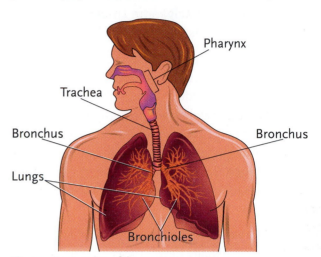

Fig. 9-11. An overview of the respiratory system.

COMMON DISORDERS
Respiratory System

Asthma is a chronic inflammatory disease. It occurs when the respiratory system is hyper-reactive (that is, it reacts quickly and strongly) to irritants, infection, cold air, or to allergens such as pollen and dust. Strenuous exercise and stress can also bring on asthma attacks. The bronchi become irritated and constrict, making it difficult to breathe. As a response to irritation and inflammation, the mucous membrane produces thick mucus that further inhibits respiration. As a result, air is trapped in the lungs, producing coughing and wheezing.

Upper respiratory infection (URI) is commonly called a cold. It is the result of a bacterial or viral infection of the nose, sinuses, and throat. Symptoms usually include nasal discharge, sneezing, sore throat, fever, and fatigue. For most people, it can be dealt with by the body's immune system and by rest, fluids, and antibiotics if the infection is bacterial.

The Human Body in Health and Disease

9

cd **Bronchitis** is an irritation and inflammation of the lining of the bronchi. Acute bronchitis is usually caused by infection. It begins with an upper respiratory infection that spreads to the lungs. Mucus, dead cells, and other fluid eventually produce a discharge that results in a productive cough. Airborne irritants cause chronic bronchitis. These irritants include cigarette smoke, car exhaust, allergens, and other pollutants.

cd **Pneumonia** can be caused by a bacterial, viral, or fungal infection. Acute inflammation occurs in a portion of lung tissue. The affected person develops a high fever, chills, cough, chest pains, and rapid pulse. In the later stages, a thick discharge is produced by the mucous membrane. Recovery may take longer for older adults and persons with chronic illnesses.

cd **Emphysema** is a chronic disease of the lungs. It usually develops as a result of chronic bronchitis and smoking. People with emphysema have difficulty breathing. Other symptoms include coughing, breathlessness, and a rapid heartbeat.

cd **Lung cancer** is the development of abnormal cells or tumors in the lungs. Symptoms of lung cancer include chronic cough, shortness of breath, and bloody sputum. **Sputum** is the fluid a person coughs up.

cd **Tuberculosis** is a highly infectious (contagious) lung disease. Symptoms include coughing, low-grade fever, shortness of breath, and bloody sputum. Chapter 5 includes more information about tuberculosis.

cd **Chronic obstructive pulmonary disease** (COPD) is a chronic disease. Four chronic lung diseases are grouped under COPD. They include bronchitis, emphysema, asthma, and bronchiectasis. People with COPD have difficulty breathing, especially in getting air out of the lungs. See chapter 20 for more information.

Make sure people with acute or chronic upper respiratory conditions are not exposed to ciga-

rette smoke or polluted air. People who have difficulty breathing will usually be more comfortable sitting up than lying down.

OBSERVING AND REPORTING
Respiratory System

Report to a supervisor the following signs and symptoms:

- O&R change in respiratory rate
- O&R shallow breathing or breathing through pursed lips
- O&R coughing or wheezing
- O&R nasal congestion or discharge
- O&R sore throat, difficulty swallowing, or swollen tonsils
- O&R the need to sit after mild exertion
- O&R the need to rest on two pillows
- O&R pale or bluish color of the lips and extremities
- O&R pain in the chest area
- O&R discolored sputum (green, yellow, blood-tinged, or gray)

6. Describe the urinary system

The urinary system is composed of two kidneys, two ureters, one urinary bladder, and a single urethra. Urine passes out of the body through the meatus, the opening at the end of the urethra (Figs. 9-12 and 9-13). The urinary system has two important functions. Through urine,

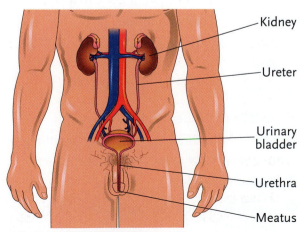

Kidney

Ureter

Urinary bladder

Urethra

Meatus

***Fig. 9-12.** The male urinary system.*

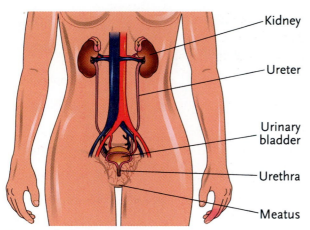

Kidney

Ureter

Urinary bladder

Urethra

Meatus

Fig. 9-13. The female urinary system.

the urinary system eliminates waste products created by the cells. The urinary system also maintains the water balance in the body.

Home health aides may play an important role in helping clients maintain fluid balance. This is done by measuring intake of fresh fluids and output of waste fluids. See chapter 13 for more information.

COMMON DISORDERS
Urinary System

- **Urinary tract infection** (UTI) causes inflammation of the bladder and the ureters. This results in a painful burning during urination and the frequent feeling of needing to urinate. UTI or **cystitis** (*sis-TYE-tis*), also inflammation of the bladder, may be caused by bacterial infection. Certain situations, such as confinement to bed, cause urine to stay in the bladder too long. This provides an ideal environment for bacteria to grow.

  Cystitis is more common in women because the urethra is much shorter in women (three to four inches) than in men (seven to eight inches). To avoid infection, women should wipe the perineal (*payr-i-NEE-al*) area from front to back after bladder and bowel elimination.

- **Calculi** (*KAL-kyoo-lye*), or kidney stones, form when urine crystallizes in the kidneys. Kidney stones can block the kidneys and ureters, causing severe pain. Kidney stones

can be caused by some of the same conditions that cause cystitis. They can also be the result of a vitamin deficiency, mineral imbalance, structural abnormalities of the urinary tract, or infection.

- **Nephritis** is an inflammation of the kidneys. Symptoms include a decrease in urine output, rusty-colored urine, and a burning feeling during urination. A person with nephritis often has a swollen face, eyelids, and hands because she is retaining fluid. Children and young adults usually recover without problems. Older people can develop a chronic form of nephritis.

- **Renovascular hypertension** is a condition in which a blockage of arteries in the kidneys causes high blood pressure.

- **Chronic kidney failure**, or **uremia** (*you-REE-mee-a*), occurs because the kidneys become unable to eliminate certain waste products from the body. This disease can develop as the result of chronic urinary tract infections, nephritis, or diabetes. Excessive salt in the diet can also cause damage to the kidneys. Over time, the disease becomes worse.

  Kidney dialysis (*dye-AL-i-sis*), an artificial means of removing the body's waste products, can improve and extend life for several years. Clients will be on fluid restrictions of different degrees. Some clients may receive a kidney transplant.

- **Benign prostatic hypertrophy** (*be-NINE pros-TAT-ik HIGH-per-troh-fee*) is an enlargement of the prostate gland. It is an illness of the endocrine system that can affect a man's urinary tract. This condition causes frequent urination, dribbling of urine, and difficulty in starting the flow of urine. Urinary retention (urine remaining in the bladder) may also occur, causing urinary tract infection. Urine can also back up into the ureters and kidneys, causing damage to these organs. Benign prostatic hypertrophy can be treated with medications.

9

The Human Body in Health and Disease

Report to a supervisor the following signs and symptoms:

- O&R weight loss or gain
- O&R swelling in the upper or lower extremities
- O&R painful urination or burning during urination
- O&R changes in the characteristics of urine, such as cloudiness, odor, or color
- O&R changes in frequency and amount of urination
- O&R swelling in the abdominal/bladder area
- O&R client complaining that bladder feels full or painful
- O&R incontinence/dribbling
- O&R pain in the kidney or back/flank region
- O&R inadequate fluid intake

7. Describe the gastrointestinal or digestive system

The gastrointestinal system or digestive system is made up of the alimentary (*al-i-MEN-tayr-ee*) canal and the accessory digestive organs (Fig. 9-14). The gastrointestinal system has two functions: **digestion** and **elimination**. Digestion is the process of preparing food physically and chemically so that it can be absorbed into the cells. Elimination is the process of expelling solid wastes made up of the waste products of food that are not absorbed into the cells.

COMMON DISORDERS
Gastrointestinal System

- cd **Heartburn** is the result of a weakening of the **sphincter** (*SFINK-ter*) **muscle** which joins the esophagus and the stomach. When healthy and strong, this muscle prevents the leaking of stomach acid and other contents back into the esophagus. Stomach acid causes a burning sensation, commonly called heartburn, in the esophagus. If heartburn occurs frequently and remains untreated, it can cause scarring or **ulceration** (*ul-ser-AY-shun*).

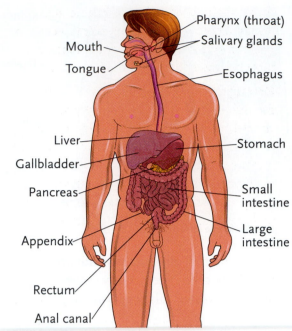

Fig. 9-14. The gastrointestinal tract consists of all the organs needed to digest food and process waste.

- cd **Gastric reflux** occurs when stomach contents pass through the esophagus into the lungs. If it occurs frequently, aspiration into the lungs is a serious problem. It can cause deterioration of lung tissue leading to asthma, pneumonia, and even death.

  Heartburn and gastric reflux must be reported to your supervisor. These conditions are usually treated with medications. Make your clients comfortable by having the evening meal served three to four hours before bedtime. Provide an extra pillow so the body is more upright during sleep. Do not allow client to lay down until at least 2-3 hours after eating. Serving the largest meal of the day at lunchtime, serving several meals of small portions throughout the day, and reducing fast foods, fatty foods, and spicy foods may also help.

- cd **Peptic ulcers** are raw sores in the stomach or the small intestine. A dull or gnawing pain occurs one to three hours after eating, accompanied by belching or vomiting. Food, antacids, and medications temporarily relieve the pain. Ulcers are caused by excessive acid production. Clients with peptic ulcers should avoid smoking and drinking too much alcohol and caffeine, which

increase the production of gastric acid. Peptic ulcers may cause bleeding. Feces, or bowel movements, may appear black and tarry because of the bleeding.

- **Constipation** is the difficult and often painful elimination of a hard, dry stool (bowel movement). Constipation occurs when the feces move too slowly through the intestine as the result of decreased fluid intake, poor diet, inactivity, medications, aging, certain diseases, or ignoring the urge to eliminate. Treatment often includes increasing the amount of fiber eaten, increasing the activity level, and possibly medication.

- **Diarrhea** is frequent elimination of liquid or semi-liquid feces. Abdominal cramps, urgency, nausea, and vomiting can accompany diarrhea, depending on the cause. Bacterial and viral infections, microorganisms in food and water, irritating foods, and certain medications can cause diarrhea. Treatment of diarrhea usually involves medications and a change of diet. A diet of bananas, rice, apples, and tea/toast (BRAT diet) is often recommended.

- **Hepatitis** means inflammation of the liver. It begins with symptoms that resemble the flu (fever, fatigue, nausea, vomiting) but eventually **jaundice** (*JAWN-dis*) appears. Jaundice is a condition in which the skin, whites of the eyes, and mucous membranes appear yellow. Different types of hepatitis have different causes. The virus causing hepatitis A is a result of fecal-oral contamination. For example, a person washes her hands improperly after having a bowel movement. She then prepares and eats food that has been contaminated by the fecal material left on her hands and/or under her nails. Hepatitis B is contracted through blood or needles that are contaminated with the virus, or by sexual contact with an infected person. Hepatitis C is also transmitted through blood and possibly sexual intercourse. Hepatitis B and C can lead to cirrhosis and liver cancer. Good nutrition

and rest are important in the treatment. Because hepatitis is an infectious disease, follow Standard Precautions when caring for a client with hepatitis.

- **Ulcerative colitis** (*UL-ser-a-tiv koh-LYE-tis*) is a chronic inflammatory disease of the large intestine. Symptoms include cramping diarrhea, with pain occurring to one side of the lower abdomen, and loss of appetite. Ulcerative colitis is a serious illness that can cause intestinal bleeding and death if left untreated.

   Medications can relieve symptoms, but they cannot cure ulcerative colitis. Surgical treatment may include a **colostomy** (*koh-LOS-toh-mee*), which is the diversion of waste to an artificial opening (**stoma**) through the abdomen. All bowels are diverted through the stoma instead of the anus. See chapter 14 for more information on colostomy care.

- **Colitis**, or irritable bowel syndrome, has symptoms similar to but milder than those of ulcerative colitis. Diet and/or medication can usually control colitis.

- **Colorectal** (*koh-loh-REK-tal*) **cancer** is cancer of the gastrointestinal tract. Signs and symptoms include changes in normal bowel patterns, cramps, abdominal pain, and rectal bleeding. Colorectal cancer must be treated surgically.

- **Hemorrhoids** are enlarged veins in the rectum that may also be visible outside the anus. Rectal itching, burning, pain, and bleeding are signs and symptoms of hemorrhoids. Treatment may include medications and compresses. Surgery may be necessary to correct hemorrhoids. When cleaning the anus, be very careful to avoid causing pain and bleeding from hemorrhoids.

OBSERVING AND REPORTING
Gastrointestinal System

Report to a supervisor the following signs and symptoms:

- difficulty swallowing or chewing (including denture problems or mouth sores)

9

The Human Body in Health and Disease

9

The Human Body in Health and Disease

- fecal incontinence (losing control of bowels)
- weight gain/weight loss
- anorexia (loss of appetite)
- abdominal pain and cramping
- diarrhea
- nausea and vomiting (especially vomitus that looks like coffee grounds)
- constipation
- flatulence
- hiccups, belching
- abnormally colored stool (bloody, black, or hard)
- heartburn
- poor nutritional intake

8. Describe the endocrine system

The endocrine system is made up of glands that secrete hormones. **Hormones** are chemicals that control many of the organs and body systems (Fig. 9-15). They are carried in the blood to the various organs, where they perform the following functions:

- maintain homeostasis
- influence growth and development
- regulate levels of sugar in the blood
- regulate levels of calcium in the bones
- determine how fast cells burn food for energy

The function of the endocrine system is to secrete hormones that regulate essential body processes.

COMMON DISORDERS
Endocrine System

- **Hyperthyroidism** (*high-per-THIGH-royd-ism*). When the thyroid produces too much thyroid hormone, the cells burn too much food. Weight loss, nervousness, and hyperactivity occur. Hyperthyroidism is usually treated with medication. Occasionally, part of the thyroid is surgically removed.

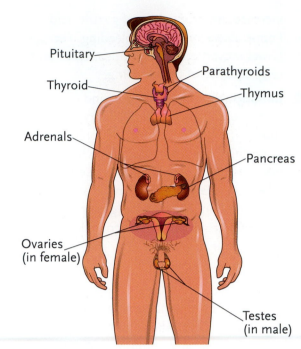

Fig. 9-15. The endocrine system includes organs that produce hormones that regulate body processes.

- **Hypothyroidism** (*high-poh-THIGH-royd-ism*). When the thyroid produces too little thyroid hormone, the body processes slow down. Weight gain and physical and mental sluggishness result. Hypothyroidism is sometimes treated with medication.

- **Diabetes Mellitus** (*mel-EYE-tus*) occurs when the pancreas produces too little insulin; as a result, sugar builds up in the blood and cannot get to the cells. This makes it difficult for the body to process carbohydrates, fats, and proteins. Diabetes is a chronic disease that has two forms: Type I, or insulin-dependent diabetes mellitus (IDDM); and Type II, or non-insulin-dependent diabetes mellitus (NIDDM).

Signs and symptoms of diabetes include increased thirst and urine production, hunger, and weight loss. Urine tests show the presence of sugar in the urine. Blood tests indicate a high level of sugar in the blood.

If not controlled, diabetes can affect other organ systems. Uncontrolled diabetes can lead to any of the following health problems:

- blindness
- diseases of the kidney

- diseases of the nerves
- diseases of the circulatory system, including stroke, heart attack, and slow healing
- frequent infections
- gangrene, which can lead to amputation of an affected body part

See chapter 20 for more information on the disease and care guidelines.

Many endocrine illnesses can be treated with hormone supplements. These supplements must be given very precisely. For example, too much insulin administered to a diabetic can cause the sudden onset of insulin shock.

Endocrine System

Report to a supervisor the following signs and symptoms:

- O&R headache*
- O&R weakness*
- O&R blurred vision*
- O&R dizziness*
- O&R hunger*
- O&R irritability*
- O&R sweating*
- O&R change in "normal" behavior*
- O&R weight gain/weight loss
- O&R loss of appetite/ increased appetite
- O&R increased thirst
- O&R frequent urination
- O&R dry skin
- O&R sluggishness or fatigue
- O&R increased confusion
- O&R hyperactivity

* indicates signs and symptoms that should be reported immediately

9. Describe the reproductive system

The reproductive system is made up of the re-

productive organs, which are different in men and women (Figs. 9-16 and 9-17). The reproductive system allows human beings to **reproduce**, or create new human life. Reproduction begins when a man's and woman's sex cells (sperm and ovum) join. These sex cells are formed in the male and female sex glands. These sex glands are called the **gonads**.

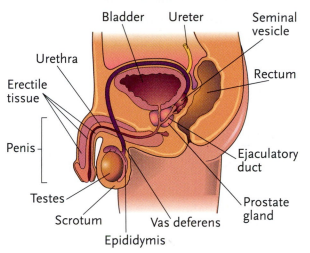

Fig. 9-16. The male reproductive system.

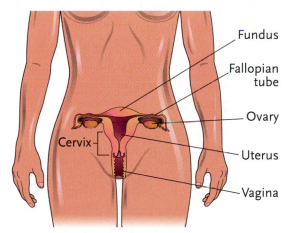

Fig. 9-17. The female reproductive system.

Reproductive System

- cd **Vaginitis**, an infection of the vagina, may be caused by a bacteria, protozoa (one-celled animals), or fungus (yeast). It may also be the result of hormonal changes in vaginal secretions after menopause. Women who have vaginitis have a white vaginal discharge, accompanied by itching and burning.

- cd **Benign prostatic hypertrophy** is a disor-

9

The Human Body in Health and Disease

der that occurs in men as they age. The prostate becomes enlarged and causes pressure on the urethra. The pressure on the urethra leads to urinary problems described earlier in this chapter. Benign prostatic hypertrophy is treatable with medications or surgery. A test is also available to screen for cancer of the prostate. As men age, they are at increased risk for prostate cancer. Prostate cancer is usually slow-growing and responsive to treatment if detected early.

Sexually Transmitted Diseases (STDs)

Sexually transmitted diseases, also called **venereal** (*ven-EER-ee-al*) **diseases**, are passed through sexual contact with an infected person. This contact includes sexual intercourse, contact of the mouth with the genitals or anus, and contact of the hands to the genitals. Using latex condoms during sexual contact can reduce the chances of being infected or passing on some STDs. The human immunodeficiency virus (HIV), acquired immunodeficiency syndrome (AIDS), and some kinds of hepatitis can be sexually transmitted. (HIV/AIDS is discussed in detail in chapter 5 and chapter 20.) STDs are very common. They can have serious health consequences. Clients may be unaware of or embarrassed by symptoms that indicate an STD.

Chlamydia infection is caused by organisms introduced into the mucous membranes of the reproductive tract. Chlamydia can cause serious infection, including pelvic inflammatory disease (PID) in women. PID can lead to sterility. Symptoms of chlamydia infection include yellow or white discharge from the penis or vagina and a burning sensation during urination. It is treated with antibiotics.

Syphilis can be treated effectively in the early stages, but if left untreated can cause brain damage, mental illness, and even death. Babies born to mothers infected with syphilis may be born blind or with other serious birth defects. Syphilis is easier to detect in men than in women, due to open sores called **chancres**

(*KAYN-kers*) that develop on the penis soon after infection.

However, the chancres are painless and can go unnoticed. If untreated, the infection progresses to the heart, brain, and other vital organs. Common symptoms at this stage include rash, sore throat, or fever. When detected, syphilis can be treated with penicillin or other antibiotics. The sooner the disease is treated, the better the person's chances of preventing long-term consequences and avoiding infection of sexual partners.

Gonorrhea, like syphilis, can be treated with antibiotics and is easier to detect in men than in women. If untreated, gonorrhea can cause sterility in both men and women. A baby born to a woman infected with gonorrhea can suffer permanent damage to the eyes. For this reason, all babies' eyes are treated with eyedrops shortly after birth to kill any infection.

Most women infected with gonorrhea show no early symptoms. This makes it easy for women to spread the disease. Men infected with gonorrhea will typically show a greenish or yellowish discharge from the penis within a week after infection. Burning during urination is another common symptom in men.

Herpes simplex II, unlike the other STDs discussed here, is caused by a virus and therefore cannot be treated with antibiotics. Once infected with the herpes virus, a person cannot be cured. The person may suffer repeated outbreaks of the disease for the rest of his or her life. A herpes outbreak includes burning, painful, red sores on the genitals that heal in about two weeks. The sores are infectious, but a person with herpes virus can spread the infection even when sores are not present.

Some people infected with herpes never experience repeated outbreaks, or the later episodes may not be as painful as the initial outbreak. Treatment with antiviral drugs can help people stay symptom-free for longer periods of time. Babies born to women infected with herpes

simplex II can be infected during birth. Pregnant women experiencing a herpes outbreak are usually delivered by cesarean (*se-SAYR-ee-an*) section, or C-section.

OBSERVING AND REPORTING
Reproductive System

Report to a supervisor the following symptoms:

- discomfort or difficulty with urination
- discharge from the penis or vagina
- swelling of the genitals
- changes in menstruation
- blood in urine or stool
- breast changes, including size, shape, lumps, or discharge from the nipple
- presence of sores on the genitals
- client reports of impotence, or inability of male to have sexual intercourse
- client reports of painful intercourse

10. Describe the immune and lymphatic systems

The immune system protects the body from disease-causing bacteria, viruses, and organisms in two ways. **Nonspecific immunity** protects the body from disease in general. **Specific immunity** protects against a particular disease that is invading the body at a given time.

The lymphatic (*lim-FAT-ik*) system removes excess fluids and waste products from body tissues and helps the immune system fight infection. Closely related to both the immune and the circulatory systems, the lymphatic system consists of lymph vessels and lymph capillaries in which a fluid called **lymph** circulates (Fig. 9-18). Lymph is a clear yellowish fluid that carries disease-fighting cells called **lymphocytes** (*LIM-foh-sytes*).

Unlike the circulatory system, in which the heart functions as a pump to move the blood, the lymph system has no pump. Lymph fluid is circulated by muscle activity, massage, and breathing.

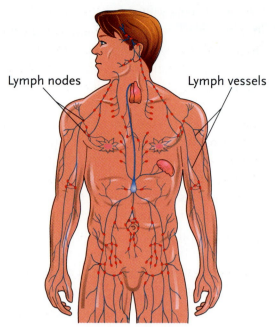

Fig. 9-18. Lymph nodes work to fight infection and are located throughout the body.

COMMON DISORDERS
Immune System

- **AIDS** is an example of immune system failure. It is caused by a massive infection of the immune system by HIV. The virus invades the body, multiplies, and disables the cells of the immune system so that it cannot protect the body from disease. People with AIDS usually die of pneumonia or other infections that their bodies are unable to fight. See chapter 20 for more information.

- **Lymphoma** (*lim-FOH-ma*) is cancer of the lymphatic system. One specific form of lymphoma is **Hodgkin's Disease**. Treatment for lymphomas may include radiation therapy or chemotherapy. See chapter 20 for more information on caring for clients with cancer.

OBSERVING AND REPORTING
Immune System

Report to a supervisor the following signs and symptoms:

- recurring infections (such as pneumonia, diarrhea, and fevers)
- swelling of the lymph nodes
- increased fatigue

OBSERVING AND REPORTING
Lymphatic System

O&R swelling of the lymph nodes

Summary

The human body is complicated. The few signs and symptoms mentioned in this chapter may seem overwhelming. This is why it is so important to note and report any change in your client. From the color of a patch of skin to changes in a client's abilities—your observations could reveal signs of a significant problem! You are in the best position to observe and report changes in a client's health and well-being. Make noticing these changes a mission!

Chapter Review

1. Why is prevention of pressure sores very important?

2. List five signs and symptoms to observe and report about the integumentary system.

3. How many bones make up the skeleton of the human body?

4. What type of exercises can help prevent contractures and muscle atrophy?

5. List five signs and symptoms to observe and report about the musculoskeletal system.

6. What are two functions of the nervous system?

7. List nine signs and symptoms to observe and report about the nervous system.

8. List three signs and symptoms to observe and report about the eyes and ears.

9. What are four functions of the circulatory system?

10. List seven signs and symptoms to observe and report about the circulatory system.

11. What does respiration mean? What are the two parts involved in respiration?

12. List seven signs and symptoms to observe and report about the respiratory system.

13. What are two functions of the urinary system?

14. Why is it important for a woman to wipe from front to back after elimination?

15. List seven signs and symptoms to observe and report about the urinary system.

16. What does digestion mean? What does elimination mean?

17. List nine signs and symptoms to observe and report about the gastrointestinal system.

18. List eight signs and symptoms to observe and report about the endocrine system immediately.

19. What is the function of the reproductive system?

20. What are three types of sexual contact that can transmit STDs?

21. Why can't Herpes simplex II be treated with antibiotics?

22. List seven signs and symptoms to observe and report about the reproductive system.

23. What is nonspecific immunity? What is specific immunity?

24. What is the function of the lymphatic system?

25. List three signs and symptoms to observe and report about the immune system.

10
Human Development and Aging

Throughout their lives, people change physically and psychologically. Physical changes occur in the body. Psychological changes occur in the mind and also in the person's behavior. These changes are called human growth and development.

Everyone will go through the same stages of development during their lives, but no two people will follow the exact same pattern or rate of development. Each client must be treated as an individual and a whole person who is growing and developing rather than someone who is merely ill or disabled.

1. Describe the stages of human development and identify common disorders for each group

Infancy, Birth to Twelve Months

Infants grow and develop very quickly. In one year a baby moves from total dependence on the caregiver to the relative independence of moving around, communicating basic needs, and feeding himself.

Physical development in infancy moves from the head down. For example, infants gain control over the muscles of the neck before they are able to control the muscles in their shoulders. Control over muscles in the trunk area, such as the shoulder, develops before control of the

arms and legs (Fig. 10-1). This head-to-toe sequence should be respected when caring for infants. For example, newborns must be supported at the shoulders, head, and neck, and babies who cannot sit or crawl should not be encouraged to stand or walk.

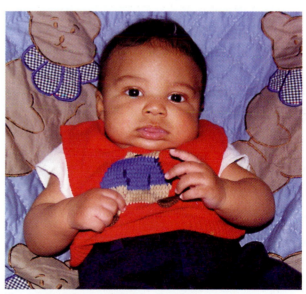

Fig. 10-1. An infant's physical development moves from the head down.

COMMON DISORDERS
Infancy

(cd) Babies who are born before 37 weeks gestation (more than three weeks before the due date) are considered **premature**. These babies may weigh from one to six pounds, depending on how early they are born. Often, premature babies will remain in the hospital for some time after birth. At home, prema-

ture babies may need special care. This includes medication, heart monitoring, and frequent feedings to ensure weight gain.

- Babies born at full term but weighing less than five pounds are called **low birth weight** babies. Low birth weight babies can have many of the same problems premature babies have. They are cared for in much the same way as premature babies.

- The term "**birth defects**" is very general. It includes many different conditions that affect an infant from birth. Some birth defects are inherited from parents. Injury or disease during pregnancy causes others. Some of the conditions you may see include cerebral palsy, Down syndrome, and cystic fibrosis. See chapter 17 for more information.

- **Viral** or **bacterial infections** can cause fever, runny nose, coughing, rash, vomiting, diarrhea, or secondary infections of the sinuses or ears. Bacterial infections can be treated with antibiotics. Viral infections are treated with extra rest, fluids, and sometimes over-the-counter medications for cough or congestion.

- **Sudden infant death syndrome** (SIDS) or crib death, is a condition in which babies stop breathing and die for no known reason while asleep. Doctors do not know how to prevent SIDS. However, studies have shown that putting the baby to sleep on its back can reduce the chances of SIDS. Because SIDS is more common among premature or low birth weight babies, these infants often wear **apnea** (*AP-nee-a*) **monitors** to alert parents if breathing stops. Another factor that may contribute to SIDS is second-hand smoke. Parents and caregivers should never smoke around infants or children.

Childhood

The Toddler Period, Ages One to Three

During the toddler years, children gain independence. One part of this independence is new control over their bodies. Toddlers learn to speak, gain coordination of their limbs, and gain control over their bladders and bowels (Fig. 10-2).

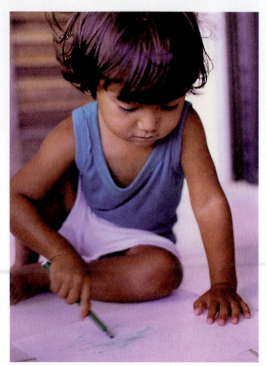

Fig. 10-2. Toddlers gain coordination of their limbs.

Toddlers assert their new independence by exploring further and further from the caregiver. Poisons and other hazards, such as sharp objects, must be locked away.

Psychologically, toddlers learn that they are individuals, separate from their parents. Children at this age may try to control their parents. They may try to get what they want by throwing tantrums, whining, or refusing to cooperate. This is a key time for parents to establish rules and standards.

The Preschool Years, Ages Three to Six

Children in their preschool years develop skills that help them become more independent and have social relationships (Fig. 10-3). They develop a vocabulary and language skills. They learn to play cooperatively in groups. They become more physically coordinated, and learn to care for themselves. Preschoolers also develop ways of relating to family members. They begin to learn right from wrong.

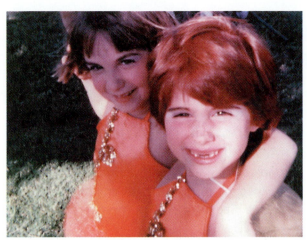

Fig. 10-3. Children in preschool years develop social relationships.

School-Age Children, Ages Six to Twelve

From ages six to about eight years, children's development is centered on **cognitive** (*KOG-ni-tiv*) development (developing thinking and learning skills) and social development. As children enter school, they also explore the environment around them and relate to other children through games, peer groups, and classroom activities (Fig. 10-4). In these years, children learn to get along with each other. They also begin to behave in a way that is common among their sex, and they develop a conscience, morals, and self-esteem.

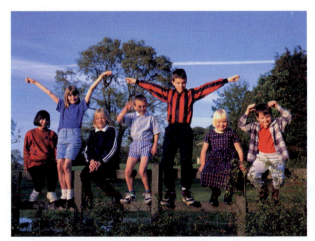

Fig. 10-4. School-age children on a field trip.

COMMON DISORDERS
Childhood

- Chicken pox is a highly contagious, viral illness that strikes nearly all children. It generally has no serious effects for healthy children. However, in adults or in anyone with a weakened immune system it can have more serious effects. Taking the varicella-zoster vaccine, commonly called the chickenpox vaccine, can prevent chicken pox.

- Children, as well as infants, may be susceptible to infections caused by viruses or bacteria. Bacterial infections can be treated with antibiotics. Viral infections are treated with extra rest, fluids, and over-the-counter medications for cough or congestion.

- **Leukemia** (*loo-KEE-mee-a*) is a form of cancer. It refers to the inability of the body's white blood cells to fight disease. Children with leukemia may be susceptible to infections and other disorders. Chemotherapy can be used to fight this disease. See chapter 20 for more information on cancer.

- **Child abuse** refers to physical, emotional, and sexual mistreatment of children, as well as neglect and maltreatment. **Physical abuse** includes hitting, kicking, burning, or intentionally causing injury to a child. **Emotional abuse** includes withholding affection, constantly criticizing, or ridiculing a child. **Sexual abuse** includes engaging in or allowing another person to engage in a sexual act with a child. **Neglect** and **maltreatment** include not providing adequate food, clothing, or support. They also include allowing children to use alcohol or drugs, leaving children alone, or exposing them to danger. See chapter 19 for more information.

- Measles, mumps, rubella, diphtheria, smallpox, whooping cough, and polio are diseases that were once common during childhood. They can all be prevented now with vaccinations.

Adolescence

Puberty

Puberty (*PYOO-ber-tee*) is the stage of growth when secondary sex characteristics, such as body hair, appear. Also, reproductive organs begin to function due to the secretion of the

reproductive hormones. The onset of puberty occurs between the ages of ten and sixteen for girls and twelve and fourteen for boys.

Adolescence, Ages Twelve to Eighteen

Many teenagers have a hard time adapting to the rapid changes that occur in their bodies after puberty. Peer acceptance is important to them. Because they see images of perfection in the media, adolescents (*ad-o-LES-ents*) may be afraid that they are unattractive or abnormal.

This concern for body image and peer acceptance, combined with changing hormones that influence moods, can cause adolescents to swing from one mood to another. Conflicting pressures develop as they remain dependent on their parents and yet need to express themselves socially and sexually. This causes conflict and stress. Social interaction between members of the opposite sex becomes very important (Fig. 10-5).

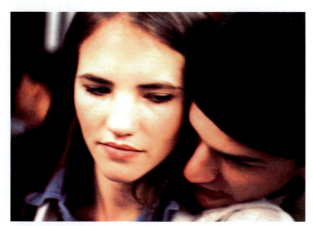

Fig. 10-5. During adolescence, people express themselves socially and sexually.

COMMON DISORDERS
Adolescence

- As their bodies change, adolescents, especially girls, may develop eating disorders. **Anorexia** (*an-or-EX-ee-a*) is a disease in which a person does not eat or exercises excessively to lose weight. A person with **bulimia** (*boo-LIM-ee-a*) **binges**, eating huge amounts of foods or very fattening foods, and then **purges** or eliminates the food by vomiting, using laxatives or exercising excessively. Eating disorders can be serious and even life-threatening. These disorders must be treated with therapy and, in some cases, hospitalization.

- Teenagers can contract **sexually transmitted diseases** (STDs) such as chlamydia (*kla-MID-ee-a*), herpes (*HER-peez*), and AIDS if they are sexually active. If teenagers are sexually active, only condoms offer some protection from sexually transmitted diseases. See chapter 9 for more information on STDs.

- Girls who are sexually active and do not use birth control, or do not use it properly, can become pregnant. **Teenage pregnancy** can have terrible consequences for adolescents, their families, and the babies born to teenage parents. Teenagers should understand that they can avoid pregnancy by using birth control or by not having sexual intercourse. Teenagers who choose to be sexually active should know what birth control methods are available and how to use them.

Pregnancy puts a great deal of stress on teenage bodies. Adolescent girls are still children. Their bodies are still developing. In most cases they are not physically ready to bear a child. It is common for teenage mothers to give birth to premature or low birth weight babies.

- Because of the many physical and emotional changes they are experiencing, adolescents may become depressed and even attempt suicide. Parents, teachers, and friends should watch for the signs of depression. These include withdrawal, loss of appetite, weight gain or loss, sleep problems, moodiness, and apathy. Teenagers who are depressed should see a doctor, counselor, therapist, minister, or other trusted adult who can get them the help they need.

- Adolescents can sustain **trauma** (*TRAW-ma*), or severe injury, to the head or spinal cord in car accidents or sports injuries. These injuries can be temporarily or permanently disabling or even fatal.

Adulthood

Young Adulthood, Ages Eighteen to Forty

By the age of eighteen, most young adults have stopped growing. Adopting a healthy lifestyle in these years can make life better now and prevent health problems in later adulthood. Psychological and social development continues, however. The developmental tasks of these years include the following:

- selecting an appropriate education and an occupation or career
- selecting a mate (Fig. 10-6)
- learning to live with a mate or others
- raising children
- developing a satisfying sex life

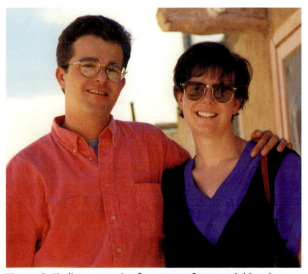

Fig. 10-6. Finding a mate is often a part of young adulthood.

Middle Adulthood, Ages Forty to Sixty-five

In general, people in middle adulthood are more comfortable and stable than they were in previous stages. Many of their major life decisions have already been made. In the early years of middle adulthood people sometimes experience a "mid-life crisis." This is a period of unrest centered on an unconscious desire for change and fulfillment of unmet goals.

Physical changes related to aging also occur in middle adulthood. Adults in this age group may notice that they have difficulty maintaining their weight or notice a decrease in strength and energy. Metabolism and other body functions slow down. Wrinkles and gray hair appear. Vision and hearing loss may begin. Women experience **menopause** (*MEN-o-paws*), the end of menstruation. This occurs when the ovaries stop secreting hormones. Many diseases and illnesses can develop in these years. These disorders can become chronic and life-threatening.

Late Adulthood, Ages Sixty-five Years and Older

Persons in late adulthood must adjust to the effects of aging. These effects or changes can include the loss of physical strength and health, the death of loved ones, retirement, and preparation for their own death. Although the developmental tasks of this age appear to deal entirely with loss, solutions often involve new relationships, friendships, and interests.

Because so many of the people receiving home care are older adults, in the rest of this chapter you will learn more about aging and the needs of elderly clients.

The disorders you are most likely to see (AIDS, arthritis, Alzheimer's disease, cancer, diabetes, and stroke) are discussed in chapter 20.

2. Distinguish between fact (what is true) and fallacy (what is not true) about the aging process

Because later adulthood covers an age range of as many as 25 to 35 years, people in this age category can have very different capabilities, depending on their health (Fig. 10-7). Some 70-year-old people still enjoy active sports, while others are not active. Many 85-year-old people can still live alone, though others may live with family members or in nursing homes.

Generalizations or stereotypes about older people are often false. They create prejudices against the elderly that are as unfair as prejudices against racial, ethnic, or religious groups.

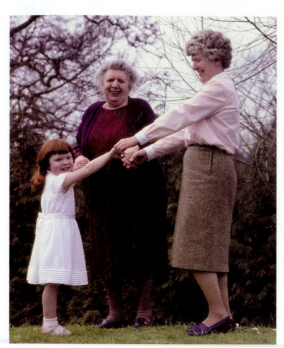

Fig. 10-7. Older adults often remain active and engaged.

On television or in the movies older people are often shown as helpless, lonely, disabled, slow, forgetful, dependent, or inactive. However, research indicates that most older people are active and engaged in work, volunteer activities, learning programs, and exercise regimens. Aging is a normal process, not a disease. Most older people live independent lives and do not need assistance (Fig. 10-8).

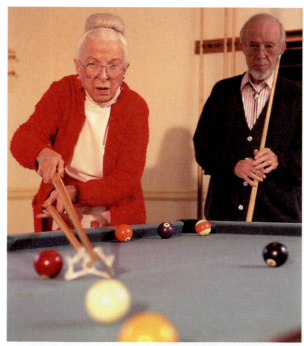

Fig. 10-8. Most older people lead active lives.

You are likely to spend much of your time working with elderly clients. You must be able to know what is true about aging and what is not true. While aging causes many physical, psychological, and social changes, normal changes of aging do not mean an older person must become dependent, ill, or inactive. Knowing normal changes of aging from signs of illness or disability will allow you to better help your elderly clients.

3. Discuss normal changes of aging and list care guidelines

Each person ages in a unique way, influenced by genetics and lifestyle. Although we cannot choose our genetic makeup, we can choose the lifestyle we lead. Habits of diet, exercise, attitude, social and physical activities, and health maintenance affect our well-being later in life.

Some of your older clients will need assistance in performing activities of daily living (ADLs). Clients who are chronically ill and need a lot of help still benefit from living at home. You perform an important role in letting older clients stay in familiar surroundings while getting the help they need. Remembering the changes that occur in the elderly will help you provide the right care. Over the next several pages, you will learn about normal and abnormal changes of aging in each body system.

Integumentary system

Changes: Skin is thinner, drier, and more fragile. Much of the fatty layer beneath the skin is lost. Hair thins and may turn gray. Wrinkles and brown spots, or "liver spots" appear. Nails are harder and more brittle. Reduced circulation to the skin can cause dryness, itching, and irritation.

Care:

• Older adults perspire less and do not need to bathe as often. Most elderly people generally need a complete bath only twice a week, with sponge baths every day.

- Use lotions as ordered for moisture to relieve dry skin. Be gentle; elderly clients' skin can be fragile and tear easily.

- Hair also becomes drier and needs to be shampooed less often. Brush dry hair to stimulate and distribute the natural oils (Fig. 10-9).

- Layer clothing and bed covers for additional warmth.

- Encourage fluids.

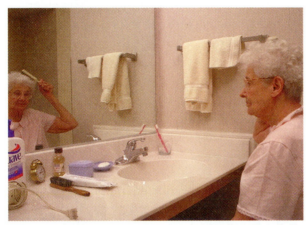

Fig. 10-9. Brushing hair helps stimulate and distribute natural oils.

Musculoskeletal system

Changes: Muscles weaken and lose tone. Bones may become more brittle. Joints may stiffen and become painful. Body movement slows. There is a gradual loss of height.

Care:

- Encourage regular movement and self-care. Assist with range of motion (ROM) exercises as needed. See chapter 15 for more information on ROM exercises. Encourage the client to perform as many ADLs as possible. For example, encourage clients to eat in the kitchen and walk to the bathroom until these activities are no longer possible. Encourage clients to make decisions and dress themselves, with assistance if necessary, no matter how long it takes.

- To prevent or slow **osteoporosis** (*os-tee-oh-po-RO-sis*), the condition that is responsible for fragile bones, encourage clients to walk and do other light exercise. Exercise can strengthen the bones as well as muscles.

- Falls can cause life-threatening complications, including fractures. Prevent falls by keeping items out of clients' paths. Keep furniture in the same place. Keep walkers and canes where clients can easily reach them.

Nervous system

Changes: Aging affects the ability to think logically and quickly. How much ability is lost depends on the individual. Aging can also affect concentration and memory. Elderly clients may experience memory loss of recent events. This short-term memory loss may cause anxiety in older clients. Long-term memory, or memory for past events, usually remains sharp. Elderly clients usually have slower responses and reflexes, too.

Care:

- Help with memory loss by suggesting clients make lists or write notes about things they want to remember. Placing a calendar nearby may help (Fig. 10-10).

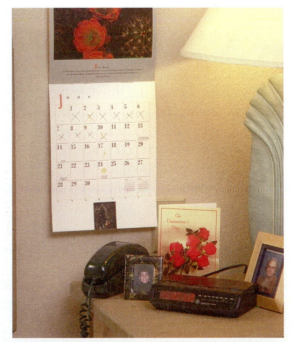

Fig. 10-10. Writing notes and placing a calender nearby may help a client with short-term memory loss.

10

Human Development and Aging

- If your clients enjoy reminiscing, take an interest in their past by asking to see photos or hear stories.

- Allow time for decision-making and avoid sudden changes in schedule.

- Allow plenty of time for movement; never rush the person.

- Encourage reading, thinking, and other mental activities.

Changes in vision, hearing, taste, and smell:
Failing vision of many elderly clients may make reading or other activities difficult. Failing hearing may make it frustrating for older adults to try to communicate. Weakened sense of smell, taste, and touch may present dangers for older adults.

Care:

- Many books and some magazines are available printed in large type. Books on tape are available at libraries and bookstores.

- Keep clients' eyeglasses clean. Bright colors and good light will also help clients with poor eyesight. When going into another room, be sure the lights are on before your client enters.

- If your client is having trouble hearing, speak in a low-pitched voice. For some people, low-pitched sounds are easier to hear. You may also need to repeat words to help the client understand them. Some clients need hearing aids and should be encouraged to use them. Excess earwax can make hearing difficult. If you suspect excess earwax, tell your supervisor. A nurse can treat this problem.

- If a client has difficulty hearing, face him or her and speak slowly, simply, and clearly. Do not shout. Do not assume that all your elderly clients are hard of hearing. Speaking loudly or oversimplifying your speech when it is not necessary can make clients feel they are being treated like children.

- Because we lose taste buds as we age, older people often cannot taste as well. Decreased sense of smell may contribute to the altered sense of taste. Make sure the food in the house is fresh because older clients may not be able to smell or taste that food is spoiled. Older clients should always have smoke and carbon monoxide detectors in their homes, since they may not smell leaking gas or smoke.

- The sense of touch is also affected by aging. Be careful with hot drinks and hot bath water. Clients sometimes cannot tell if something is too hot for them. The elderly client who is confined to bed may not feel uncomfortable, but because of decreased circulation and dry skin, he or she is at risk for developing pressure sores. The sense of pain may also be diminished in the elderly. Be alert to changes in your clients' health.

Circulatory system

Changes: As we age, our hearts pump less efficiently. Increased activity places greater demand on the heart, which it may not be able to meet. Older people may need more rest to reduce demand on the heart. They may not be able to walk long distances, climb stairs, or exert themselves. Less efficient circulation of blood in older people causes older adults to be more sensitive to the cold.

Care:

- Moderate exercise is necessary and helpful (Fig. 10-11). Walking, stretching, and even lifting light weights can help older people maintain strength and mobility.

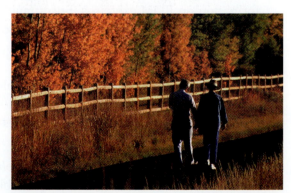

Fig. 10-11. Moderate exercise can help older adults maintain strength and mobility.

- Active or passive ROM exercises are important for clients who cannot get out of bed. Your clients' care plans will specify what kinds of exercise they should be doing. Abilities can vary a great deal from client to client.

- Clients with heart conditions, particularly heart failure, must avoid vigorous activity or exercise. This includes carrying heavy objects. Some clients may experience dizziness when they stand up too quickly.

Encourage clients to rise slowly and to stand still for a few moments, supporting themselves by holding onto a piece of furniture (Fig. 10-12).

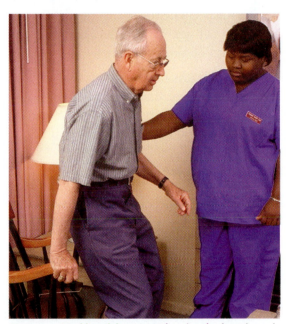

Fig. 10-12. An older adult may need to rise slowly and stand still for a moment to keep from getting dizzy.

- Houses may need to be kept at a higher temperature than normal. Layer clothing to keep clients warm. Some clients who are concerned about the cost of heating may actually lower the thermostat to a dangerous level.

- Poor circulation causes the feet to feel cold. Be sure your client wears slippers or shoes and socks.

- Do not use hot water bottles or heating pads. Poor circulation causes dry skin that is fragile and can burn easily. In addition, because of the dulled sense of pain, an older person may not realize he or she is being burned until it is too late.

Respiratory system

Changes: As the body ages, the lungs have fewer alveoli in which oxygen/carbon dioxide exchange can take place. Shortness of breath is a common problem for older adults. Older clients may also have a harder time coughing up mucus.

Care:

- You may need to provide frequent rest periods when assisting a client with ADLs.

- Follow the care plan carefully for exercise and activity instructions. Moderate exercise is helpful, but overdoing it can be very dangerous for an older adult. If you have a question about the activity specified in the care plan, talk to your supervisor.

- Assist with deep breathing exercises.

Urinary system

Changes. The bladder is not able to hold the same amount of urine as it did when clients were younger. Older clients may need to urinate more frequently. Many elderly persons awaken several times during the night to urinate. The bladder may not empty completely, causing susceptibility to infection.

Care:

- Encourage clients to drink plenty of fluids. Offer frequent trips to the bathroom.

- **Incontinence** (*in-KON-ti-nens*) is the inability to control the bladder. Incontinence is *not* a normal part of aging. Always report incontinence. It may be a sign and symptom of an illness. Cleanliness and good skin care are important for clients who are incontinent. Keep clients clean and dry.

Gastrointestinal system

Changes:. Older people may have a dulled sense of taste. This is often made worse by side

effects of medications, and may result in a poor appetite. Decreased saliva production affects the ability to chew and swallow. Digestion takes longer and is less efficient in older adults. Many older adults have trouble with indigestion, or an upset stomach. Body waste moves more slowly through the intestines. Constipation, or the inability to have a bowel movement, may occur.

Care:

- Encourage fluids and nutritious, appealing meals.

- Older people who have trouble chewing may require soft foods. Make sure dentures fit properly and are cleaned regularly.

- Clients who have trouble chewing and swallowing are at risk of choking. Provide plenty of fluids with meals. Cut food into bite-sized pieces.

- Some clients need to eat several small meals a day or have the large meal in the middle of the day.

- Clients should eat a diet that contains fiber and drink plenty of fluids to help prevent constipation.

Dehydration is a condition that results from inadequate fluid in the body. It is not a normal sign of aging. However, many older people do not feel thirsty and may not be aware that they are dehydrated. Dehydration can cause constipation, weight loss, dry skin, infection, dizziness and weakness, and other illnesses that require medical attention. See chapter 22 for more information on dehydration.

Endocrine system

Changes: Levels of reproductive hormones are lower. Pancreas function lessens, which may lead to diabetes for some clients.

Care:

- Older clients may need to take insulin or eat certain foods to regulate blood sugar. The client's doctor or nurse will teach the client what to do. Any special instructions on care will be included in the care plan.

Reproductive system

Changes: Genital areas may become dry and uncomfortable. In males, the prostate gland increases in size. In females, fatty tissue in the breasts may diminish. Mucous secretions in the vagina decrease. Though the reproductive organs change, sexual needs and desires do not necessarily change.

Care:

- Avoiding too many hot baths can help prevent discomfort in the genital area.

- Despite changes in the reproductive organs, older adults remain sexual beings. Provide privacy whenever necessary for sexual activity. Respect clients' sexual needs. Do not make any generalizations about the sexual feelings of older adults.

- Do report any behavior that makes you uncomfortable or that seems inappropriate. Inappropriate behavior is not a normal sign of aging, and could be a sign of illness.

Immune and lymphatic systems

Changes: As we age, our immune system gradually weakens. It also may take longer to recover from an illness. Bone marrow activity (which produces white blood cells that fight infections) decreases as we age. Changes in the respiratory system's protective surface may result in increased respiratory infections. The number and size of lymph nodes is reduced. This results in the body being less able to contract a fever to fight infection.

Care:

- Vaccines against common infections, such as influenza (flu), are very important. Encourage proper nutrition and fluid intake to help older clients stay healthy.

- An older adult fighting an infection may not experience a fever. Even a slight temperature increase may indicate that the person is fighting an infection. Taking accurate vital signs is very important. See chapter 14 for more information.

- Follow rules for preventing infection. Wash your hands often. Keep the client's environment clean.

Psychological Changes

Some forgetfulness is a normal part of aging, but constant memory lapses or forgetting basic information such as family members' names are not normal changes of aging.

Any of the following signs should be reported immediately. They may indicate illness.

OBSERVING AND REPORTING
Psychological Changes

- **disorientation**, or change in ability to remember who they are, what month or season of the year it is, or other basic facts
- difficulty concentrating
- depression
- dementia, or a loss of mental abilities that interferes with ADLs
- confusion
- suicidal thoughts
- insomnia (inability to sleep)

Depression is very common among the elderly, but it is not a normal sign of aging. Elderly persons may not admit feelings of depression to themselves or others. According to the National Center for Health Statistics, the elderly are at higher risk for suicide than all other age groups. Report any signs of depression in your clients to your supervisor. In many cases, depression may be successfully treated. See chapter 18 for more information.

OBSERVING AND REPORTING
Depression

Report any of the following to your supervisor:
- anorexia or loss of appetite
- insomnia
- acting moody or withdrawn
- other changes in appearance, speech, movement, and behavior

- Sleep disorders and emotional changes, such as hopelessness, anxiety, apathy, agitation, restlessness, withdrawal, and demanding or violent behavior, are particularly important to report.

Lifestyle Changes: Aging brings many social, physical, and mental changes. Friends, colleagues, and relatives die. Physical strength and stamina diminish. Fears of illness, injury, and death may increase. Retirement causes changes in what and how much people do each day. Living arrangements may also change. These changes require adjustment, which can become more difficult as people age.

Care:
- You can help your clients adjust to change by listening to them and caring about their feelings.
- Ensuring that clients are safe is another way you help them adapt to changing lifestyles. See chapter 6 for information on how to help make clients' homes safe for them.

4. Identify attitudes and living habits that good health

Staying active, maintaining self-esteem, and living independently promote good physical and mental health for older adults. Encourage your clients in these attitudes and habits in the following ways:

Encourage your clients to pursue activities they enjoy and can succeed in. Many older people enjoy reading, playing checkers, gardening, doing crafts, or listening to music (Fig. 10-13). Working with others on charity or community service projects can allow older people to share their knowledge and experience. Senior centers or community centers offer classes, hobby groups, exercise, and field trips that some older clients may enjoy. Many older people are involved in activities through a church or synagogue. Encourage your clients by asking them about what they are doing, admiring their work,

10

Human Development and Aging

or even participating in games or crafts when time permits.

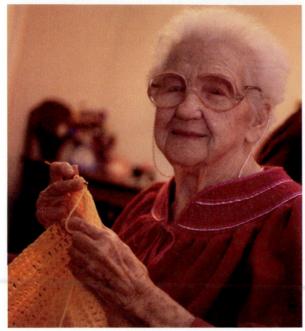

Fig. 10-13. Continuing to participate in activities they enjoy promotes good mental and physical health for older adults.

Help clients develop a routine for the day. Structuring the day around meals, activities, rest, and self-care can help fight depression and give older people a sense of purpose. Older people who do not have a routine may simply stay in bed or become bored and lonely.

Encourage self-care. Your clients should do as much for themselves as they possibly can. Your job is to assist with or perform activities the client cannot do alone. The more your clients can care for themselves, the better they will feel about themselves. Follow the care plan. Keep in touch with your supervisor about changes in the client's abilities.

Help your clients be well-groomed. Appearance affects the way we feel about ourselves. Help your clients style hair, dress neatly, use cosmetics, or shave (Fig. 10-14).

Address your clients respectfully. Do not call your clients by their first names unless they ask you to. Use their last names with whatever title they prefer (Mr., Ms., Miss, Mrs., or Dr.). Speak to them with respect. Ask for their opinions and

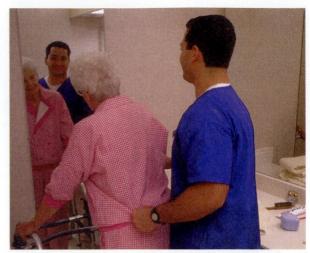

Fig. 10-14. A well-groomed appearance helps people of all ages feel good about themselves.

let them make their own decisions as much as possible. The more independent and capable they feel, the more independent and capable they will be. Never treat a client like a child or talk about a client as if he or she were not there.

Respect the needs for privacy and for social interaction. Let your client be alone to read, study, pray, or work if he or she seems to want this. Knock before you enter the room, even if the door is open (Fig. 10-15). Remember that

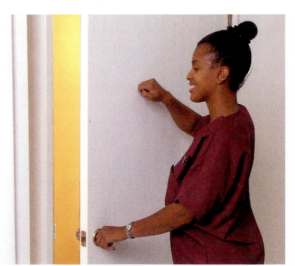

Fig. 10-15. Respect your clients' privacy. Knock before entering any room, even if the door is open.

clients may not want to talk all the time. When visitors come by, let your client visit undisturbed. Do not try to participate in the conversation. Treat visitors respectfully and make them feel welcome. Even if an unannounced visit dis-

rupts your schedule, remember how important social contact is. Try to be flexible.

5. List ways to recognize and report elder abuse and neglect

The healthcare community has become aware of the growing problem of elder abuse and neglect. The National Center on Elder Abuse published the first-ever "National Elder Abuse Incidence Study" in 1998. This study estimates that at least 500,000 older persons in domestic settings were abused and/or neglected during 1996. It also found that for every reported incident of elder abuse or neglect, approximately five go unreported. As the elderly population grows, this problem may become worse.

Elderly people may be abused intentionally or unintentionally, through ignorance, inexperience, or inability to care for them. People who abuse elders may mistreat them physically, psychologically, sexually, verbally, financially, and/or materially. They may deprive them of their rights or they may neglect them by failing to provide food, clothing, shelter, or medical care. Some older adults may also become self-abusive or neglect their own needs.

You will be in an excellent position to observe and report abuse or neglect. Home health aides have an ethical and legal responsibility to observe for signs of abuse and report suspected cases to a supervisor. Give your supervisor as much information as possible. Take this responsibility seriously. Help end this disturbing trend.

OBSERVING AND REPORTING
Abuse and Neglect

- Old and new bruises, contusions and welts
- Scars
- Fractures, dislocation
- Burns of unusual shape and in unusual locations
- Scalp tenderness and patches of missing hair
- Teeth marks
- Scratches and puncture wounds
- Swelling in the face, broken teeth, nasal discharge
- Bruises, bleeding, or discharge from the vaginal area
- Withdrawal or apathy
- Agitation or anxiety; signs of stress
- Low self-esteem
- Constant pain
- Client or family reports of questionable care
- Fear, vigilance, apprehension; afraid of being alone
- Mood changes, confusion, disorientation
- Weight loss, poor appetite
- Dehydration
- Living conditions that are unsafe, unclean, or inadequate
- Private conversations are not allowed, or the family member/caregiver is present during all conversations

6. Identify community resources available to help the elderly

Government and private agencies exist in most areas to serve the needs of the elderly. These agencies may have counselors to work with victims of abuse or neglect, and other programs to protect senior citizens' rights and contribute to their quality of life. Look in the phone book under community services, senior citizens, aging, or elder services. Local churches or synagogues may also have programs for seniors.

In the United States, many elder services can be found using a service sponsored by the Administration on Aging. The toll-free Eldercare Locator Service operates Monday through Friday, 9:00 a.m. to 8:00 p.m., Eastern time, and can be reached at 1-800-677-1116. Their web site is www.eldercare.gov.

Be familiar with programs available in your area, or refer clients or families to your supervisor or a social worker.

Chapter Review

1. Name at least two common disorders for each stage of human development.

2. What stereotypes about older people do you think are most common? What can you do to avoid being prejudiced by these stereotypes?

3. What should you do if your client has dry, itchy, irritated skin?

4. How can you prevent or slow osteoporosis?

5. Name five signs and symptoms you need to report about a client's psychological health.

6. How can you help a client who is hard of hearing?

7. What can you do to help clients with a poor sense of touch?

8. What should you do if your client experiences dizziness when he stands up?

9. Why might older clients need to urinate more frequently?

10. What should you do if you think your client is becoming dehydrated?

11. What are possible signs of depression?

12. How can you help your clients adjust to lifestyle changes due to aging?

13. What are two things that can help prevent constipation?

14. Why should you encourage clients to do as much for themselves as possible?

15. Name one way you can show respect for your clients' privacy.

16. List ten signs of elder abuse.

11

Dying, Death and Hospice

1. Discuss the stages of dying

Death can occur suddenly and without warning, or it can be expected. Older people, or people with terminal illnesses, may have time to prepare for death. A **terminal illness** is a disease or condition that will eventually cause death. Preparing for death is a process that affects the dying person's emotions and behavior.

Dr. Elisabeth Kubler-Ross researched and wrote about the process of dying. Her book, *On Death and Dying*, describes five stages that dying people and their families or friends may experience before death. These five stages are described below. Not all clients go through all the stages. Some may stay in one stage until death occurs. Clients may move back and forth between stages during the process.

Denial. People in the denial stage may refuse to believe they are dying. They often believe a mistake has been made. They may talk about the future and avoid any discussion about their illnesses. This is the "No. Not me." stage.

Anger. Once they start to face the possibility of their death, people become angry that they are dying. Anger is a normal and healthy reaction. The caregiver must learn not to take anger personally. This is the "Why me?" stage.

Bargaining. Once people have begun to believe that they really are dying, they may make prom-

ises to God or somehow try to bargain for their recovery. This is the "Yes me, but..." stage.

Depression. As dying people become physically weaker and symptoms of the illness get worse, they may become deeply sad or depressed. They may cry or withdraw or be unable to perform even simple activities. They need physical and emotional support. Listen to and be understanding of clients.

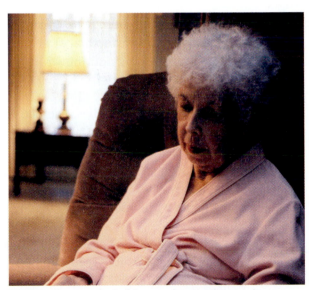

Fig. 11-1. A person who is dying may become depressed.

Acceptance. Most people who are dying are eventually able to accept death and prepare for it. They may make plans for their last days or for the ceremonies that may follow. At this stage, people who are dying may seem emotionally detached.

2. Describe the grief process

Dealing with grief after the death of a relative or friend is a process as well. Grieving is an individual process. No two people will grieve in exactly the same way. Clergy, counselors, or social workers can provide help for people who are grieving. Family members or friends may have any of the following reactions to the death of a loved one:

Shock. Even when death was expected, family members and friends may still be shocked after death occurs. Many of us do not know what to expect after the death of a relative or friend. We may be surprised by our feelings.

Denial. Sometimes we want to believe that everything will quickly return to normal after a death. Denying or refusing to believe we are grieving can help people deal with the hours or days after a death. But eventually we must face our feelings. Grief can be so overwhelming that some people may take years to face their feelings. Professional help can be very valuable.

Anger. Although it is hard to admit it, many of us feel angry after a death. We may be angry with ourselves, at God, at the doctors, or even at the person who died. There is nothing wrong with feeling anger as part of grief.

Guilt. It is very common for families, friends, and even caregivers to feel guilty after a death. We may wish we had done more for the dying person. We may simply feel that he or she did not deserve to die any more than we did. We may feel guilty that we are still living.

Regret. Often we have regrets about what we did or did not do for the dying person. We may regret things we said or did not say to a person who has died. Many people carry regrets with them for years.

Sadness. Feeling depressed is very common after a death. We may cry or feel emotionally unstable. We may suffer headaches or insomnia when we cannot express our sadness.

Loneliness. Missing someone who has died is very normal. It can bring up other feelings, such as sadness or regret. Many things may remind us of the person who died. The memories may be painful at first. With time, we usually feel less lonely and memories are less painful.

3. Discuss how feelings and attitudes about death differ

Death is a very sensitive topic. Many people find it hard to discuss death. Feelings and attitudes about death can be influenced by many factors.

Experience with death. Someone who has been through other deaths may have a different understanding of death than someone who has never experienced the death of someone close.

Personality type. Open, expressive people may have an easier time talking about and coping with death than people who are very reserved or quiet. Expressing feelings is a way of working through fears and concerns.

Religious beliefs. Religious practices and beliefs influence the experience with death (Fig. 11-2). This includes the process of dying, rituals at the

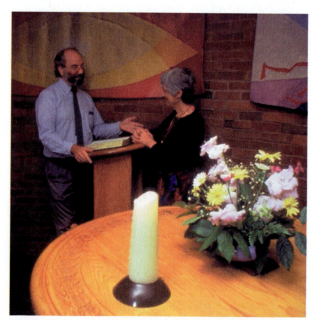

Fig. 11-2. Religious beliefs influence a person's feelings about death.

11

Dying, Death and Hospice

time of death, burial or cremation practices, services held after death, and mourning customs. For example, some Catholics do not believe in cremation. Orthodox Jews may not believe in viewing the body after death. Beliefs about what happens to people after death can also influence grieving. People who believe in an afterlife, such as heaven, may be comforted by this belief.

Cultural background. The practices we grow up with will affect how we deal with death. Different cultural groups may have different practices to deal with death and grieving. Some groups provide meals and other services but say very little about a person's death. In other cultures, talking about and remembering the person who has died may be a way of comforting family and friends (Fig. 11-3).

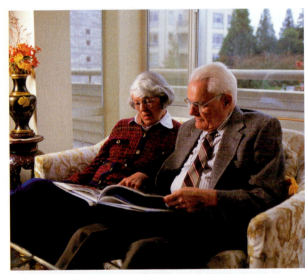

Fig. 11-3. Cultural practices affect the way a family grieves.

4. Explain common signs of approaching death

Death can be sudden or gradual. Certain physical changes occur that can be recognized as signs and symptoms of approaching death. Vital signs and skin color are often affected. Disorientation, confusion, and reduced responsiveness may occur. Vision, taste, and touch usually diminish. However, hearing is often present until death occurs.

Common signs of approaching death include the following:

- blurred and failing vision
- unfocused eyes
- impaired speech
- diminished sense of touch
- loss of movement, muscle tone, and feeling
- a rising or below-normal body temperature
- decreasing blood pressure
- weak pulse that is abnormally slow or rapid
- slow, irregular respirations or rapid, shallow respirations
- a "rattling" or "gurgling" sound as the person breathes
- cold, pale skin
- mottling, spotting, or blotching of skin caused by poor circulation
- perspiration
- incontinence
- disorientation or confusion

5. Discuss how to care for a dying client

Follow the care plan when caring for a client who is dying. However, keep the following guidelines in mind to help you make the client as comfortable as possible:

GUIDELINE
Caring for the Dying Client

- **Diminished Senses**. Keep the room softly lighted and without glare (Fig. 11-4). Hearing is usually the last sense to leave the body, so speak in a normal tone. Tell them about any procedures that are being done or what is happening in the room. Do not expect an answer. Ask few questions. Encourage family to speak to the client, but to avoid subjects that are disturbing. Observe body language to anticipate a client's needs.

134

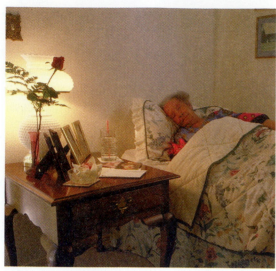

Fig. 11-4. Keep a dying client's room softly lighted without glare.

Care of the Mouth. Give mouth care frequently. If the client is unconscious, give mouth care every two hours. Apply lubricant, such as lip balm, to lips.

Skin Care. Give bed baths and incontinence care as needed. Bathe perspiring clients often. Their skin should be kept clean and dry. Sheets and clothes should be changed for their comfort. Keep sheets wrinkle-free. Skin care to prevent pressure sores is important.

Comfort. Pain relief is very important. Clients may not be able to communicate that they are in pain. Observe your clients for signs of pain and report them. Frequent changes of position, back massage, skin care, mouth care, and proper body alignment may help. This type of care is discussed more in chapters 12 and 13. Body temperature usually increases. Many clients are more comfortable with light covers.

Environment. Display favorite objects and photographs where the client can easily see them. They may provide comfort. Make sure the room is comfortable, appropriately lighted, and well ventilated.

Emotional and Spiritual Support. Listening may be one of the most important things you can do for a client who is dying. They may also need the quiet, reassuring, and loving presence of another person. Touch can be very important. Holding your client's hand as you sit quietly can be very comforting. Some clients who are dying may also seek spiritual comfort from clergy.

Postmortem care means care of the body after death. Be sensitive to the needs of the family after death occurs. Family members or friends may wish to sit by the bed to say goodbye. Be aware of religious practices that the family wants to observe. Home health agencies will also have different policies on postmortem care. Always follow your agency's policies and procedures. Perform assigned tasks.

GUIDELINES
Postmortem Care

Bathe the body. Be gentle to avoid bruising. Place drainage pads where needed, most often under the head and/or under the **perineum** (*payr-i-NEE-um*, or the area between the genitals and anus). Be sure to follow Standard Precautions.

Check with family about how to dress the client and whether to remove jewelry.

Do not remove any tubes or other equipment. A nurse or the funeral home will do it later.

Put dentures back in the mouth and close the mouth. You may need to place a rolled towel under the chin to support the closed mouth position. Or you can place dentures in a denture cup near the client's head.

Close the eyes carefully.

Position the body on the back, with legs straight, arms folded across the abdomen. Place a small pillow under the head.

Strip the bed after the body has been removed.

Open windows to air the room, as appropriate, and straighten up.

Arrange personal items carefully so they are not lost.

Document according to your agency's policy.

Ask family members or friends how you can be of help. If you are working with a hospice pro-

gram, you may be asked to answer the phone, make coffee or a meal, supervise children, or keep family members company. Do not leave the home until the client's body has been removed or until your supervisor says you may leave.

6. Define the goals of a hospice program

Hospice care is the term used for the special care that a dying person needs. Hospice care may be provided in a hospital, at a special care facility, or in the home. A hospice can be any location where a person who is dying is treated with dignity by caregivers who provide for their physical, emotional, social, and spiritual needs.

Any caregiver may provide hospice care, but often specially trained nurses, social workers, and volunteers provide hospice care. The hospice team may include doctors, nurses, social workers, counselors, home health aides, therapists, clergy, dietitians, and volunteers.

In home care, goals include a focus on the client's recovery, or on the client's ability to care for him- or herself as much as possible. In hospice care, however, the goals of care are the comfort and dignity of the client (Fig. 11-5). This is an important difference. You will need to adjust your mind-set when caring for hospice clients. Focus on relieving their pain and making them comfortable, rather than on teaching them to care for themselves. Clients who are dying also need to feel some independence for as long as possible. Caregivers should allow clients to retain as much control over their lives as possible. Eventually, caregivers may have to meet all of the client's basic needs.

Family members or friends who are caregivers for the dying person will appreciate your help. You are providing them with a break. This kind of care is sometimes referred to as **respite** (*RES-pit*) **care**. You must be aware of the feelings of family caregivers. Encourage them to take breaks and take care of themselves.

However, do not insist that they do so. Many want to do all they can for their loved one during his or her last days. Do observe family caregivers for signs of excessive stress. Report any signs to your supervisor. Your agency may be able to refer them to local support services.

I have the right to:

be treated as a living human being until I die.

maintain a sense of hopefulness, however changing its focus may be.

be cared for by those who can maintain a sense of hopefulness, however changing this might be.

express my feelings and emotions about my approaching death in my own way.

participate in decisions concerning my care.

expect continuing medical and nursing attention even though "cure" goals must be changed to "comfort" goals.

to die alone.

be free from pain.

have my questions answered honestly.

not be deceived.

have help from and for my family in accepting my death.

die in peace and dignity.

retain my individuality and not be judged for my decisions which may be contrary to beliefs of others.

discuss and enlarge my religious and/or spiritual experiences, whatever these may mean to others.

expect that the sanctity of the human body will be respected after death.

be cared for by caring, sensitive, knowledgeable people who will attempt to understand my needs and will be able to gain some satisfaction in helping me face my death.

Fig. 11-5. The Dying Person's Bill of Rights. (This was created at a workshop on "The Terminally Ill Patient and the Helping Person," sponsored by Southwestern Michigan In-service Education Council, and appeared in the *American Journal of Nursing*, Vol. 75, January, 1975, p. 99.)

7. Identify special skills and attitudes helpful in hospice work

The most important attitude for hospice work is the focus on providing comfort for the dying client, rather than on promoting wellness or recovery. Other attitudes and skills useful when providing hospice care include the following:

Be a good listener. It is hard to know what to say to someone who is dying or to his or her relatives and friends. Most often, people need someone to listen to them (Fig. 11-6). Review the listening skills discussed in chapter 4. A good listener can be a great comfort. Recognize that some people will not want to confide in you. Never push someone to talk.

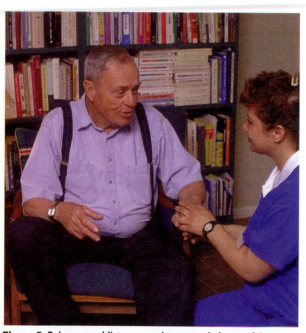

Fig. 11-6. Being a good listener can be a great help to a dying client and his or her family.

Respect privacy and independence. Relatives, friends, clergy, or others may visit a dying client. Make it easy for these difficult visits to take place. Stay out of the way when you can. Do not join in the conversation unless you are asked to do so. Dying clients can hold on to some independence even when they need total care. Let the client make choices when possible, such as whether to bathe now or later, or what to eat or drink.

Be sensitive to individual needs. Different clients and families will have different needs. The more you know what is needed from you, the more helpful you will be. Some clients need a quiet and calm atmosphere. Others appreciate a cheery presence and might like you to make small talk or stay close by. If you are not sure what you can do to help, ask someone.

Be aware of your own feelings. Caring for people who are dying can be draining. Know your limits and respect them. Discuss your feelings of frustration or grief with your supervisor or another care team member. Request a change of assignment when you need a break.

Be sure to follow the plan of care. Know whom to call and when to call them.

8. Describe the role of the hospice volunteer

According to the National Hospice and Palliative Care Organization, there are now more than 3,200 hospices across the country. They provided care to more than 775,000 people in 2001. Approximately 200,000 hospice volunteers give more than 10 million hours of their time each year to help people who are dying. Hospice volunteers go through a training program to prepare them for hospice work. The volunteers provide a variety of services. This includes caring for the home or family of a dying person, driving or doing errands, and providing emotional support.

9. Discuss the importance of caring for yourself when working in hospice care

Hospice care can be very draining physically and psychologically. Caregivers must keep their own needs in mind and learn to take care of themselves while taking care of others. It is easy to get "burned out" when working in hospice care, especially if you ignore your own needs.

Recognize the stress. Just realizing how stressful it is to work with clients who are dying is a first step toward caring for yourself. Talking with a counselor about your experiences at work can help you understand and work through your feelings. Remember, however, you must keep clients' specific information confidential. Your supervisor may be able to refer you to a counselor or support group.

Take good care of yourself. Eating right, exercising, and getting enough rest are ways of taking care of yourself. Remember to care for your emotional and spiritual health, too. Talk about and acknowledge your feelings. Take time out to do things for yourself, such as reading a book, taking a bubble bath, or whatever you enjoy. Spiritual needs may be met by attending religious services, reading, praying, meditating, or just taking a quiet walk. Meeting your needs allows you to best meet other people's needs.

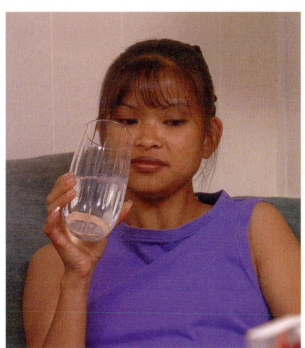

Fig. 11-7. Recognize the stress of caring for a dying client, and take good care of yourself.

Take a break when you need to. Find ten minutes to sit down and relax or stand up and stretch. These ideas may be enough of a break in some situations. There may come a time when the demands of hospice care are too great. You may need to request a change of assignment from your supervisor. Do not feel guilty about doing this when you need to.

Chapter Review

1. Describe one kind of behavior you might see at each stage of dying.

2. Describe five possible feelings/emotions in the grief process.

3. How would you describe your personality type? What helps you work through difficult feelings like those associated with grief?

4. Which sense is generally present until death occurs?

5. What are some of the ways you might provide emotional and spiritual support for a dying client?

6. What measures may help a dying client who is in pain?

7. What is the focus in dealing with hospice clients? How does it differ from the usual care you provide?

8. Why is it important to be aware of your feelings as you provide hospice care?

9. What are some of the services provided by hospice volunteers?

10. It's not always easy to recognize when we are feeling stress. How do you recognize signs of stress in yourself? What helps you relieve your stress?

11

Dying, Death and Hospice

12

Transfers, Ambulation, and Positioning

1. Explain the guidelines for safely transferring and positioning clients

Review the principles of body mechanics in chapter 6. Always use good body mechanics when moving or positioning a client. Avoid lifting whenever possible. Instead, push, roll, slide, or pivot, so that you are not bearing the client's weight. Using good body mechanics helps protect both you and your clients.

Before a client who has been lying down moves to a standing position, she should **dangle**. To dangle means to sit up with the feet over the side of the bed for a moment to regain balance. For some clients who are unable to walk, sitting up and dangling the legs for a few minutes may be ordered.

Assisting a client to a dangling position

1. Wash your hands.

2. Explain the procedure to the client, speaking clearly, slowly, and directly, maintaining face-to-face contact whenever possible.

3. Provide privacy if the client desires it.

4. If the bed is adjustable, adjust bed to a safe working level, usually waist high. If the bed is movable, lock bed wheels (Fig. 12-1).

5. Fanfold (fold into pleats) the top covers to the foot of the bed. Ask the client to roll onto

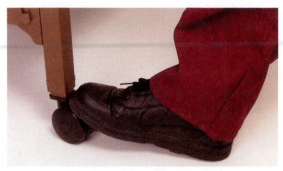

Fig. 12-1. Always lock bed wheels if bed is movable before repositioning or transferring a client.

her side, facing you. Assist as needed (A procedure later in this chapter describes how to help a client roll over).

6. Tell the client to reach across her chest with her top arm and place her hand on the edge of the bed near her opposite shoulder. Ask her to push down on that hand to raise her shoulders up while swinging her legs over the side of the bed (Fig. 12-2).

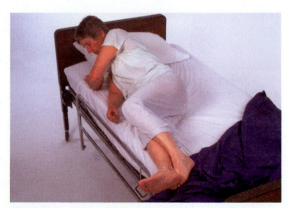

Fig. 12-2.

7. Always allow the client to do all she can for herself. However, if the client needs assistance, have her lie on her back propped up on pillows or with the head of the bed raised. With the client bending her knees and assisting as able, reach your arm under the client's neck and grasp her far shoulder. Slip your other arm under her knees and grasp her far knee. Stand with your legs about 12 inches apart, with one foot 6-8 inches in front of the other. Bend your knees and pull your body a quarter turn backward. In a smooth movement, swing the client's knees toward you and over the side of the bed (Fig. 12-3). The weight of the client's legs hanging down from the bed helps the client sit up (Fig. 12-4).

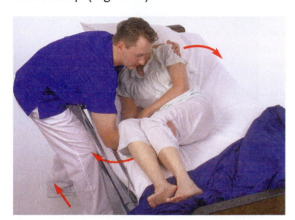

Fig. 12-3.

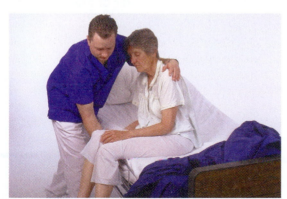

Fig. 12-4.

8. Allow the client to sit on the edge of the bed to gain her balance. This procedure is called **dangling**. It gives the client time to adjust to being in an upright position after lying down.

9. Put non-skid shoes on the client while she is dangling. Do not leave the client alone. If the client is dizzy for more than a minute,

have her lie down again. Take her pulse and respirations and report to your supervisor according to your agency's policy (you will learn how to take vital signs in chapter 14).

10. The care plan may direct you to allow the client to dangle for several minutes and then return her to lying down, or it may direct you to allow the client to dangle in preparation for walking or a transfer. Follow the instructions in the care plan.

11. If you raised an adjustable bed, be sure to return it to its lowest position. Wash your hands after the transfer is completed.

12. Document the procedure and your observations. How did the client tolerate sitting up? Did the client become dizzy?

Helping a client sit up using the arm lock

1. Wash your hands.

2. Explain the procedure to the client, speaking clearly, slowly, and directly, maintaining face-to-face contact whenever possible.

3. Provide privacy if the client desires it.

4. If the bed is adjustable, adjust bed to a safe working level, usually waist high. If the bed is movable, lock bed wheels.

5. Stand facing the head of the bed, with your legs about 12 inches apart and your knees bent. The foot that is further from the bed should be slightly ahead of the other foot (Fig. 12-5).

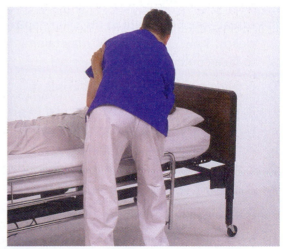

Fig. 12-5.

1. Explain guidelines for transferring and positioning clients

6. Place your arm under the client's armpit and grasp the client's shoulder. Have the client grasp your shoulder in the same manner. This hold is called the **arm lock** or **lock arm** (Fig. 12-6).

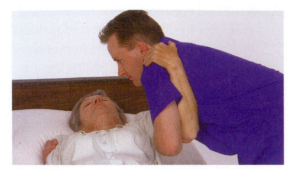

Fig. 12-6.

7. Reach under the client's head and place your other hand on the client's far shoulder. Have the client bend her knees. Bend your knees.

8. At the count of three, rock yourself backward and pull the client to a sitting position. Use pillows or a bed rest to support the client in the sitting position.

9. Check the client for dizziness or weakness.

10. If you raised an adjustable bed, be sure to return it to its lowest position.

11. Wash your hands.

12. Document the procedure and any observations. Was the client able to help at all? Did the client become dizzy?

Helping a client stand up

1. Wash your hands.

2. Explain the procedure to the client, speaking clearly, slowly, and directly, maintaining face-to-face contact whenever possible.

3. Provide privacy if the client desires it.

4. If the bed is adjustable, adjust bed to a safe working level, usually waist high. If the bed is movable, lock bed wheels.

5. Assist the client to a dangling position (see procedure earlier in this chapter).

6. Put non-skid footwear on client.

7. If the client is able, have her place her hands on the edge of the bed and push to stand-

ing, while you stay nearby to steady her or offer support if needed.

8. Always allow your client to do whatever she is able to do for herself. If the client is unable to stand without help, place one foot between the client's feet. If the client has a weak knee, brace it against your knee (Fig. 12-7).

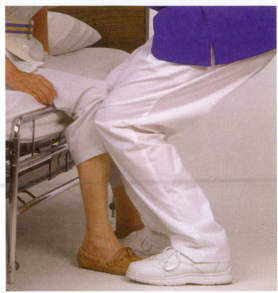

Fig. 12-7.

9. Have the client place her stronger leg directly under herself.

10. Bending your knees and leaning forward, put both arms around the client's waist and hold her close to your center of gravity (Fig. 12-8).

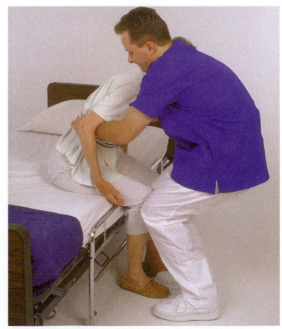

Fig. 12-8.

11. Tell the client to lean forward, push down on the bed with her hands, and stand, on the count of three. When you start to count, begin to rock. At three, rock your weight onto your back foot and assist the client to a standing position.

12. Check the client for dizziness before you allow her to stand alone. If you raised an adjustable bed, be sure to return it to its lowest position.

13. Wash your hands.

14. Document the procedure and any observations. How did the client tolerate standing? How much help did you offer?

If the client starts to fall, widen your stance. Bring the client's body close to you to break the fall (Fig. 12-9). Bend your knees and support the client as you lower her to the floor. You may need to drop to the floor with the client to avoid injury to you or the client. Do not try to reverse or stop a fall. You or the client can suffer worse injuries if you try to stop a fall than if you just break the fall.

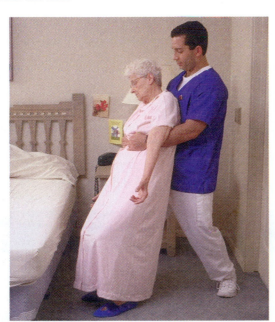

Fig. 12-9. Maintaining a wide base of support will help you assist a falling client.

If the client has fallen, call for help if a family member is around. Do not attempt to get the client up unless you are certain the client is not injured. Many agencies do not allow helping a client up after a fall until she has been evaluated by a nurse. Follow your agency's policies and procedures. Always call your supervisor if you are unsure of what to do. If you do help the client up, get her in bed, take vital signs, then report the fall to your supervisor.

Adaptive Equipment

Clients who have difficulty walking may use canes, walkers, or crutches to help themselves (Fig. 12-10). Understanding the purpose of each device will help you know how to use it properly. The purpose of a cane is to help with balance. A **straight cane** is not designed to bear weight. A **quad cane**, with four rubber-tipped feet, is designed to bear a little weight. Clients using canes should be able to bear weight on both legs. If one leg is weaker, the cane should be held in the hand on the strong side.

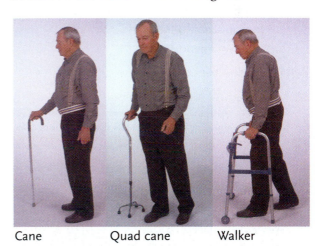

Cane   Quad cane   Walker

Fig. 12-10. Clients who have difficulty walking may use canes, walkers, or crutches to help themselves.

A **walker** is used when the client can bear some weight on the legs. The walker provides excellent stability for clients who are unsteady or lack balance. The metal frame of the walker may have rubber-tipped feet and/or wheels. Crutches are used for clients who can bear no weight or limited weight on one leg. Some people use one crutch, and some use two.

Whichever device is being used, your role is to ensure safety. Stay near the person, on the weak side. Make sure the equipment is in proper condition. It must be sturdy, and it must have rubber tips or wheels on the bottom.

1. Explain guidelines for transferring and positioning clients

Ambulation is walking. A client who is **ambulatory** is one who can get out of bed and walk. Many older clients are ambulatory, but need assistance to walk safely. Several tools, including transfer or gait belts, canes, walkers, and crutches, assist with ambulation.

A **transfer belt**, or **gait belt**, is used to assist clients who are able to walk but are weak, unsteady, or uncoordinated. The belt is made of canvas or other heavy material. It sometimes has handles and fits around the client's waist outside the clothing. The transfer belt is a safety device that gives you something firm to hold on to. When placing the belt on a client, leave enough room to insert two fingers into the belt (Fig. 12-11).

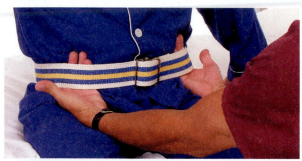

Fig. 12-11. Leave enough room to insert two fingers into a transfer belt.

Using a transfer belt to assist with ambulation

1. Wash your hands.

2. Explain the procedure to the client, speaking clearly, slowly, and directly, maintaining face-to-face contact whenever possible.

3. Provide privacy if the client desires it.

4. If the bed is adjustable, adjust bed to a safe working level, usually waist high. If the bed is movable, lock bed wheels.

5. Place the belt around the client's waist. Always apply the belt over clothing. Never place it next to skin.

6. Put non-skid footwear on client.

7. Help the client stand up, as described in the earlier procedure. Observe the client for strength and coordination.

8. Stand behind and to the side of the client as you hold onto the belt. If the client has a weaker side, stand on that side. Use the hand that is not holding the belt to offer support on the weak side (Fig. 12-12).

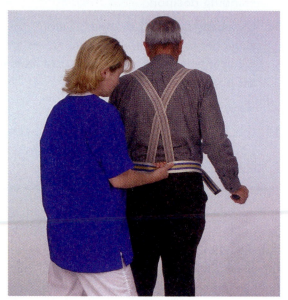

Fig. 12-12.

9. Observe the client's strength while you walk together. Provide a chair if the client becomes dizzy or tired.

10. Return the client to the bed or chair and be sure he is comfortable. If you raised an adjustable bed, be sure to return it to its lowest position.

11. Wash your hands.

12. Document the procedure and your observations. How far did the client walk? How did the client appear or say he felt while walking? How much help did you give?

Assisting with ambulation for a client who uses a cane or walker

1. Wash your hands.

2. Explain the procedure to the client, speaking clearly, slowly, and directly, maintaining face-to-face contact whenever possible.

3. Provide privacy if the client desires it.

4. If the bed is adjustable, adjust bed to a safe working level, usually waist high. If the bed is movable, lock bed wheels.

5. Fasten the transfer belt around the client's waist.

6. Put non-skid footwear on client.

7. Assist the client to a standing position.

8. Assist as necessary with ambulation.

a   Cane: Client places cane about 12 inches in front of his stronger leg. He brings weaker leg even with cane. He then brings stronger leg forward slightly ahead of cane (Fig. 12-13). Repeat.

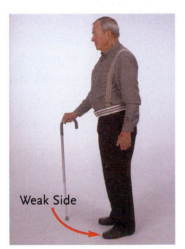

Weak Side

Fig. 12-13.

b   Walker: Client picks up or rolls the walker and places it about 12 inches in front of him. All four feet or wheels of the walker should be on the ground before client steps forward to the walker. The walker should not be moved again until the client has moved both feet forward and is in a steady position (Fig. 12-14). The client should never put his feet ahead of the walker.

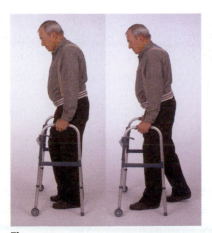

Fig. 12-14.

9. Whether the client is using a cane or walker walk slightly behind the client, on the weak side if the client has one. Hold the transfer belt unless you think the client is steady on his own.

10. Watch for obstacles in the client's path, and encourage the client to look ahead, rather than down at his feet.

11. Encourage the client to rest if tired. Allowing a client to become too tired increases the chance of a fall. Let the client set the pace. Discuss how far he plans to go based on the physician's orders.

12. Settle the client back into a safe and comfortable position after ambulation. If you raised an adjustable bed, be sure to return it to its lowest position.

13. Wash your hands.

14. Document the procedure and your observations. How did the client feel or appear while walking? How far did the client walk? How much help did the client need?

Clients should be fitted for crutches and taught to use them correctly by a physical therapist or nurse. The client may use the crutches several different ways, depending on what his weakness is. No matter how the client is using the crutches, weight should be on the client's hands and arms rather than on the underarm area (Fig. 12-15).

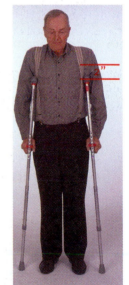

Fig. 12-15. When a client uses crutches, weight should be on his hands and arms, not on the underarm area.

GUIDELINES
Assisting a client in using a wheelchair

Ⓖ   Learn how each wheelchair works. Know how to apply and release the brake and how to operate the footrests. Always lock a wheelchair before assisting a resident into or out of it (Fig. 12-16). After a transfer, unlock the wheelchair.

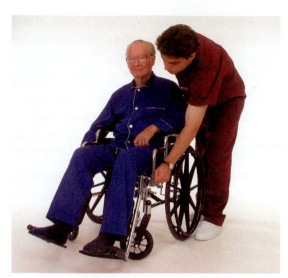

Fig. 12-16. You must always lock the wheelchair before a client gets into or out of it.

ⓖ To transfer to or from a wheelchair, the client must use the side or areas of the body that can bear weight to support and lift the side or areas that cannot bear weight. Clients who can bear no weight with their legs may use leg braces or an overhead trapeze to support themselves during transfers.

ⓖ During wheelchair transfers make sure the client is safe and comfortable. Ask the client how you can assist. Some may only want you to bring the chair to the bedside. Others may want you to be more involved. Always be sure the chair is as close as possible to the client and is locked in place. Use a transfer belt if you are going to assist in the transfer. Be sure the transfer is done slowly, allowing time for the client to rest. Check the client's alignment in the chair when the transfer is complete.

ⓖ If the client needs to be moved back in the wheelchair, go to the back of the chair. Reach forward and down under the client's arms. Ask the client to place his feet on the ground and push up. Pull the client up in the chair while the client pushes.

Helping a client move from a bed to a chair

Equipment: robe and non-skid footwear, transfer belt, chair or wheelchair, sheet or blanket

1. Wash your hands.

2. Explain the procedure to the client, speaking clearly, slowly, and directly, maintaining face-to-face contact whenever possible.

3. Provide privacy if the client desires it. Check the area to be certain it is uncluttered and safe.

4. Assist the client to the dangling position, as in earlier procedure.

5. Place the chair or wheelchair at the side of the bed on the client's **stronger** side. The chair should be at an angle slightly facing the client. If using a wheelchair, lock the brakes and raise or remove the foot and leg rests so they are not in the way. Cover plastic seats with a bath blanket or a soft pillow.

6. Help the client stand up, as in earlier procedure (Fig. 12-17).

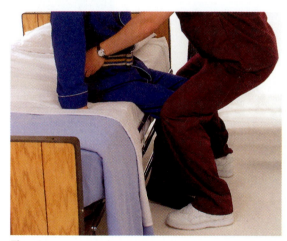

Fig. 12-17.

7. Tell the client to take small steps in the direction of the chair while turning his back toward the chair. If more assistance is needed, have the client pivot on the foot that is farther away from the chair. Always allow the client to do all he can for himself.

8. Have the client use one arm to grasp the arm of the chair. When the chair is touching the back of the client's legs, help the client lower himself into the chair.

9. If using a wheelchair, lower the footrests and help the client place his feet on them. Check that the client is in good alignment. Place a lap robe, folded blanket, or sheet over the client's lap as appropriate.

10. Wash your hands.

11. Document the procedure and your observations. How did the client feel or appear during the transfer? How much assistance was required?

A **slide board** may be used to help transfer clients who are unable to bear weight on their legs. Slide boards can be used for almost any transfer that involves moving from one sitting or reclining position to another. For example, slide boards can be helpful for transfers from bed to chair, wheelchair to bathtub, or wheelchair to car.

Helping a client transfer using a slide board

1. Follow steps 1 through 5 of the procedure for helping a client move from a bed to a chair.

2. Have the client lean away from transfer side to take the weight off her thigh (Fig. 12-18). Place one end of the sliding board under the buttocks and thigh. Take care not to pinch the client's skin between the bed and the board. Place the other end of the sliding board on the surface to which the client is transferring.

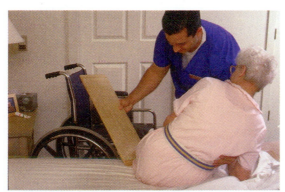

Fig. 12-18.

3. If the client is able, have her push up with her hands and scoot herself across the board. Stay close so you can provide support if needed. Always allow the client to do all she can for herself.

4. If the client needs assistance, stand in front of her and put your knees in front and a little

to the outside of her knees to keep them from buckling during the transfer. Make sure your back is straight.

5. Get as close to the client as possible and have her lean into you as you grasp the transfer belt from behind. Lean back with your knees bent. Using your legs rather than your back, pull the client up slightly and toward you to help her scoot across the board (Fig. 12-19).

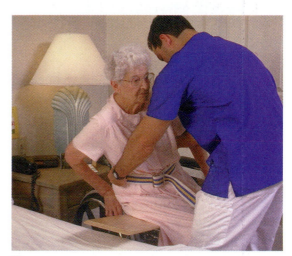

Fig. 12-19.

6. Complete the transfer in two or three lifting and scooting movements. Never drag the client across the board. Friction from the client's skin dragging across the slide board can cause skin breakdown that can lead to pressure sores.

7. After the client is safely transferred, remove the sliding board. Make sure the client is positioned safely and comfortably.

8. Wash your hands.

9. Document the procedure and any observations. How did the client feel or appear during the transfer? How much assistance was required?

Some clients may have a mechanical lift in the home. If you are trained to do so, you may assist the client with many types of transfers using the mechanical or hydraulic lift. This equipment avoids wear and tear on your body. Lifts help prevent injury to you and the client. Never use equipment you have not been trained

to use. You or your client could get hurt if you use lifting equipment improperly. There are many different types of mechanical lifts (Fig. 12-20). You must be trained on the specific lift you will be using.

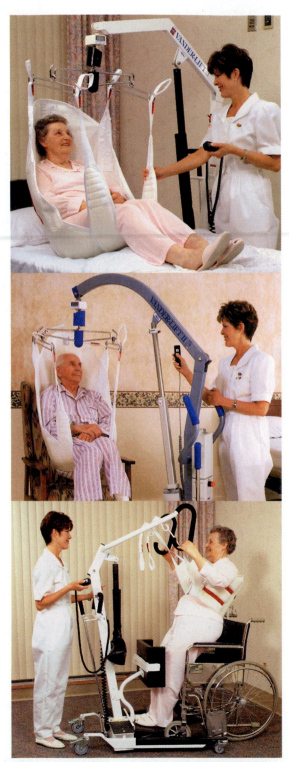

Fig. 12-20. Today, there are lifts that transfer completely dependent clients and clients who can bear some weight. (Photos courtesy of VANCARE Inc., 800-694-4525)

Transfers, Ambulation, and Positioning

Transferring a client using a mechanical lift

The following is a basic procedure for transferring using a mechanical lift. Ask someone to help you before starting.

Equipment: wheelchair or chair, lifting partner (if available), mechanical or hydraulic lift

1. Wash your hands.

2. Explain the procedure to the client, speaking clearly, slowly, and directly, maintaining face-to-face contact whenever possible.

3. Provide privacy if the client desires it.

4. Position wheelchair next to bed. Lock brakes.

5. Help the client turn to one side of the bed. Position the sling under the client, with the edge next to the client's back fanfolded if necessary, and the bottom of the sling even with the client's knees. Help the client roll back to the middle of the bed, and then spread out the fanfolded edge of the sling.

6. Roll the mechanical lift to bedside. Make sure the base is opened to its widest point, and push the base of the lift under the bed.

7. Position the overhead bar directly over the client (Fig. 12-21).

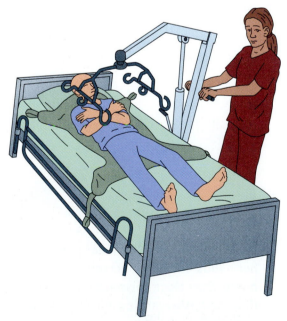

Fig. 12-21.

8. With the client lying on his back, attach one set of straps to each side of the sling, and

one set of straps to the overhead bar (Fig. 12-22). If available, have a lifting partner support the client at the head and shoulders and at the knees while the client is being lifted. The client's arms should be folded across her chest (Fig. 12-23). If the device has "S" hooks, they should face away from client (Fig. 12-24).

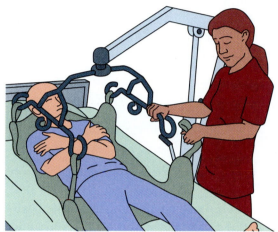

Fig. 12-22.

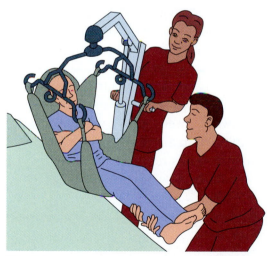

Fig. 12-23.

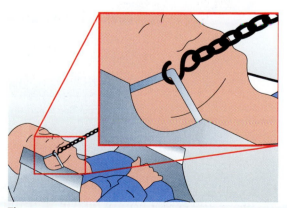

Fig. 12-24.

9. Following manufacturer's instructions for operating the lift, raise the client two inches above the bed. Pause a moment for the client to gain equilibrium.

10. If available, a lifting partner can help support and guide the client's body while you roll the lift so that the client is positioned over the chair or wheelchair.

11. Slowly lower the client into the chair or wheelchair. Push down gently on the client's knees to help the client into a sitting, rather than reclining, position.

12. Undo the straps from the overhead bar to the sling. Leave the sling in place for transfer back to bed.

13. Be sure the client is seated comfortably and correctly in the chair or wheelchair.

14. Wash your hands.

15. Document the procedure and any observations. How did the client tolerate the transfer? Were there any problems? Did the equipment operate properly?

2. Explain the guidelines for safely positioning a client in each of the five basic positions

Clients who spend a lot of time in bed often need help getting into comfortable positions. They also need to change positions periodically to avoid muscle stiffness and skin breakdown or pressure sores. **Positioning** means helping clients into positions that will be comfortable and healthy for them. Bed-bound clients should be repositioned every two hours. Document the position and time every time there is a change.

Which positions a client uses will depend on the diagnosis, the condition, and the client's preference. The care plan will give specific positioning instructions. Remember, even immobile clients may not stay in the position you put them in. Recheck them periodically. Always keep principles of body mechanics and alignment in mind when positioning clients. Also, check skin for

whiteness or redness, especially around bony areas, each time you reposition a client.

The following are guidelines for positioning clients in the five basic body positions:

1. **Supine** (*SUE-pine*): In this position, the client lies flat on his back. To maintain correct body position, support the client's head and shoulders with a pillow (Fig. 12-25). You may also use pillows or rolled towels or washcloths to support his arms (especially a weak or immobilized arm) or hands. The heels should be "floating." This is done by placing a very firm pillow under the calves so the heels do not touch the bed. Pillows or a footboard can be used to keep feet flexed slightly.

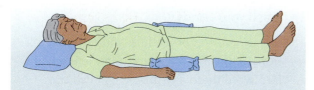

Fig. 12-25. A person in the supine position is lying flat on his or her back.

2. **Lateral/Side**: A client in the lateral position is lying on either side. There are many variations in this position. Pillows can be used to support the arm and leg on the upper side, the back, and the head (Fig. 12-26). Ideally, the knee on the upper side of the body should be flexed, with the leg brought in front of the body and supported on a pillow. There should be a pillow under the bottom foot so that the toes are not touching the bed. If the top leg cannot be brought forward and instead rests on the bottom leg, pillows should be used between the two legs to relieve pressure and avoid skin breakdown.

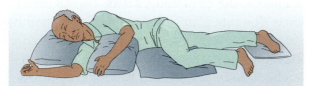

Fig. 12-26. A person in the lateral position is lying on his or her side.

3. **Prone**: A client in the prone position is lying on the stomach, or front side of the body (Fig. 12-27). This is not a comfortable position for many people, especially elderly people. Never leave a client in a prone position for very long. Always check the care plan before using the prone position. In this position, the arms are either at the sides or raised above the head. The head is turned to one side and a small pillow may be used under the head.

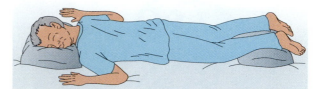

Fig. 12-27. A person lying in the prone position is lying on his or her stomach.

4. **Fowler's**: A client in the Fowler's position is in a semi-sitting position, with the head and shoulders elevated. The client's knees may be flexed and elevated using a pillow or rolled blanket as a support (Fig. 12-28). The feet may be flexed and supported using a footboard or other support. The spine should be straight. In a true Fowler's position the upper body is raised to a point halfway between sitting straight up and lying flat. In a semi-Fowler's position the upper body is not raised as high.

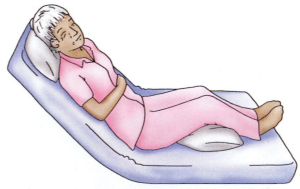

Fig. 12-28. A person lying in the Fowler's position is partially reclined.

5. **Sims'**: The Sims' position is a variation on the lateral, or side, position. The lower arm is behind the back and the upper knee is flexed and raised toward the chest, using a

pillow as support. There should be a pillow under the bottom foot so that the toes are not touching the bed (Fig. 12-29).

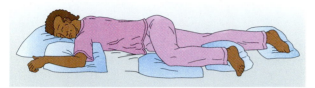

Fig. 12-29. A person lying in the Sims' position is lying on his or her side with one leg drawn up.

Use the positions indicated in the care plan. If you have questions about how to position a client, ask your supervisor. In general, use positions that are natural and comfortable for the client. Always check the skin for signs of irritation whenever you reposition a client.

Turning a client in bed

1. Wash your hands.

2. Explain the procedure to the client, speaking clearly, slowly, and directly, maintaining face-to-face contact whenever possible.

3. Provide privacy if the client desires it.

4. If the bed is adjustable, adjust bed to a safe working level, usually waist high. If the bed is movable, lock bed wheels.

5. With the client in supine position and centered in the bed, stand at the side of the bed client will face. Place the client's near hand palm-up under her hip.

6. Lift the client's far leg over her near leg, flexing the knee (Fig. 12-30).

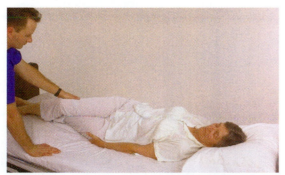

Fig. 12-30.

7. Assume a good stance. your feet hip width apart, your knees bent, and one foot slightly in front of the other.

8. Grasp the client's far shoulder and far hip. Count to three, rocking your weight forward and back on each count. On three, roll the client onto her side (Fig. 12-31).

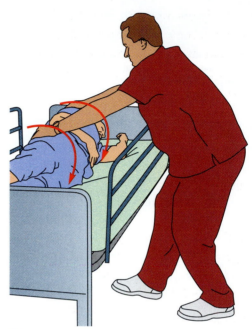

Fig. 12-31.

9. Use whatever pillows or supports are necessary to be sure the client is in a comfortable position, with good body alignment. Arrange the bed covers so that the client is comfortable. If you raised an adjustable bed, be sure to return it to its lowest position.

10. Wash your hands.

11. Document the procedure and any observations.

Helping a client move up in bed helps prevent skin irritation that can lead to pressure sores. You can use a helper if one is available. You may have to help a client move up in bed by yourself. If the client is unable to assist you, use a **draw sheet** or **turning sheet** (Fig. 12-32). A draw sheet is an extra sheet placed on top of the bottom sheet when the bed is made. It allows a caregiver to reposition the client without causing **shearing**, or friction and pressure on the skin from rubbing or dragging it across another surface (the bottom sheet)

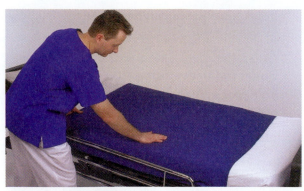

Fig. 12-32. A draw sheet is a special sheet (or a regular bed sheet folded in half) that is used to help move clients in bed without causing shearing on the skin.

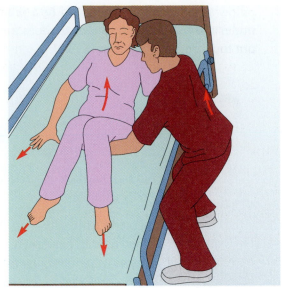

Fig. 12-33. Keep your back straight and your knees bent.

Moving a client up in bed

Always allow the client to do all she can for herself. Following is the procedure for clients who can help you move them up in bed.

1. Wash your hands.

2. Explain the procedure to the client, speaking clearly, slowly, and directly, maintaining face-to-face contact whenever possible.

3. Provide privacy if the client desires it.

4. If the bed is adjustable, adjust bed to a safe working level, usually waist high. Lower the head of bed to make it flat. If the bed is movable, lock bed wheels. If side rails are available, raise the rail on the far side of the bed. Remove the pillow and set it aside for later use.

5. Place one arm under the client's shoulders and the other under the client's buttocks.

6. Ask the client to bend her knees and push down on the mattress with her feet and hands on the count of three (Fig. 12-33).

7. Keeping your back straight and bending at the knees, help the client move toward the head of the mattress on the count of three. As always, allow the client to do all she can for herself.

8. Help the client into a comfortable position and arrange the pillow and blankets for her. If you raised an adjustable bed, be sure to return it to its lowest position.

9. Wash your hands.

10. Document the procedure and any observations.

When the client cannot assist and there is no one else around to help you move her up in bed, take the following steps:

1. Follow steps 1 through 3 above.

2. If the bed is adjustable, adjust bed to a safe working level, usually waist high. Lower the head of bed to make it flat. If the bed is movable, lock bed wheels. Raise both side rails.

3. Stand behind the head of the bed with your feet shoulder width apart and one foot slightly in front of the other.

4. Roll and grasp the top edge of the draw sheet.

5. With your knees bent and your back straight, rock your weight from the front foot to the back foot in one smooth motion (Fig. 12-34).

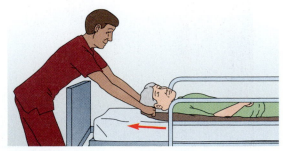

Fig. 12-34.

6. Help the client into a comfortable position and arrange the pillow and blankets for her. Unroll the draw sheet and leave it in place for the next repositioning. If you raised an adjustable bed, be sure to return it to its lowest position.

7. Wash your hands.

8. Document the procedure and any observations.

When you have help from another person, you can modify the procedure as follows:

1. Follow steps 1 through 3 above.

2. If the bed is adjustable, adjust bed to a safe working level, usually waist high. Lower the head of bed to make it flat. If the bed is movable, lock bed wheels.

3. Stand on the opposite side of the bed from your helper. Each of you should be turned slightly toward the head of the bed. For each of you, the foot that is closest to the head of the bed should be pointed that direction.

4. Roll the draw sheet up to the client's side, and have your helper do the same on his side of the bed. Grasp the sheet with your palms up, and have your helper do the same.

5. Shift your weight to your back foot (the foot closer to the foot of the bed) and have your helper do the same (Fig. 12-35). On the count of three, you and your helper both shift your weight to your forward feet as you slide the draw sheet toward the head of the bed (Fig. 12-36).

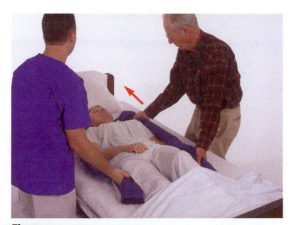

Fig. 12-35.

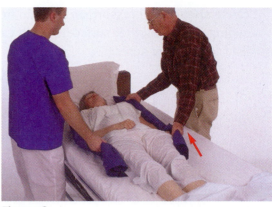

Fig. 12-36.

6. Help the client into a comfortable position and arrange the pillow and blankets for her. Unroll the draw sheet and leave it in place for the next repositioning. If you raised an adjustable bed, be sure to return it to its lowest position.

7. Wash your hands.

8. Document the procedure and any observations.

Some clients' spinal columns must be kept in alignment. To turn these clients in bed, you will use a procedure called **logrolling**.

Logrolling a client

1. Wash your hands.

2. Explain the procedure to the client, speaking clearly, slowly, and directly, maintaining face-to-face contact whenever possible.

3. Provide privacy if the client desires it.

4. If the bed is adjustable, adjust bed to a safe working level, usually waist high. Lower the head of bed to make it flat. If the bed is movable, lock bed wheels.

5. Move the client to the side of the bed you are standing on. To do this, assume a good stance, with feet hip width apart, knees bent, and one foot slightly in front of the other. Slip your arms under the client's shoulders and move her toward you by rocking your weight backwards onto your back foot (Fig. 12-37). Keep your knees bent. Be careful not to slide the client across the sheets and

cause **shearing** (pressure on the skin from sliding across another surface), which can lead to pressure sores.

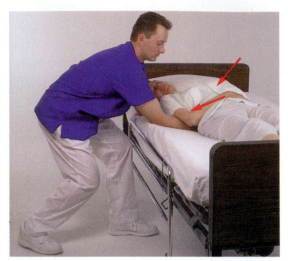

Fig. 12-37.

6. Keeping the same good stance, slide your arms under the client's hips and shift them toward you, as you did her shoulders (Fig. 12-38). Make sure the client's head and legs are in alignment with her shoulders and hips before continuing with the procedure.

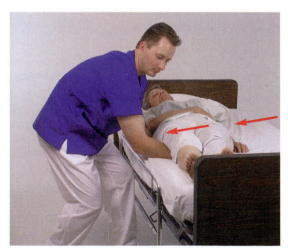

Fig. 12-38.

7. If available, raise the side rail on the side of the bed the client is now closest to. If no side rail is available, be sure the client is safe and stable before moving to the next step.

8. Move to the other side of the bed and lower the side rail if there is one. Assume a good stance.

9. With your knees bent, grasp the client with one hand on the far hip and one on the far shoulder. Roll the client toward you onto her side (Fig. 12-39).

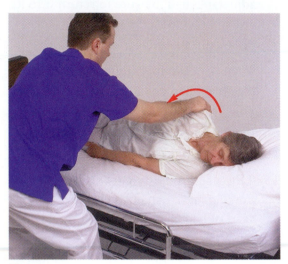

Fig. 12-39.

10. Check the client's body alignment. Arrange pillows and covers for comfort. Raise the side rail if available and if necessary for client's safety. If you raised an adjustable bed, be sure to return it to its lowest position.

11. Wash your hands.

12. Document the procedure and any observations.

3. List things you can do to help make your client comfortable

There are several things you can do to provide for the comfort and safety of your client in and around the bed:

• Have plenty of pillows available to provide support in the various positions.

• Use positioning devices (such as backrests, bed cradles and tables, footboards, and handrolls).

• Give back rubs for comfort and relaxation.

• Change positions frequently (every two hours) and as directed in the care plan.

• Always maintain the client's body alignment.

3. List things you can do to help make your client comfortable

A back rub can help relax your client and make him or her more comfortable. Back rubs increase circulation, too. They are often given after baths. Follow instructions in the care plan for when to give back rubs and for how long.

Giving a back rub

Equipment: cotton blanket or towel, lotion, gloves if client's skin is broken

1. Wash your hands.

2. Explain the procedure to the client, speaking clearly, slowly, and directly, maintaining face-to-face contact whenever possible.

3. Provide privacy if the client desires it.

4. If the bed is adjustable, adjust bed to a safe working level, usually waist high. Lower the head of the bed. If the bed is movable, lock bed wheels.

5. Have the client lie in a prone position (Fig. 12-40). If this is uncomfortable, have the client lie on his side. Cover the client with a cotton blanket, then fold back the bed covers. Expose the client's back to the top of the buttocks. If the client is positioned on the side, place the towel on the bed along the length of his back. Back rubs can also be given with the client sitting up.

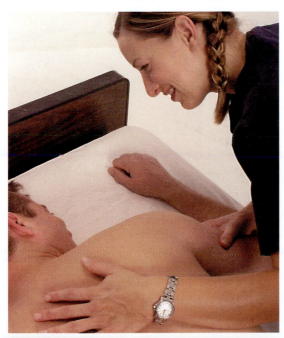

Fig. 12-40.

6. Warm the lotion bottle in warm water for five minutes. Run your hands under warm water to warm them. Pour the lotion on your hands. Rub them together to spread it. Warn the client that the lotion may still feel cool. Always put the lotion on your hands rather than directly on the client's skin.

7. Place your hands on each side of the upper part of the buttocks. Make long, smooth upward strokes with both hands along each side of the spine, up to the shoulders (Fig. 12-41). Circle your hands outward. Then move back along the outer edges of the back. At the buttocks, make another circle and move your hands back up to the shoulders. Without taking your hands from the client's skin, repeat this motion for three to five minutes.

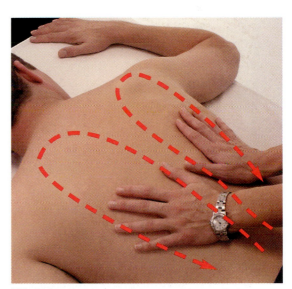

Fig. 12-41.

8. Make kneading motions with the first two fingers and thumb of each hand. Place them at the base of the spine. Move upward together along each side of the spine, applying gentle downward pressure with the fingers and thumbs. Follow the same direction as with the long smooth strokes, circling at shoulders and buttocks (Fig. 12-42).

9. Gently massage bony areas (spine, shoulder blades, hip bones) with circular motions of your fingertips. Gentle massage stimulates circulation and helps prevent skin damage. However, if any of these areas are red,

3. List things you can do to help make your client comfortable

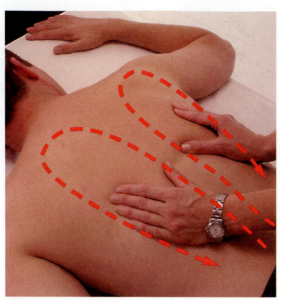

Fig. 12-42.

massage around them rather than on them. The redness indicates that the skin is already irritated and fragile.

10. Let your client know when you are almost through. Finish with some long smooth strokes, like the ones you used at the beginning of the massage.

11. Dry the back if extra lotion remains on it. If appropriate, apply powder to the back to allow better movement against the sheets.

12. Remove the cotton blanket and towel.

13. Assist the client with getting dressed.

14. Help the client into a comfortable position. If you raised an adjustable bed, be sure to return it to its lowest position.

15. Store the lotion and put dirty linens in the hamper.

16. Wash your hands.

17. Document the procedure and your observations. Did the client appear comfortable during the back rub? Did you observe any discolored areas or broken skin?

Many positioning devices are available to make clients more comfortable. Some can be inexpensively made in the client's home. Check with your supervisor on the use of positioning devices for each client.

GUIDELINES
Positioning Devices

g Backrests can be made of pillows, cardboard or wood covered by pillows, or special wedge-shaped foam pillows (Fig. 12-43).

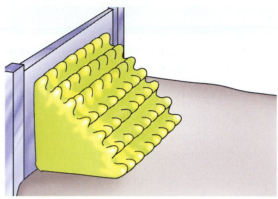

Fig. 12-43. A backrest.

g Bed cradles are used to keep the bed covers from pushing down on clients' feet. Metal frames that work like a tent when the bed covers are over them can be purchased (Fig. 12-44). A cardboard box can be used as a bed cradle by placing the client's feet inside the box underneath the covers (Fig. 12-45). The box should be at least **two inches above** the toes.

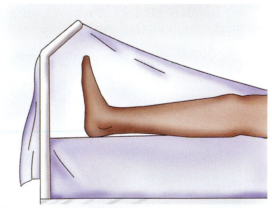

Fig. 12-44. A bed cradle.

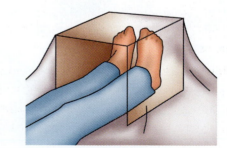

Fig. 12-45. A homemade bed cradle.

g Bed tables are available commercially. You can also make one by cutting openings in each of the longer sides of a sturdy cardboard box (Fig. 12-46).

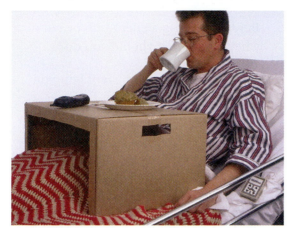

Fig. 12-46. A bed table.

g Draw sheets may be placed under a client to help move clients who are unable to assist with turning in bed, lifting, or moving up in bed. Draw sheets also help prevent skin damage that can be caused by shearing. A regular bed sheet folded in half can be used as a draw sheet.

g Footboards are padded boards placed against the client's feet to keep them flexed and prevent footdrop (Fig. 12-47). Rolled blankets or pillows can also be used as footboards.

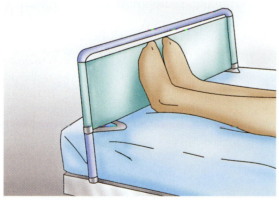

Fig. 12-47. A footboard.

g Handrolls keep the fingers from curling tightly. A rolled washcloth, gauze bandage, or a rubber ball placed inside the palm may be used to keep the hand in a natural position (Fig. 12-48).

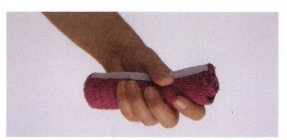

Fig. 12-48. A handroll.

g Splints may be prescribed by a doctor to keep a client's joints in the correct position (Fig. 12-49).

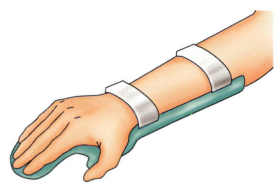

Fig. 12-49. A splint.

g Trochanter rolls are used to keep the client's hips from turning outward. A rolled towel works well as an improvised trochanter roll (Fig. 12-50).

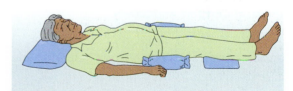

Fig. 12-50. Trochanter rolls.

GUIDELINES
Physical Restraints

Throughout this book, we discuss ways to protect your clients' physical safety. For example, using side rails when available can prevent a client from rolling out of bed. Your supervisor may train you to use other devices to protect your clients in the home.

As discussed earlier in this book (chapters 3 and 6), physical restraints have been used in the past. These restraints were intended to safeguard clients who wander, are violent, or are at risk of hurting themselves.

However, due to client abuse and injury, new laws restrict the use of restraints. In many states, restraints are illegal. If restraint use is legal, a doctor must prescribe it. Never use physical restraints unless a doctor has ordered it in the care plan and you have been trained in their use. It is against the law for a caregiver to apply a restraint for convenience or to discipline a client.

When a client is restrained, he or she has to be monitored continuously. The client must be checked at least every 30 minutes. Every two hours, or as needed, the following must be done:

- 🅖 Release the restraint for at least ten minutes.
- 🅖 Offer assistance with toileting. Check for episodes of incontinence. Provide incontinence care.
- 🅖 Offer fluids.
- 🅖 Check the skin for irritation. Report any red or discolored areas to your supervisor immediately.
- 🅖 Reposition the client.
- 🅖 Ambulate client if he or she is able.

OBSERVING AND REPORTING
Physical Comfort and Safety

Your observations about your clients' physical comfort and safety can be very helpful to the care team. Report the following:

- how well clients tolerate positioning, transferring, and ambulation
- any signs of skin breakdown (whiteness, redness, rashes, or broken skin)
- changes that could be made in the home environment to improve comfort or safety
- any change in client's ability

Chapter Review

1. What is dangling?

2. Describe what you should you do if a client has fallen.

3. What is one difference between a straight cane and a quad cane?

4. Which side should you stay by when a client is using adaptive equipment?

5. Before assisting a client into or out of a wheelchair, what should you do?

6. In which position is a client lying on his/her side?

7. In which position is a client lying on his/her stomach?

8. In which position is a client lying flat on his/her back?

9. In which position is a client lying on his/her side with the lower arm behind the back and the upper knee flexed and raised toward the chest?

10. In which position is a client in a semi-sitting position with the head and shoulders elevated?

11. What is a draw sheet?

12. List four comfort and safety measures for a client who is in bed.

13. List five types of positioning devices that can make clients more comfortable.

14. If a client is restrained, how often must he or she be checked?

13

Personal Care Skills

1. Describe the home health aide's role in assisting clients with personal care

Hygiene (*HIGH-jeen*) is the term used to describe practices to keep our bodies clean and healthy. Bathing and brushing teeth are two examples. **Grooming** refers to practices like caring for fingernails and hair. Hygiene and grooming activities, as well as dressing, preparing meals, and eating, are called **activities of daily living (ADLs)**.

Some people who are ill may not have the energy to care for themselves. These clients may need assistance with their personal care, or they may need you to provide it for them entirely. You may provide any or all of the personal care, including bathing, **perineal** (*payr-i-NEE-al*) care (care of the area around and between the genitals and anus), mouth care, shampooing and combing the hair, nail care, shaving, dressing, and changing bed linens.

Some clients may never be able to care for themselves. However, many clients will regain strength and be able to perform their own personal care. An important part of your job is to help clients be as independent as possible. This means teaching clients with disabilities to care for themselves, and encouraging other clients to perform self-care as soon as they are able.

Promoting independence is an important part of care.

We all have routines for personal care and activities of daily living. We also have preferences for how they are done. These routines remain important even when we are elderly, sick, or disabled. Be aware of your clients' individual preferences concerning their personal care (Fig. 13-1). Clients may prefer certain soaps or skin care products. They may choose to bathe in the morning or at night. It is important to ask clients about their routines and preferences.

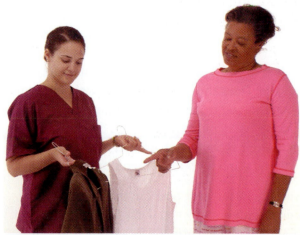

Fig. 13-1. Asking a client which outfit she would like to wear promotes independence and shows respect.

Before you begin any task, explain to the client exactly what you will be doing. Ask if he or she

would like to use the bathroom or bedpan first. Provide the client with privacy. Let him or her make as many decisions as possible about when, where, and how a procedure will be done. This promotes dignity and independence. During the procedure, if the client appears tired, stop and take a short rest. Never rush a client. After care, always ask if the client would like anything else.

Personal care gives you the opportunity to observe your client's skin, mental state, mobility, flexibility, comfort level, and ability to perform ADLs. For example, as you bathe a client, observe the skin for color, texture, temperature, and whether it is dry or moist. Is it pale, yellow, ashen, or flushed? Are there blotches or a rash? Is there redness around bony areas? Is the skin dry and flaky?

Personal care offers you an opportunity to talk with clients. Some clients will talk about symptoms they are experiencing during personal care. They may tell you that they have been itching or their skin feels dry. They may complain of numbness and tingling in a certain part of the body. Keep a small note pad in a pocket to jot down exactly how the client describes these symptoms. Make notes right after the procedure. Report these comments to your supervisor and document them properly.

Observe the client's mental and emotional state at this time. Is the client depressed or confused? Can the client concentrate on the activity or hold a conversation? Is the client short of breath? Does the client tremble or shake? Is the client having trouble using certain muscles or joints? Focus on changes from the client's normal state. Is there a change in behavior, level of activity, skin color, movement, or anything else?

You are in the best position to observe, report, and document any small change in your client. No matter what care task is assigned to you, performing it is only half the job. For example, when bathing a client, observe changes in the client's skin, in his ability to move, reach, or help himself, and in his willingness to help himself.

Noticing and reporting change

Licensed nurses once performed much of the care you are learning to give. Nurses have completed years of education to notice signs of illnesses and health problems. Because you will be performing these care tasks, nurses lose an opportunity to discover early signs of illness or disease. Your role is to make certain small changes in a client do not go unnoticed. Noticing and reporting change is one of the most important parts of your job!

After you have finished a procedure, check the client's room. Is it a comfortable temperature? Is it well-ventilated, but free from drafts? Can the client easily signal for help? Does the room have good lighting? Are there electrical cords or other objects in the walkways? Is the room cluttered and unsafe? Also, make certain your client does not smoke in bed.

2. Explain guidelines for assisting with bathing

Bathing promotes good health and well-being. It removes perspiration, dirt, oil, and dead skin cells that collect on the skin. Taking a bath or having a bed bath can also be relaxing. The bed bath is an excellent time for moving arms and legs and increasing circulation.

Only give a client a tub bath if it is assigned. Many agencies have rules against helping clients into the bathtub. These rules are for the client's safety, as well as the home health aide's. Follow your agency's policies and procedures.

Many people prefer a daily bath or shower, but this is not really necessary. The face, hands, **axillae** (*AK-sil-eye*, or underarms), and perineum should be washed every day. A complete bath or shower can be taken every other day or even less frequently. Older skin produces less perspiration and oil. Elderly people whose skin is dry and fragile should bathe only once or twice a week. Be gentle with the skin when bathing older clients.

Before any bathing task, make sure the room is warm enough. Remove any loose rugs that do not have slip-resistant, rubber backings. Be familiar with available safety and assistive devices. Never leave an elderly person or young child alone in the bathtub. Never use bath oils. They make the tub slippery and can cause a fall.

Wearing gloves is sometimes recommended for assisting clients with bathing. Some agencies only require that you wear gloves for perineal care or if broken skin is present. As always, follow your agency's policies and procedures.

GUIDELINES
Using assistive devices in bathing

🄖 Assistive devices, such as a transfer belt or lift, tub chair, and safety bars, can make bathing easier and safer. An occupational therapist (OT) may teach you and the client transfer techniques for getting safely in and out of the bathtub. Occupational therapists help clients improve their abilities to perform ADLs.

🄖 A **tub** or **shower chair** (Fig. 13-2) is a sturdy chair designed to be placed in a bathtub. It is water- and slip-resistant. The chair or bench enables a client who is unable to get into a tub or is too weak to stand in a shower to bathe in the tub rather than in bed. Safety bars/grab bars are often installed in and near the tub and toilet to give the client something to hold on to while changing position.

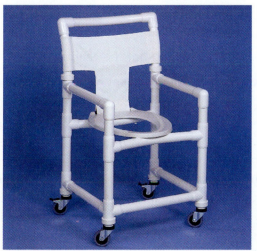

Fig. 13-2. One type of shower chair. (Photo courtesy of Innovative Products Unlimited)

🄖 You will not find the same adaptive equipment in each client's home. Become familiar with the tools you have to work with. Learn how to use them before trying to assist the client. Report any need for equipment to your supervisor.

Helping the client transfer to the bathtub

You may have to adapt this procedure to work with your clients' different strength levels.

Equipment: chair, transfer belt (if appropriate), shirt or robe to wear under transfer belt, slide board (if appropriate), tub or shower chair, bath supplies (as listed in next procedure), gloves

1. Wash your hands.

2. Explain the procedure to the client, speaking clearly, slowly, and directly, maintaining face-to-face contact whenever possible.

3. Help the client to the bathroom.

4. Provide privacy for the client.

5. Seat the client in a chair facing the bathtub and centered between the grab bars. If using a wheelchair, lock brakes and raise footrests (Fig. 13-3).

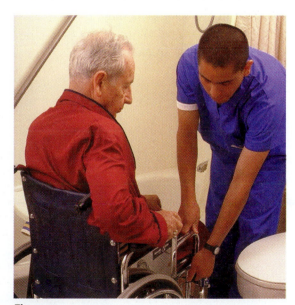

Fig. 13-3.

6. Ask the client to place one leg at a time over the sides of the tub.

7. Have client hold onto the grab bars or the edge of the tub to bring himself to a sitting

position on the edge of the tub (Fig. 13-4). A slide board may also be used to help the client move from the chair to the tub.

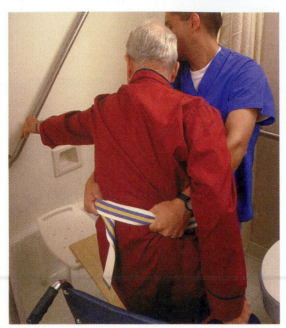

Fig. 13-4.

8. Help the client lower himself into the tub or onto the tub chair while holding onto the edge of the tub or grab bars (Fig. 13-5). If necessary, assist by holding him around the waist or by having him wear a transfer belt. If using a transfer belt to get in and out of the tub, the client will need to wear a shirt or robe while transferring, so the belt is not placed directly against his skin.

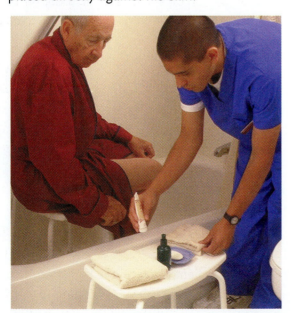

Fig. 13-5.

9. Reverse this procedure to help the client out of the tub when the bath is over. If the client has trouble getting out of the tub, help him to his hands and knees. From that position, he can use the grab bar or the edge of the tub to help pull himself up. You can also help by putting the transfer belt back on the client (over a robe).

10. Wash your hands.

11. Document the procedure and your observations.

Helping the ambulatory client take a shower or tub bath

Clients who can get out of bed to take a shower or bath will need different assistance and supervision. Follow the instructions in the care plan.

Equipment: two bath towels, washcloth, soap or other cleanser, bath thermometer (if available), rubber bath mat, tub or shower chair (if appropriate), table for bath supplies and bell (for clients who bathe without assistance), non-skid bath rug, deodorant, lotion and other toiletries, clean clothes or a robe, shoes or non-skid slippers, disposable gloves

1. Wash your hands.

2. Explain the procedure to the client, speaking clearly, slowly, and directly, maintaining face-to-face contact whenever possible.

3. Clean tub or shower if necessary. Place rubber mat on tub or shower floor. Set up tub or shower chair. Place non-skid bath rug on the floor next to the tub or shower.

4. Provide privacy for the client.

5. Put on gloves if client has broken skin.

6. Fill the tub with warm water (105° to 110°F on the bath thermometer, or test the water on the inside of your wrist to see if it is comfortable) or adjust the shower water temperature. Have the client test water temperature to see if it's comfortable.

7. Ask the client to undress, and assist as needed. Help client transfer to bathtub or step in the shower.

8. If the care plan allows you to leave the client to bathe alone, place the bathing supplies on a small table within the client's reach. Place a bell or other signal on the table (Fig. 13-6). Tell the client to signal when you are needed. Ask the client not to add more hot or warm water and not to remain in the tub more than 20 minutes. Do not lock the bathroom door. Check on your client every five minutes. If the client is weak, remain in the bathroom. Otherwise, you can make the client's bed while he is in the tub.

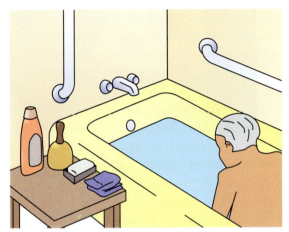

Fig. 13-6.

9. For a shower, stay with the client and assist with washing hard-to-reach areas. Observe for signs of fatigue.

10. If the client needs more assistance in the bath or shower, help him wash himself. Always wash from clean areas to dirty areas, so you don't spread dirt into areas that have already been washed. Make sure all soap is rinsed off so the client's skin does not become dry or irritated.

11. Assist the client with shampooing hair, if necessary (see procedure below). Make sure all shampoo is rinsed out of hair.

12. When the bath or shower is finished, help the client get out of the tub. Wrap him in a towel. Have the client sit in a chair or on the toilet seat, and provide him with another towel for drying himself (Fig. 13-7). Offer assistance in drying hard-to-reach places. The client may need help applying powder, deodorant, or lotion. If necessary, help the client get dressed.

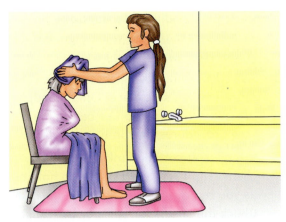

Fig. 13-7.

13. If your client is tired after the bath or shower, help him back to the bed. Other personal care, such as mouth care, can be done later or while the client is in bed.

14. Clean the tub and place soiled laundry (towels, washcloths, dirty clothes) in the laundry hamper.

15. Wash your hands.

16. Put away supplies.

17. Document the procedure and your observations. Did you observe any redness or whiteness on the skin? Was there any broken skin? How did the client tolerate bathing or showering? Has there been a change in the client's abilities since the last bath or shower?

    Talk with your supervisor if the client makes a request that is not included in the care plan.

Assisting with a bed bath

Equipment: basin, bath thermometer (if available), soap, two washcloths, two or three towels, orangewood stick or nail brush (if available), lotion, deodorant, soft cotton blanket or large towel, clean clothes, clean bed linens, gloves

1. Wash your hands.

2. Explain the procedure to the client, speaking clearly, slowly, and directly, maintaining face-to-face contact whenever possible.

3. Provide privacy for the client. Be sure the room is a comfortable temperature and there are no drafts.

162

13

Personal Care Skills

4. If the bed is adjustable, adjust bed to a safe working level, usually waist high. If the bed is movable, lock bed wheels.

5. Ask client to remove glasses and jewelry and put them in a safe place. Offer a bedpan or urinal for the client to use before the bath (see procedures later in this chapter).

6. Place a soft cotton blanket or towel over client (Fig. 13-8) and ask him to hold onto it as you remove the top sheet and blanket. Check the sheets for spills or body discharges.

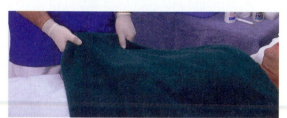

Fig. 13-8.

7. Fill the basin with warm water and check the temperature with a bath thermometer or against the inside of your wrist. Water temperature should be between 105° and 110°F on a thermometer. Allow the client to check the temperature to see if it is adequate. During the bath, change the water when it becomes too cool, soapy, or dirty.

8. If the client has open wounds or broken skin, put on gloves.

9. Ask and assist the client to participate in washing.

10. Uncover only one part of the body at a time. Place a towel under the body part being washed.

11. Wash, rinse, and dry one part of the body at a time. Start at the head, work down, and complete the front first. Fold the washcloth over your hand like a mitt and hold it in place with the thumb (Fig. 13-9).

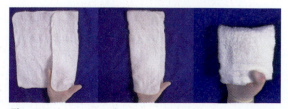

Fig. 13-9.

Eyes and Face: Wash face with wet washcloth (no soap), beginning with the eye farther away from you, and wash inner aspect to outer aspect (Fig. 13-10). Use a different area of the washcloth for each eye. Wash the face from the middle outward using firm but gentle strokes. Wash the neck and ears and behind the ears. Rinse and pat dry.

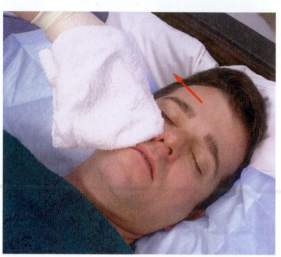

Fig. 13-10.

Arms: Remove the client's top clothing, and cover him with the bath blanket or towel. With a soapy washcloth, wash the upper arm and the underarm. Use long strokes from the shoulder down to the elbow. Rinse and pat dry. Wash the elbow. Wash, rinse, and dry from the elbow down to the wrist (Fig. 13-11).

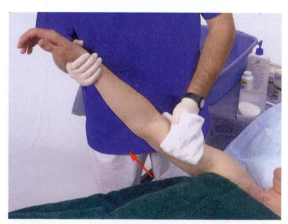

Fig. 13-11.

Wash the hand in a basin: Clean under the nails with an orangewood stick or nail brush if available (Fig. 13-12). Rinse and pat dry. Provide nail care (see procedure later in this

chapter) only if it has been assigned. Do not provide nail care for a diabetic client. Repeat for the other arm. Put lotion on the client's elbows and hands if ordered.

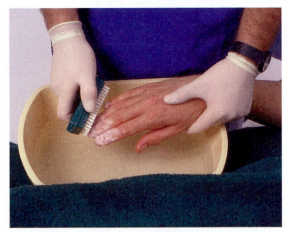
Fig. 13-12.

Chest: Place the towel again across the client's chest. Pull the blanket down to the waist. Lift the towel only enough to wash the chest, rinse it, and pat dry. For a female client, wash, rinse, and dry breasts and under breasts. Check the skin in this area for signs of irritation and chafing.

Abdomen: Fold the blanket down so that it still covers the pubic area. Wash the abdomen, rinse, and pat dry. If the client has an **ostomy** (*AH-stoh-mee*), or opening in the abdomen for getting rid of body wastes, provide skin care around the opening (Chapter 14 includes more information about ostomies). Cover with the towel. Pull the cotton blanket up to the client's chin and remove the towel.

Legs: Expose one leg and place a towel under it. Wash the thigh. Use long downward strokes. Rinse and pat dry. Do the same from the knee to the ankle (Fig. 13-13). Place another towel under the foot and transfer the basin to the towel. Place the foot into the basin. Wash the foot and between the toes in a basin (Fig. 13-14). Rinse foot and pat dry, making sure area between toes is dry. Provide nail care (see procedure later in this chapter) only if it has been assigned. Do not perform nail care for a diabetic client. Never clip a client's toenails.

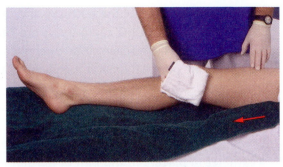
Fig. 13-13.

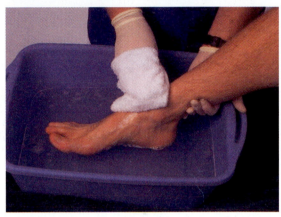
Fig. 13-14.

Apply lotion to the foot if ordered, especially at the heels. Repeat steps for the other leg and foot.

Back: Help client move to the center of the bed, then turn onto his or her side so his or her back is facing you. If the bed has rails, raise the rail on the opposite side for safety. Fold the cotton blanket away from the back. Place a towel lengthwise next to the back. Wash the back, neck, and buttocks with long, downward strokes. Rinse and pat dry (Fig. 13-15). Apply lotion if ordered.

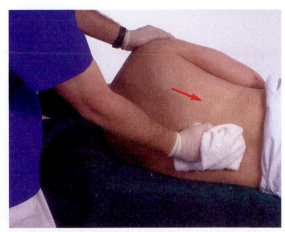
Fig. 13-15.

12. Place the towel under the buttocks and upper thighs. Help the client turn onto his or her back. Ask the client if he or she is able to wash the perineal area. If the client is able to do this, place a basin of clean, warm water within reach, along with a washcloth and towel. Leave the room if the client would like privacy. If the client has a urinary catheter in place, remind him or her not to pull it.

13. If the client is unable to provide perineal care, you must do so. Put on gloves (if you haven't already done so) before washing perineal area. Provide privacy at all times.

14. Change bath water. Wash, rinse, and dry perineal area, working from front to back.

    For a female client: Wash the perineum with soap and water from front to back, using single strokes (Fig. 13-16). Do not wash from the back to the front. This may cause infection. Use a clean area of washcloth or a clean washcloth for each stroke. First wipe the center of the perineum, then each side. Then spread the labia majora, the outside folds of perineal skin that protect the urinary meatus and the vaginal opening. Wipe from front to back on each side. Rinse the area in the same way. Dry entire perineal area moving from front to back, using a blotting motion with towel. Ask client to turn on her side. Wash, rinse, and dry buttocks and anal area. Cleanse the anal area without contaminating the perineal area.

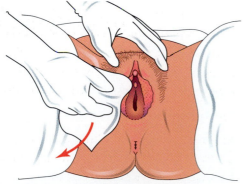

Fig. 13-16.

For a male client: If the client is uncircumcised, retract the foreskin first. Gently push skin towards the base of penis.

Hold the penis by the shaft and wash in a circular motion from the tip down to the base. Use a clean area of washcloth or clean washcloth for each stroke (Fig. 13-17). Rinse the penis. Then wash the scrotum and groin. The **groin** is the area from the pubis (area around the penis and scrotum) to the upper thighs. Rinse and pat dry. If client is uncircumcised, gently return foreskin to normal position. Ask the client to turn on his side. Wash, rinse, and dry buttocks and anal area. Cleanse the anal area without contaminating the perineal area.

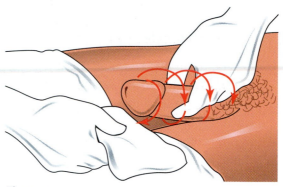

Fig. 13-17.

15. Cover the client with the cotton blanket.

16. Place soiled washcloths and towels in the hamper or laundry basket. Dispose of the dirty bath water in the toilet. Discard gloves into a trash receptacle.

17. If time permits, a bed bath is a good time to give the client a back rub if he wants one (Chapter 12 explains how to give a back rub).

18. Provide the client with deodorant. Place a towel over the pillow and brush or comb the client's hair (see procedure later in this chapter). Help the client put on clean clothing and get into a comfortable position with good body alignment. If you raised an adjustable bed, be sure to return it to its lowest position.

19. If the client uses a signaling device, place it within reach. Take the bath supplies away, and wash and store everything. Change bed sheets and blanket. Place used bed linens in the hamper or laundry basket.

20. Wash your hands.

21. Document the procedure and your observations. Did you observe any redness or whiteness on the skin? Was there any broken skin? How did the client tolerate bathing? Did the client tell you about any symptoms? Has there been a change in the client's abilities since the last bath or shower?

Nail care should only be provided if it has specifically been assigned. Never cut a client's toenails. In some clients, poor circulation can lead to infection if skin is accidentally cut while caring for nails. In a diabetic client, such an infection can lead to a severe wound or even amputation. If you are directed to provide nail care, know exactly what care you need to provide.

Providing fingernail care

Equipment: orangewood stick, emery board, small basin or bowl, washcloth, lotion, cuticle softener, bath towel, soap, gloves if client has broken skin

1. Wash your hands.

2. Explain the procedure to the client, speaking clearly, slowly, and directly, maintaining face-to-face contact whenever possible.

3. Provide privacy for the client.

4. If the bed is adjustable, adjust bed to a safe working level, usually waist high. If the bed is movable, lock bed wheels.

5. Put on gloves if the client has any broken skin.

6. If necessary, remove nail polish with a cotton ball soaked with nail polish remover.

7. Fill the basin halfway with warm water. Test water temperature with the bath thermometer or with your wrist to ensure it is safe. Water temperature should be 105°F. Have the client check the water temperature. Adjust if necessary.

8. Soak the client's nails in the water. If you need to soften cuticles to push them back (step 10, below), add a cuticle softener to the water or apply to the cuticles. Soak all ten fingertips for two to four minutes.

9. Remove hands from water. Wash hands with soapy washcloth. Rinse. Dry the client's hands with a towel, including between the fingers. Remove the hand basin.

10. Place the client's hands on the towel. Gently push back the cuticles using the flat end of the orangewood stick or a towel.

11. Use the pointed end of the orangewood stick or a nail brush to remove dirt from under the nails (Fig. 13-18). Wipe orangewood stick on towel after cleaning under each nail. Wash the hands again. Dry them thoroughly.

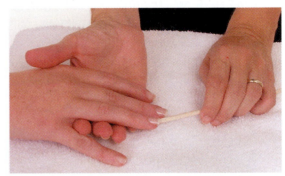
Fig. 13-18.

12. Shape fingernails with an emery board or nail file. Apply lotion.

13. Discard the water and clean the basin. Dispose of the towels in the laundry hamper and store supplies. If you raised an adjustable bed, be sure to return it to its lowest position.

14. Wash your hands.

15. Document procedure and any observations.

Providing foot care

Equipment: basin, pumice stone (optional), two bath towels, washcloth, lotion, soap, clean socks, bath thermometer, gloves if client has broken skin

1. Wash your hands.

2. Explain the procedure to the client, speaking clearly, slowly, and directly, maintaining face-to-face contact whenever possible.

3. Provide privacy for the client.

4. Put on gloves if the client has any broken skin.

13

Personal Care Skills

5. Fill the basin halfway with warm water. Test water temperature with the bath thermometer or with your wrist to ensure it is safe. Water temperature should be 105°F. Have the client check the water temperature. Adjust if necessary. Place basin on a bath towel on the floor (if the client is sitting in a chair) or on a towel at the foot of the bed (if the client is in bed).

6. Soak the client's feet for ten minutes. Add warm water to the basin as necessary.

7. Remove one foot from basin. Smooth any rough areas with the pumice stone or a washcloth. Wash entire foot, including between the toes and around nail beds, with a soapy washcloth (Fig. 13-19).

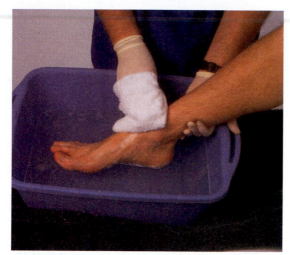

Fig. 13-19.

8. Rinse entire foot, including between the toes. Thoroughly dry entire foot, including between the toes. Apply lotion. Do not attempt any further care of the toenails.

9. Repeat steps 7-8 for other foot.

10. While you are giving foot care, observe the feet for sores, irritated or reddened areas (especially on the heels), any discoloration or darkening on the foot, discoloration of the toes or toenails, swelling, infection, or differences in temperature. Even if another person gives your client foot care, you should still observe for these signs of problems or illness on a regular basis.

11. Assist client to replace socks.

12. Discard the water and clean the basin. Dispose of the towels in the laundry hamper and store supplies.

13. Wash your hands.

14. Document procedure and any observations. Was there any redness, whiteness, or broken or discolored skin? Were there any differences in temperature?

Clients who can get out of bed may have their hair shampooed in the sink, tub, or shower. For clients who cannot get out of bed, special troughs exist for shampooing hair in bed. Troughs fit under the client's head and neck and have a spout or hose that drains the water into a basin at the side of the bed. Your agency should be able to provide this equipment. You may also use a plastic garbage bag formed around a rolled towel.

Shampooing hair

Equipment: shampoo, hair conditioner (if requested), washcloth, pitcher, plastic cup or hand-held shower or sink attachment, chair (for washing hair in sink), large garbage bag or plastic sheet (for washing hair in sink), towel (two towels if washing hair in bed), cotton blanket (for washing hair in bed), waterproof mat (for washing hair in bed), trough or garbage bag and extra towel (for washing hair in bed), catch basin (for washing hair in bed)

1. Wash your hands.

2. Explain the procedure to the client, speaking clearly, slowly, and directly, maintaining face-to-face contact whenever possible.

3. Provide privacy for the client.

4. Position the client and wet the client's hair.

a. For washing hair in the sink, seat the client in a chair covered with plastic. Use a pillow under the plastic to support the head and neck. Have the client lean her head back toward the sink. Give the client a folded washcloth to hold over her forehead or eyes. Wet hair using a plastic cup or a hand-held sink attachment (Fig. 13-20).

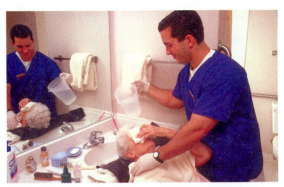

Fig. 13-20.

b. For washing hair in the tub, have the client tilt her head back. Give the client a folded washcloth to hold over her forehead or eyes. Wet hair using a plastic cup or hand-held shower attachment.

c. For washing hair in the shower, have the client turn so her back is toward the shower-head. Ask the client to tilt her head backwards. Direct the flow of water over the hair to wet it.

d. For washing hair in bed, arrange the supplies within reach on a nearby table. Remove all pillows, and place the client in a flat position. If the bed is adjustable, adjust bed to a safe working level, usually waist high. If the bed is movable, lock bed wheels. Place a waterproof sheet or mat beneath the client's head and shoulders. Cover the client with the cotton blanket, and fold back the top sheet and regular blankets. Place the trough under the client's head and connect trough to the catch basin (Fig. 13-21). Using the pitcher, pour enough water on the client's hair to make it thoroughly wet.

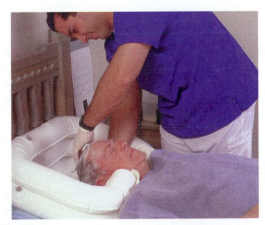

Fig. 13-21.

5. Apply a small amount of shampoo to your hands and rub them together. Using both hands, massage the shampoo to a lather in the client's hair. With your fingertips, massage the scalp in a circular motion, from front to back (Fig. 13-22).

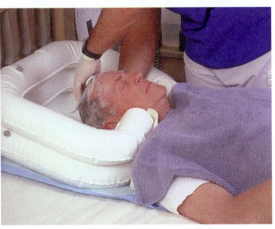

Fig. 13-22.

6. Rinse the hair in the same way you wet it. Repeat the shampoo, rinse again, and use conditioner if the client wants it. Be sure to rinse the hair thoroughly to prevent the client's scalp from getting dry and itchy.

7. Wrap the client's hair in a towel. If shampooing at the sink, return the client to an upright position. If shampooing in the bath or shower, assist the client from the tub or shower. If shampooing in bed, remove the trough. Using the washcloth or a face towel, wipe water from the head and neck.

8. Remove the hair towel and comb or brush hair (see procedure later in the chapter).

9. Dry hair with a hair dryer on the low setting. Style hair as the client prefers.

10. Wash and store equipment. Put soiled towels and washcloth in the hamper or laundry basket. If you raised an adjustable bed, be sure to return it to its lowest position.

11. Wash your hands.

12. Document the procedure and your observations. How did the client tolerate having her hair washed? Was the client able to help? Have the client's abilities changed since the last time her hair was washed?

13

Personal Care Skills

13

Personal Care Skills

3. Describe guidelines for assisting with grooming

When assisting a client with grooming, always allow the clients to do all they can for themselves. Follow the instructions in the care plan. Some clients may have particular ways of grooming themselves. Try to work with the client to establish a routine that includes everything in the care plan and satisfies the client. Check with your supervisor if you have any questions or problems.

Some clients may be embarrassed or depressed because they need help with grooming tasks they have performed for themselves all their lives. Be professional, respectful, and cheerful while assisting your clients with grooming. Your attitude can go a long way toward helping your clients maintain self-respect and feel good about themselves.

Types of Razors

A safety razor has a sharp blade, but with a special safety casing to help prevent cuts. This type of razor requires shaving cream or soap.

An electric razor is the safest and easiest type of razor to use. It does not require soap or shaving cream.

A disposable razor requires shaving cream or soap. It is discarded after use.

Helping a client shave

Equipment: a clean safety or electric razor, shaving cream or gel (if using a safety razor), basin filled with warm water (if using a safety razor), bath towel, washcloth, mirror, aftershave lotion, gloves

Be sure the client wants you to shave him or help him shave before you begin.

1. Wash your hands.

2. Explain the procedure to the client, speaking clearly, slowly, and directly, maintaining face-to-face contact whenever possible.

3. Provide privacy for the client.

4. Put on gloves. Place the equipment on a table within reach of the client if he will shave himself. If the client is confined to bed, use pillows or a backrest to help the client sit up in a comfortable position. If the bed is adjustable, adjust bed to a safe working level, usually waist high. If the bed is movable, lock bed wheels. If the client wears dentures, be sure they are in place. Place the towel across the client's chest.

5. If using an electric razor, use a small brush to clean it. Do not use an electric razor near any water source, when oxygen is in use, or if client has a pacemaker. Turn on the razor and shave the face, pulling the skin tight over the mouth and cheeks if necessary to shave more smoothly (Fig. 13-23). Shave the chin and under the chin.

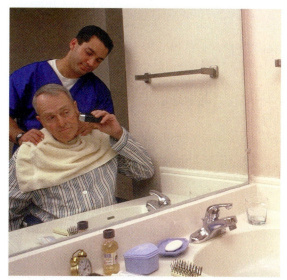

Fig. 13-23.

6. If using a safety or disposable razor, use a blade that is sharp. A dull blade is hard on the skin. Soften the beard with a warm wet towel on the face for a few minutes before shaving. Lather the face with shaving cream or gel and warm water. Warm water and lather make shaving more comfortable. Shaving in the direction of hair growth is also more comfortable. It will result in a more even shave (Fig. 13-24). Use short strokes on the chin and longer strokes on

the cheeks. Rinse the blade frequently in the basin.

7. When you have finished, rinse the client's face with a warm, wet washcloth or let him use the washcloth himself. Offer a mirror to the client.

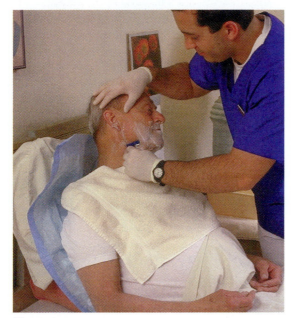

Fig. 13-24.

8. If the client wants aftershave, moisten your palms with aftershave lotion and pat it onto the client's face.

9. Clean the equipment and store it. Dispose of the used razor blade or disposable razor. Put the towel and washcloth in the hamper or laundry basket. Remove and discard gloves. If you raised an adjustable bed, be sure to return it to its lowest position.

10. Wash your hands.

11. Document the procedure and any observations.

Combing or brushing hair

Equipment: comb, brush, or hair pick, bath towel, mirror, hair care items requested by the client, gloves if client has broken skin on scalp or face

Use hair care products that the client prefers for his or her type of hair.

1. Wash your hands.

2. Explain the procedure to the client, speaking clearly, slowly, and directly, maintaining face-to-face contact whenever possible.

3. Provide privacy for the client.

4. If the client is confined to bed, raise the head of the bed, use a backrest, or use pillows to raise the client's head and shoulders. If the bed is adjustable, adjust bed to a safe working level, usually waist high. If the bed is movable, lock bed wheels. Place the towel under the client's head. If the client is ambulatory, provide a chair. Place the towel around client's shoulders.

5. Put on gloves only if the client has broken skin on the scalp or face.

6. Remove any hairpins, hair ties, and clips.

7. If the hair is tangled, work on the tangles first. Remove tangles by dividing hair into small sections. Hold the lock of hair just above the tangle so you don't pull at the scalp, and gently comb or brush through the tangle (Fig. 13-25). Gently comb out from ends of hair to scalp. If client agrees, you can use a small amount of detangler or leave-in conditioner on the tangle.

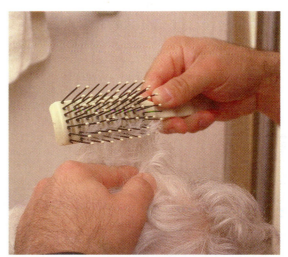

Fig. 13-25.

8. Brush two-inch sections of hair at a time. Brush from roots to ends.

9. Each client may prefer a different hairstyle. Style hair in the way the client prefers (Fig. 13-26). Avoid childish hairstyles. Offer a mirror to the client.

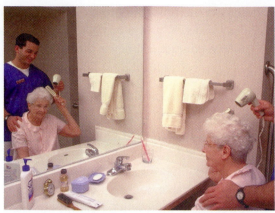

Fig. 13-26.

10. Remove the towel and shake excess hair in the wastebasket. Place the soiled towel in the hamper. Store supplies. Remove your gloves. If you raised an adjustable bed, be sure to return it to its lowest position.

11. Wash your hands.

12. Document the procedure and any observations.

When assisting a client with dressing, know what limitations he or she has. If he or she has a weakened side from a stroke or injury, that side is called the **affected side**. It will be weaker. Never refer to the weaker side as the "bad side," or talk about the "bad" leg or arm. Use the terms **weaker** or **involved** to refer to the affected side. The weaker arm is usually placed through a sleeve first (Fig. 13-27). When a leg is weak, it is easier if the client sits down to pull the pants over both legs.

GUIDELINES
Helping a client dress and undress

- As with all care, the client's preferences should be asked and followed. Remember: client-directed care is the client's right and your responsibility.

- Allow the client to choose clothing for the day. However, check to see if it is clean, appropriate for the weather, and in good condition.

- Encourage the client to dress in regular clothes rather than nightclothes. Wearing regular daytime clothing encourages more activity and out-of-bed time. Elastic-waist

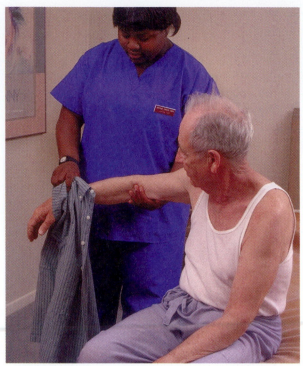

13-27. When dressing assist with the involved (weaker) side first.

pants or skirts are easy to pull on over legs and hips. Be sure the elastic waistband of underpants, slip, pantyhose, pants, or skirt fits comfortably at the waist. Clothing that is a size larger than the client would normally wear is easier to put on.

- The client should do as much to dress or undress himself as possible. It may take longer, but it helps maintain independence and regain self-care skills. Ask where your assistance is needed.

- Provide privacy. If the client has just had a bath, cover him with the bath blanket and put on undergarments first. Never expose more than you need to.

- When putting on socks or stockings, roll or fold them down so they can be slipped over the toes and foot, then unrolled up into place. Make certain toes, heels, and seams of socks or stockings are in the right place.

- For a female client, make sure bra cups fit over the breasts. Front-fastening bras are easier for clients to manage by themselves. Bras that fasten in back can be put around the waist and fastened first, then rotated around and moved up, putting arms

through the straps last. This can be done in reverse for undressing.

g For clients who have weakness or paralysis on one side, place weak arm or leg through the garment first, then the strong arm or leg. When undressing, do the opposite.

Several types of adaptive aids for dressing are available to help clients maintain independence in dressing themselves (Fig. 13-28). An occupational therapist may teach clients to perform ADLs using adaptive equipment.

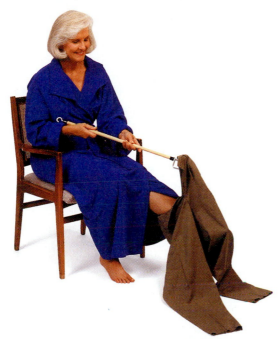

13-28. (Photo courtesy of North Coast Medical, Inc., www.ncmedical.com, 800-821-9319)

4. Identify guidelines for good oral care

Oral care, or care of the mouth, teeth, and gums, is performed at least twice each day to cleanse the mouth. Oral care should be done after breakfast and after the last meal or snack of the day. It may also be done before a client eats. Oral care includes brushing teeth and gums and tongue, flossing teeth, and caring for dentures. **Dental floss** is a special kind of string used to clean between teeth.

When you perform or assist with oral care, observe the client's mouth.

OBSERVING AND REPORTING
Oral Care

- O&R irritation
- O&R infection
- O&R raised areas
- O&R coated tongue
- O&R ulcers, such as canker sores or small, painful, white sores
- O&R flaky, white spots
- O&R dry and cracked or chapped lips
- O&R loose or decayed teeth
- O&R swollen, bleeding, or whitish gums
- O&R breath that smells bad or fruity

Assisting with mouth care

Equipment: soft-bristled toothbrush, toothpaste or powder, glass of water, two towels, moisturizer for lips, basin and a drinking straw (if the client is in bed), gloves

1. Wash your hands.

2. Explain the procedure to the client, speaking clearly, slowly, and directly, maintaining face-to-face contact whenever possible.

3. Provide privacy for the client.

4. If your client is in bed, have him sit up, propped up by pillows. If the bed is adjustable, adjust bed to a safe working level, usually waist high. If the bed is movable, lock bed wheels. Place a towel under your client's head and one across the chest.

5. Put on gloves.

6. Remove any dental bridgework or ask your client to do so. (A procedure later in this chapter explains how to remove dentures.)

7. Wet toothbrush and put a small amount of toothpaste on it.

8. Gently brush the teeth, or help the client brush teeth. Use short strokes and brush back and forth on all surfaces. Brush the tongue gently as well.

9. Give the client water to rinse the mouth and place the basin under the client's chin for

him to spit the water into (Fig. 13-29). Wipe the client's mouth and remove towels.

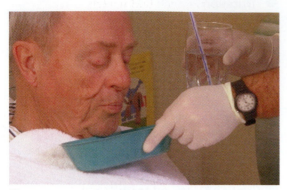

Fig. 13-29.

10. Replace any dental bridgework. (A procedure later in this chapter explains how to reinsert dentures). Apply moisturizer to the lips if the client desires.

11. Put the soiled towels in the laundry hamper. Dispose of the water in the basin by pouring it into the toilet. Clean the basin and put away supplies. Remove your gloves and discard them. If you raised an adjustable bed, be sure to return it to its lowest position.

12. Wash your hands.

13. Document the procedure and any observations. Did you observe any mouth ulcers or other broken skin? What was the condition of the mucous membrane? Did the client's breath smell unusual?

Even though unconscious clients cannot eat, breathing through the mouth causes saliva to dry in the mouth. Good mouth care needs to be performed more frequently to keep the mouth clean and moist. Swabs with a mixture of lemon juice and glycerine are sometimes used to soothe the gums. However, these may further dry the gums if used too often. Follow the care plan regarding the use of swabs.

With unconscious clients, it is important to use as little liquid as possible when performing mouth care. Because the person's swallowing reflex is weak, he or she is at risk for aspiration. **Aspiration** is the inhalation of food or drink into the lungs. Aspiration can cause pneumonia or death.

Performing mouth care for the unconscious client

Equipment: sponge swabs, lemon glycerine swabs (optional), padded tongue blade, mouthwash, emesis basin or small bowl, towel, glass of cool water, lip moisturizer, gloves

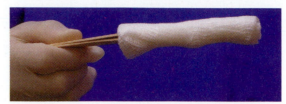

Fig. 13-30. To make a padded tongue blade, place two wooden tongue blades together and wrap the upper portion with gauze. Tape the gauze in place.

1. Wash your hands.

2. Explain the procedure to the client, speaking clearly, slowly, and directly, maintaining face-to-face contact whenever possible. Even clients who are unconscious may be able to hear you. Always speak to them as you would to any client.

3. Provide privacy for the client.

4. If the bed is adjustable, adjust bed to a safe working level, usually waist high. If the bed is movable, lock bed wheels.

5. Put on gloves.

6. Turn your client's head to the side and place a towel under his cheek and chin. Place emesis basin or bowl next to the cheek and chin so that excess fluid flows into the basin.

7. Dip the sponge swab in the mouthwash. Do not dip a lemon glycerine swab in mouthwash.

8. Separate the upper and lower teeth with the padded tongue blade. Using the swab, cleanse all surfaces in the mouth cavity, including the teeth and underneath the tongue. Remove debris with the swab (Fig. 13-31). Rinse and rewet swab as necessary. Repeat this step until the mouth is clean.

9. If ordered, swab again, this time with the lemon glycerine swab.

10. Remove the towel and basin. Pat lips or face dry if needed. Apply lip moisturizer.

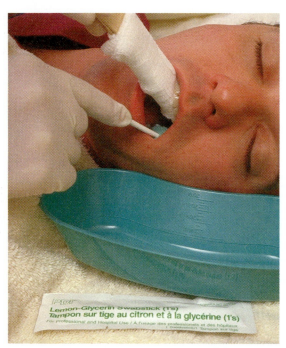

Fig. 13-31.

11. Place the towel in the laundry hamper. Clean the basin and put away supplies. Remove your gloves and discard them. If you raised an adjustable bed, be sure to return it to its lowest position.

12. Wash your hands.

13. Document the procedure and your observations. Did you observe any mouth ulcers or other broken skin? What was the condition of the mucous membrane? Did the client's breath smell unusual?

Flossing the teeth removes plaque and tartar buildup around the gum line and between the teeth. Teeth may be flossed immediately after or before they are brushed. Follow the client's preference.

Flossing teeth

Equipment: about 18 inches of dental floss, glass of water, emesis basin, face towel, gloves

1. Wash your hands.

2. Explain the procedure to the client, speaking clearly, slowly, and directly, maintaining face-to-face contact whenever possible.

3. Provide privacy for the client.

4. If the bed is adjustable, adjust bed to a safe working level, usually waist high. If the bed is movable, lock bed wheels.

5. Put on gloves.

6. Wrap the ends of the floss securely around each of your index fingers (Fig. 13-32).

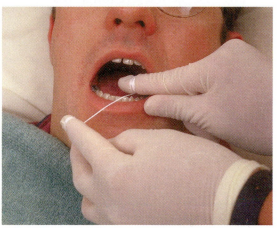

Fig. 13-32.

7. Starting with the back teeth, place the floss between teeth and move it down the surface of the tooth using a gentle sawing motion (Fig. 13-33). Continue to the gum line. At the gum line, curve the floss into a letter C, slip it gently into the space between the gum and tooth, then go back up, scraping that side of the tooth (Fig. 13-34). Repeat this on the side of the other tooth.

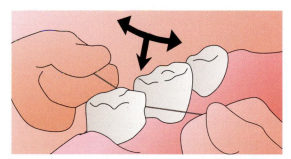

Fig. 13-33.

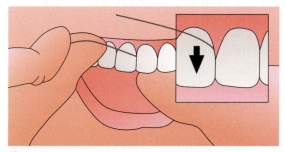

Fig. 13-34.

8. After every two or three teeth, unwind floss from your fingers and move it so you are using a clean area. Floss all teeth.

9. Occasionally offer water so that the client can rinse debris from the mouth into the basin.

10. Offer the client a face towel when done flossing all teeth.

11. Discard floss. Pour water from the basin into the toilet. Clean and store the basin. Put the soiled face towel in the laundry hamper. Remove your gloves and discard them. If you raised an adjustable bed, be sure to return it to its lowest position.

12. Wash your hands.

13. Document procedure and observations.

Ask the client how you can assist with denture care. Each person has his own preference about when and how it should be done.

Assisting with denture care

Equipment: denture cup for storage, denture cleaner or toothpaste, denture brush or soft toothbrush, two face towels, basin or sink, gauze squares, mouthwash or a sponge swab, disposable gloves

1. Wash your hands.

2. Explain the procedure to the client, speaking clearly, slowly, and directly, maintaining face-to-face contact whenever possible.

3. Provide privacy for the client.

4. Line the sink or a basin with a face towel and fill with water. The towel and water will prevent the dentures from breaking if they slip from your hands and fall into the sink.

5. Put on gloves.

6. Ask the client to remove the dentures and place them in the denture cup. If the client is unable to remove them, do it yourself. Remove the lower denture first. The lower denture is easier to remove because it floats on the gum line of the lower jaw. Grasp the lower denture with a gauze square (for a good grip) and remove it. Place it in a denture cup filled with water.

7. The upper denture is sealed by suction. Firmly grasp the upper denture with a gauze square and give a slight downward pull to break the suction. Turn it at an angle to take it out of the mouth.

8. Take the denture cup to the sink or basin. Apply denture cleanser to a denture brush or soft toothbrush, and brush the dentures under warm, running tap water to remove all material (Fig. 13-35). Do not use hot water, or dentures may warp. Rinse out the denture cup and place dentures in it.

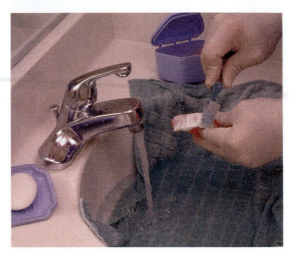

Fig. 13-35.

9. Your client may prefer to clean the dentures with a soaking solution. Read the directions on the bottle and prepare the solution. Soak the dentures for the amount of time indicated. Rinse and place in denture cup.

10. Store dentures in water or solution to prevent them from warping. To avoid accidentally throwing dentures away, always store them in a labeled denture cup when the client is not wearing them.

11. Offer the client mouthwash or a swab to cleanse the mouth.

12. Discard gauze pads and swabs. Put towels in laundry hamper. Clean out sink or basin. Rinse and store toothbrush and other supplies. Remove your gloves.

13. Wash your hands.

14. Document procedure and any observations.

Reinserting dentures

Equipment: denture cup with dentures, denture cream or adhesive, face towel, gloves
Ask if the client needs your assistance in inserting dentures.

1. Wash your hands.
2. Explain the procedure to the client, speaking clearly, slowly, and directly, maintaining face-to-face contact whenever possible.
3. Provide privacy for the client.
4. Position client as you would for brushing teeth (help him to as upright a position as possible).
5. Put on gloves.
6. Apply denture cream or adhesive to the dentures if needed.
7. Ask client to open his or her mouth. Insert the upper denture into the mouth by turning it at an angle. Straighten it and press it onto the upper gum line firmly and evenly (Fig. 13-36).

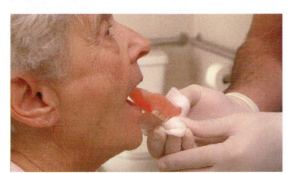

Fig. 13-36.

8. Insert the lower denture onto the gum line of the lower jaw and press firmly.
9. Offer the client the face towel.
10. Rinse and store the denture cup. Remove the gloves and discard them.
11. Wash your hands.
12. Document the procedure and any observations.

5. Explain care guidelines for hearing aids and prosthetic devices

Many different types of hearing aids exist (Fig. 13-37). Always follow manufacturer's directions for cleaning the hearing aid. In general, use a little soap and water on a cloth, cotton swab, or pipe cleaner to keep the earpiece free of wax and dirt. Do not put the hearing aid in water. Handle the hearing aid carefully. Do not drop it. Always keep it in the same safe place when it is not being worn. Remind clients it is a good idea to have an extra battery on hand.

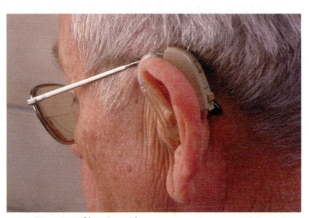

13-37. One type of hearing aid.

A **prosthesis** (*pros-THEE-sis*) is a device that replaces a body part that is missing or deformed because of an accident, injury, illness, or birth defect (Fig. 13-38). You may work with clients who have prosthetic feet, legs, hands, arms, or eyes. Because prostheses are specially fitted, expensive pieces of equipment (an artificial leg may cost from $10,000 to $20,000), only care for them as assigned. Know exactly how to care for the equipment before you begin. If you have any questions, call your supervisor.

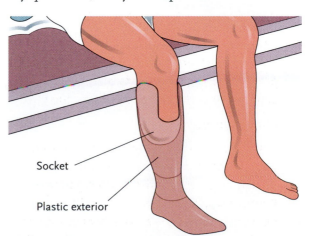

Socket

Plastic exterior

13-38. Prostheses are specially fitted, expensive pieces of equipment.

Personal Care Skills

Wash your hands, provide privacy, and put on gloves before beginning to care for an artificial eye. Artificial eyes are held in by suction. They will come out quickly when pressure is applied below the lower eyelid. Wash eye with solution and rinse in warm water. Moisten the artificial eye and place it far under upper eyelid. Pull down on lower eyelid and the eye should slide into place.

6. Explain guidelines for assisting with toileting

Clients who are unable to get out of bed to go to the bathroom may be given a bedpan, a fracture pan, or a urinal. A **fracture pan** is a bedpan that is flatter than the regular bedpan. It is used for clients who cannot assist with raising their hips onto a regular bedpan (Fig. 13-39). Women will generally use a **bedpan** for urination and bowel movements. Men will generally use a **urinal** (Fig. 13-40) for urination and a bedpan for a bowel movement.

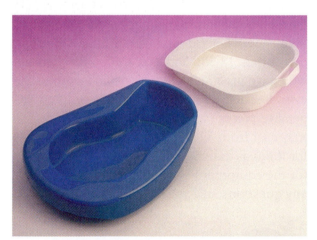

13-39. a) Standard pan and b) fracture pan.

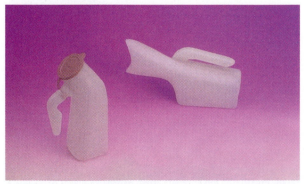

13-40. Two types of urinals.

Some clients are able to get out of bed, but may still need help walking to the bathroom and using the toilet. Others who are able to get out of bed but cannot walk to the bathroom may use a portable commode. A **portable commode** is a chair with a toilet seat and a removable container underneath (Fig. 13-41). Toilets can be fitted with raised seats to make it easier for clients to get up and down (Fig. 13-42). Hand rails can also be installed next to the toilet. Observe and report if these assistive devices are needed but not present. When clients need assistance to get to the bathroom or use the commode, offer to help often. This can avoid accidents and embarrassment.

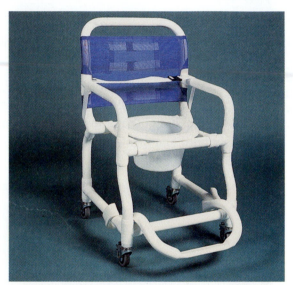

13-41. A portable commode.

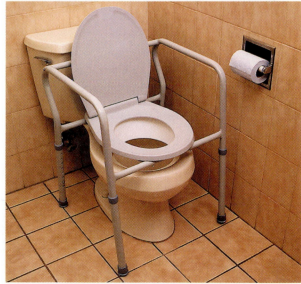

13-42. A raised toilet seat makes it easier for a client to get up and down.

Your client may ask for the bedpan, or you may need to ask if he needs it at regular times listed on the assignment sheet. Remember that clients may be embarrassed about needing assistance with bodily functions. Always be professional when providing assistance. Provide as much privacy as possible.

Assisting clients in using a bedpan

Equipment: bedpan, bedpan cover (newspaper or washable cloth), protective pad or sheet, bath blanket, toilet paper, disposable washcloths or wipes, soap, towel, plastic bag, three pair of gloves

1. Wash your hands.

2. Explain the procedure to the client, speaking clearly, slowly, and directly, maintaining face-to-face contact whenever possible.

3. Provide privacy for the client by closing doors and shades and using a covering blanket.

4. If the bed is adjustable, adjust bed to a safe working level, usually waist high. If the bed is movable, lock bed wheels. Lower the head of the bed before placing bedpan.

5. Put on gloves.

6. Warm outside of the bedpan with warm water in the bathroom and cover it when you bring it to the client. Dust the top of the bedpan with powder to prevent it from sticking to the client's skin. Do not use talcum powder if the client has open sores on the buttocks or genitals. Do not use powder if a stool or urine sample is needed. If a stool or urine sample is not needed, place a few sheets of toilet paper in the bedpan to make cleanup easier.

7. Cover the client with the bath blanket and ask him to hold it while you pull down the top covers underneath it.

8. Place a protective sheet under the client. To do this, have the client roll toward you. If the client is unable to roll toward you unassisted, you must roll the client (see chapter 12). Be sure the client cannot roll off the bed. Move to the empty side of the bed and place the protective sheet on the area where

the client will lie on his back. The side of the protective sheet nearest the client should be fanfolded (folded several times into pleats) (Fig. 13-43). Ask the client to roll onto his back, or roll him as you did before. Unfold the rest of the protective sheet so it completely covers the area under and around the client's hips (Fig. 13-44).

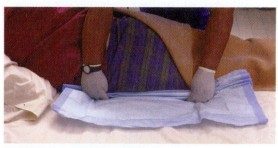
Fig. 13-43.

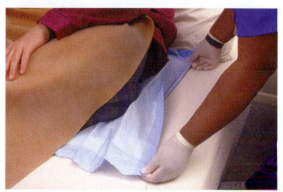
Fig. 13-44.

9. Ask the client to remove undergarments, or help him do so.

10. Place the bedpan near his hips with the open end facing the foot of the bed.

11. Ask the client to help by raising his hips at the count of three (Fig. 13-45). Slide the bedpan under his hips.

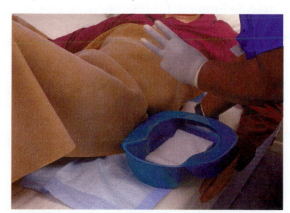
Fig. 13-45.

13

Personal Care Skills

If the client cannot do this himself, place your arm under the small of his back and tell him to push with his heels and hands on your signal as you raise his hips (Fig. 13-46). If a client cannot help you in any way, keep the bed flat and roll the client onto the far side. Slip the bedpan under the hips and roll the client back onto the bedpan. Then raise the head of the bed after placing the bedpan under the client. Prop the client into a semi-sitting position using pillows.

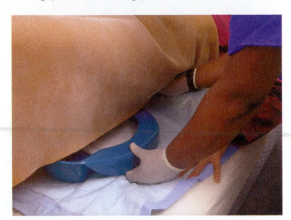

Fig. 13-46.

12. Check the bedpan to be certain it is in the correct position. Make sure the bath blanket is still covering the client. Provide the client with toilet paper, washcloths or wipes, and a bell or other way to call you. Tell the client you will return when called. Make sure the client is comfortable before you leave.

13. If the client is unable to clean the anal area and the rest of the perineum, you must do this. With gloves on, help the client to roll onto his side. Use the toilet paper to clean the perineal area first. For female clients, wipe from the front to the back. Use one washcloth to cleanse the front part of the perineum and another to cleanse the anal area.

14. Wrap the toilet paper and disposable wash-cloths in a plastic bag and discard them. Dry the perineal area with a towel. Place the towel in a hamper. Remove your gloves and discard them. Immediately replace gloves with a clean pair.

15. Offer a wet washcloth and soap and water to the client to wash hands. Cover the client and remove the bath blanket. Help the client put on undergarment.

16. Cover the bedpan and take it to the bath-room. Empty the bedpan carefully into the toilet and flush. If you notice anything un-usual about the stool or urine (for example, the presence of blood), do not discard it. Remove and discard your gloves, wash your hands, and notify your supervisor. He or she may ask you to save a specimen (Chapter 14 describes how to collect stool specimens). Put on new gloves.

17. Turn the faucet on with a paper towel. Rinse the bedpan with cold water first and empty it into the toilet. Then clean the bedpan with hot, soapy water and store.

18. Remove and discard gloves. If you raised an adjustable bed, be sure to return it to its lowest position.

19. Wash your hands.

20. Document the time of the elimination, the contents, and any observations.

Assisting clients in using a urinal

Equipment: urinal, protective pad or sheet, bath blanket, washcloth, soap, towel, gloves

1. Wash your hands.

2. Explain the procedure to the client, speaking clearly, slowly, and directly, maintaining face-to-face contact whenever possible.

3. Provide privacy for the client by closing doors and shades and using a covering blanket.

4. If the bed is adjustable, adjust bed to a safe working level, usually waist high. If the bed is movable, lock bed wheels.

5. Put on gloves.

6. Place a protective pad under the client's but-tocks and hips, as in earlier procedure.

7. Hand the urinal to the client. If the client is not able to help himself, place the urinal be-tween his legs and position the penis inside the urinal (Fig. 13-47). Replace covers.

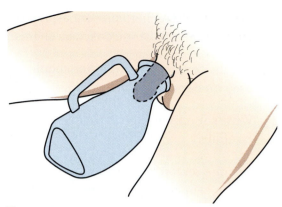

Fig. 13-47.

8. Give the client a bell or another way to call you. Leave the room and close the door.

9. When the client signals that he is finished, remove the urinal or have him hand it to you. Follow the correct procedure if a specimen has been ordered (see chapter 14). Discard urine in the toilet. Use a paper towel to turn on the faucet. Rinse the urinal with cold water and store it away.

10. Remove your gloves and discard them. Wash your hands.

11. Give the client a washcloth, soap, and water to wash his hands.

12. After taking the washcloth from the client and placing it aside (to be washed separately from other laundry), wash your hands again. If you raised an adjustable bed, be sure to return it to its lowest position.

13. Document the time, the amount of urine (if monitoring intake and output), and any other observations.

Assisting clients in using a portable commode or toilet

Equipment: toilet paper, disposable washcloths or wipes, soap, washcloth, and basin (if using portable commode), gloves

1. Wash your hands.

2. Explain the procedure to the client, speaking clearly, slowly, and directly, maintaining face-to-face contact whenever possible.

3. Provide privacy for the client by closing doors and shades and using a covering blanket.

4. If the bed is adjustable, adjust bed to a safe working level, usually waist high. If the bed is movable, lock bed wheels.

5. Put on gloves.

6. Help client out of bed and to the bathroom or portable commode.

7. If needed, help client remove clothing and sit on toilet seat.

8. Provide privacy. Leave the room or area. Close the door, but do not lock it. Provide a bell or another way for the client to call you. Don't go too far away in case you are needed soon.

9. When the client calls you, return. If assistance is needed to clean the perineal area, provide it. Remember to wipe female clients from front to back. Use disposable washcloths if necessary. Dispose of these in the toilet, or in the wastebasket if they are not flushable. If your gloves become soiled, discard them and put on fresh gloves.

10. Help the client up and be sure she washes her hands before returning to bed. Use the sink or a basin, soap, and a washcloth.

11. When using a portable commode, remove waste container and empty it into the toilet unless a specimen is needed or the client's urine is being measured for intake/output monitoring (Chapter 14 explains how to measure output). Clean the container as you would a bedpan, rinsing first with cold water and then washing with hot water and cleanser.

12. Remove your gloves and discard them. If you raised an adjustable bed, be sure to return it to its lowest position.

13. Wash your hands.

14. Document the procedure and any observations.

7. Describe how to dispose of body wastes

Remember that wastes such as urine and feces can carry infection. Always dispose of wastes in the toilet. Be careful not to spill or splash. Wear gloves when handling bedpans, urinals, or basins that contain wastes, including dirty bath water. Wash these containers thoroughly. Remove your gloves and wash your hands. Put on a new pair of gloves if you are not finished with client care.

Washcloths used to wash perineal areas must be washed in hot water. Handle such laundry carefully, and wear gloves. Washing it separately is safest. Disposable washcloths may or may not be flushable. Read the package to be sure. If they are not flushable, dispose of them in a waste container lined with a plastic bag. Remove and replace the plastic bag frequently to prevent odors.

Chapter Review

1. List four examples of activities of daily living (ADLs).

2. Give two examples of how to promote dignity and independence while giving personal care.

3. Why is it unnecessary for older clients to have a complete bath or shower every day?

4. Why should clients, as well as home health aides, test the water temperature before bathing?

5. When should gloves be worn during personal care? When should gloves NOT be worn?

6. Explain why HHAs must be especially careful while giving nail care to diabetic clients.

7. Why should gloves be worn while shaving clients?

8. If a client has an affected side due to a stroke or an injury, how should the HHA refer to that side?

9. How can HHAs help prevent aspiration during oral care of unconscious clients?

10. List the reason that hot water should not be used on dentures.

11. Why is it important to care for prostheses carefully?

12. List one reason why a fracture pan, rather than a bedpan, may be used for a client.

13. Where should wastes, such as urine and feces, be discarded?

14

Core Healthcare Skills

1. Explain the importance of monitoring vital signs

You will monitor, document, and report your clients' **vital signs**. Vital signs are important. They show how well the vital organs of the body, such as the heart and lungs, are working. They consist of the following:

- taking the body temperature
- counting the pulse
- counting the rate of respirations
- taking the blood pressure
- observing and reporting the level of pain

Watching for changes in vital signs is very important. Changes can indicate a client's condition is worsening. You should always notify your supervisor if

- the client is running a fever (temperature is above average for the client or outside the normal range listed at right)
- the client has a respiratory or pulse rate that is too rapid or too slow
- the client's blood pressure changes
- the client's pain is worse or is not relieved by pain management

Normal Ranges for Adult Vital Signs

Temperature	Fahrenheit	Celsius
Oral	97.6 - 99.6	36.5 - 37.5
Rectal	98.6 - 100.6	37.0 - 38.1
Axillary	96.6 - 98.6	36.0 - 37.0

Pulse: 60 - 100 beats per minute

Respirations: 12 - 20 respirations per minute

Blood Pressure
  Normal:
    Systolic 100 - 119
    Diastolic 60 - 79
  Prehypertension:
    Systolic 120 - 139
    Diastolic 80 - 89
  High:
    140/90 or above *

* Millions of people whose blood pressure was previously normal (120/80) now fall into the "prehypertension" range. Prehypertension means that the person does not have high blood pressure now but is likely to develop it in the future. This is based on the new, more aggressive high blood pressure guidelines from the Seventh Report of the Joint National Committee (JNC 7) on Prevention, Detection, Evaluation, and Treatment of High Blood Pressure (2003).

14

Core Healthcare Skills

Temperature

Body temperature is normally very close to 98.6°F (Fahrenheit) or 37°C (Celsius). Body temperature reflects a balance between the heat created by our bodies and the heat lost to the environment. Increases in body temperature may indicate an infection or disease.

There are four sites for taking body temperature:

1. the mouth (oral)

2. the rectum (rectal)

3. the armpit (axillary)

4. the ear (tympanic)

The different sites require different thermometers. Temperatures are most often taken orally. Do not take an oral temperature on a person who

- is unconscious

- is using oxygen

- is confused or disoriented

- is paralyzed from stroke

- has facial trauma

- is younger than six years old

Taking a rectal temperature on an uncooperative client, such as a small child, can be dangerous. A rectal temperature is considered to be the most accurate. An axillary temperature is considered the least accurate.

Using glass bulb or mercury thermometers to take oral or rectal temperatures used to be common. However, because mercury is a dangerous, toxic substance, thousands of healthcare facilities now discourage the use of products containing mercury. In fact, many states have passed laws to ban the sale of mercury thermometers.

Mercury-free thermometers are becoming more common (Fig. 14-1). They can be used to take an oral or rectal temperature, and they are considered much safer. Mercury-free thermometers can usually be purchased at your local pharmacy.

If your client still uses a mercury thermometer, check with your supervisor about replacing it

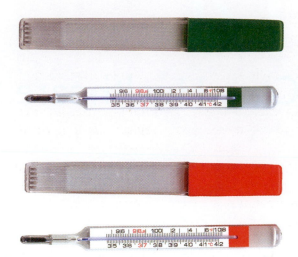

Fig. 14-1. A mercury-free oral thermometer and a mercury-free rectal thermometer. (Photos provided by RG Medical Diagnostics of Southfield, MI.)

with a mercury-free thermometer. If you must use a mercury thermometer, be careful. If you break a glass thermometer, never touch the mercury or broken glass. Know your agency's policies and procedures regarding safe disposal of mercury.

Although mercury-free thermometers are slightly larger than glass bulb thermometers, they operate identically. Numbers on the thermometer let you read the temperature after it registers. Most thermometers show the temperature in degrees Fahrenheit (F). Each long line represents one degree and each short line represents two-tenths of a degree. Some thermometers show the temperature in degrees Celsius (C), with the long lines representing one degree and the short lines representing one-tenth of a degree. The small arrow points to the normal temperature: 98.6°F and 37°C (Fig. 14-2).

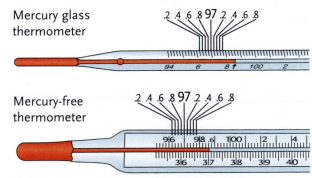

Fig. 14-2. You read a mercury-free and a mercury glass thermometer the same way.

Battery-powered, digital, or electronic thermometers are other types of thermometers (Fig. 14-3). These thermometers display the results digitally and register the temperature more quickly than mercury-free or glass bulb thermometers. Digital thermometers usually take two to sixty seconds to register the temperature. The thermometer will beep or flash when the temperature has registered. Digital thermometers may be used to take oral, rectal, or axillary temperatures. Follow the manufacturer's guide for proper use of these thermometers.

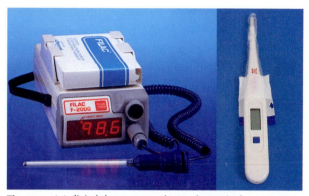

Fig. 14-3. a) A digital thermometer. b) An electronic thermometer.

The tympanic thermometer, or ear thermometer, also registers a temperature quickly (Fig. 14-4). However, these thermometers are expensive and may not be as common in the home. They also require more practice to be able to take accurate temperatures.

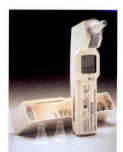

Fig. 14-4. A tympanic thermometer.

Remember that there is a range of normal temperatures. Some people's temperatures normally run low. Others in completely good health will run slightly higher temperatures. Normal temperature readings also vary according to the method used to take the temperature.

Taking and recording an oral temperature

Do not take an oral temperature on a client who has smoked, eaten or drunk fluids, or exercised in the last 10-20 minutes.

Equipment: mercury-free, glass, digital, or elec-tronic thermometer, disposable plastic sheath/cover for thermometer, tissues, pen and paper

1. Wash your hands.

2. Explain procedure to client, speaking clearly, slowly, and directly, maintaining face-to-face contact whenever possible.

3. Provide privacy for the client.

Using a mercury-free thermometer or glass thermometer:

4. Hold the thermometer by the stem.

5. Before inserting the thermometer in client's mouth, shake thermometer down to below the lowest number (at least below 96°F or 35°C). To shake the thermometer down, hold it at the side opposite the bulb with the thumb and two fingers. With a snapping motion of the wrist, shake the thermometer (Fig. 14-5). Stand away from furniture and walls while doing so.

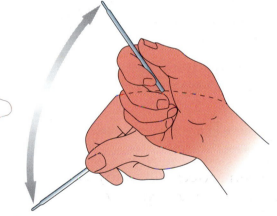

Fig. 14-5.

6. Put on disposable sheath, if available. Insert fluted tip or bulb end of the thermometer into client's mouth, under tongue and to one side (Fig. 14-6).

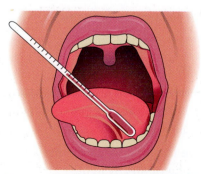

Fig. 14-6.

7. Tell the client to hold the thermometer in mouth with lips closed. Assist as necessary. Client should breathe through his or her nose. Ask the client not to bite down or talk.

8. Leave the thermometer in place for at least three minutes.

9. Remove the thermometer. Wipe with a tissue from stem to bulb or remove sheath. Dispose of the tissue or sheath.

10. Hold the thermometer at eye level. Rotate until line appears, rolling the thermometer between your thumb and forefinger. Read the temperature. Document the temperature, date, time and method used (oral).

11. Rinse the thermometer in lukewarm water and dry. Return it to plastic case or container. If using a mercury/glass thermometer, store it away from a heat source.

Using a digital thermometer:

4. Put on the disposable sheath.

5. Turn on thermometer and wait until "ready" sign appears.

6. Insert the end of digital thermometer into client's mouth, under tongue and to one side.

7. Leave in place until thermometer blinks or beeps.

8. Remove the thermometer.

9. Read temperature on display screen. Document the temperature, date, time and method used (oral).

10. Using a tissue, remove and dispose of sheath.

11. Replace the thermometer in case.

Using an electronic thermometer:

4. Remove the probe from base unit.

5. Put on probe cover.

6. Insert the end of electronic thermometer into client's mouth, under tongue and to one side.

7. Leave in place until you hear a tone or see a flashing or steady light.

8. Read the temperature on the display screen.

9. Remove the probe. Press the eject button to discard the cover (Fig. 14-7).

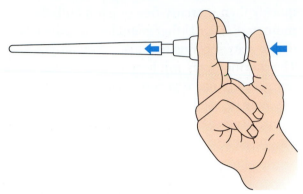

Fig. 14-7.

10. Document the temperature, date, time and method used (oral).

11. Return the probe to the holder.

Final step for all thermometers:

12. Wash your hands.

You may need to take a rectal temperature. You can use a mercury-free, digital, or glass thermometer. Rectal temperatures can be necessary when caring for unconscious clients, clients who suffer from seizures, clients with poorly-fitted dentures or missing teeth, anyone having difficulty breathing through the nose, and infants or young children. Always explain what you will do before beginning. You need the client's cooperation to take a rectal temperature. Advise the client to hold still. Reassure him or her that the procedure will only take a few minutes. Hold onto the thermometer at all times while taking a rectal temperature.

Taking and recording a rectal temperature

Equipment: rectal mercury-free, glass, or digital thermometer, lubricant, gloves, tissue, disposable plastic sheath/cover, pen and paper

1. Wash your hands.

2. Explain procedure to client, speaking clearly, slowly, and directly, maintaining face-to-face contact whenever possible.

3. Provide privacy for the client.

14

Core Healthcare Skills

4. Assist the client to a side-lying position (Fig. 14-8). An infant can be placed on his back or stomach for measuring rectal temperature.

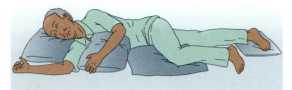

Fig. 14-8.

5. Fold back the linens to expose only the rectal area.

6. Put on gloves.

7. *Mercury-free or glass thermometer*: Hold thermometer by stem.

   Digital thermometer: Apply probe cover.

8. *Mercury-free or glass thermometer*: Shake the thermometer down to below the lowest number.

9. Apply a small amount of lubricant to tip or bulb or probe cover.

10. Separate the buttocks. Gently insert thermometer into rectum 1 inch (1/2 inch for a child). Stop if you meet resistance. Do not force the thermometer in (Fig. 14-9).

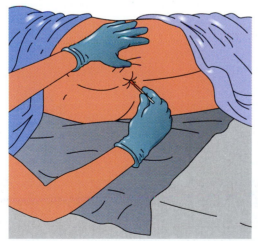

Fig. 14-9.

11. Replace the sheet over buttocks while holding onto the thermometer. Hold onto the thermometer at all times while taking a rectal temperature.

12. *Mercury-free or glass thermometer*: Hold thermometer in place for at least three minutes.

Digital thermometer: Hold thermometer in place until thermometer blinks or beeps.

13. Gently remove the thermometer. Wipe with tissue from stem to bulb or remove sheath. Dispose of tissue or sheath.

14. Read the thermometer at eye level as you would for an oral temperature. Document the temperature, date, time and method used (rectal).

15. *Mercury-free or glass thermometer*: Rinse the thermometer in lukewarm water and dry. Return it to plastic case or container. If using a mercury/glass thermometer, store it away from a heat source.

    Digital thermometer: Throw away probe cover and return thermometer to storage area.

16. Remove and dispose of gloves.

17. Assist the client to a position of safety and comfort.

18. Wash your hands.

Tympanic thermometers can be used to take a fast and accurate temperature reading. As always, explain what you will do before beginning any procedure. Tell the client that you will be taking his or her temperature by placing a thermometer in the ear canal. Reassure the client that the procedure is entirely painless. The short tip of the thermometer will only go into the ear one-quarter to one-half inch. Because thermometer models vary, follow the manufacturer's instructions.

Taking and recording a tympanic temperature

Equipment: tympanic thermometer, disposable probe sheath/cover, pen and paper

1. Wash your hands.

2. Explain procedure to client, speaking clearly, slowly, and directly, maintaining face-to-face contact whenever possible.

3. Provide privacy for the client.

4. Put a disposable sheath over earpiece of the thermometer.

14

Core Healthcare Skills

5. Position the client's head so that the ear is in front of you. Straighten the ear canal by pulling up and back on the outside edge of the ear for an adult (Fig. 14-10). Pull straight back for infants and children. Insert the covered probe into the ear canal and press the button.

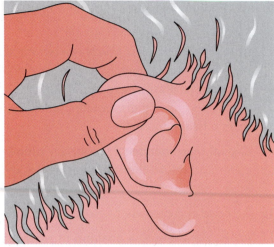

Fig. 14-10.

6. Hold thermometer in place either for one second or until thermometer beeps (depends on model).

7. Read temperature. Document the temperature, date, time and method used (tympanic).

8. Dispose of sheath. Return the thermometer to storage or to the battery charger if thermometer is rechargeable.

9. Wash your hands.

Axillary temperatures are much less reliable than temperatures taken at other sites. For this reason the axillary site should only be used as a last resort.

Taking and recording an axillary temperature

Equipment: mercury-free, glass, or digital thermometer, pen and paper

1. Wash your hands.

2. Explain procedure to client, speaking clearly, slowly, and directly, maintaining face-to-face contact whenever possible.

3. Provide privacy for the client.

4. Adjust or remove enough of the client's clothing to allow skin contact with the end of thermometer. Make sure the axilla is dry before placing the thermometer under the arm.

5. Hold the thermometer in place, with the arm close against the side, for eight to ten minutes (Fig. 14-11).

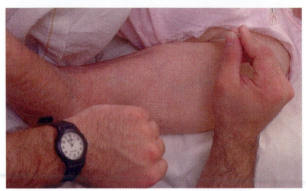

Fig. 14-11.

6. Read temperature. Document the temperature, date, time and method used (axillary).

7. Clean and store thermometer.

8. Wash your hands.

Pulse

The pulse is essentially the number of heartbeats per minute. The beat that you feel at certain pulse points in the body represents the wave of blood moving as a result of the heart pumping. The most common site for monitoring the pulse is on the inside of the wrist, where the radial artery runs just beneath the skin. This is called the **radial pulse**. The procedure for taking this pulse is located later in this chapter. The **brachial pulse** is the pulse inside of the elbow, about 1-1 1/2 inches above the elbow. The radial and brachial pulse are involved in taking blood pressure. Taking blood pressure is explained later in this chapter. Other common pulse sites are shown in Fig. 14-12.

For adults, the normal pulse rate is 60-100 beats per minute. Small children have more rapid pulses, in the range of 100-120 beats per minute. A newborn baby's pulse may be as high

as 120-140 beats per minute. Many things can affect the pulse rate, including exercise, fear, anger, anxiety, heat, medications, and pain. An unusually high or low rate does not necessarily indicate disease. However, sometimes the pulse rate can be a signal that serious illness exists. For example, a rapid pulse may result from fever, infection, or heart failure. A slow or weak pulse may indicate dehydration, infection, or shock.

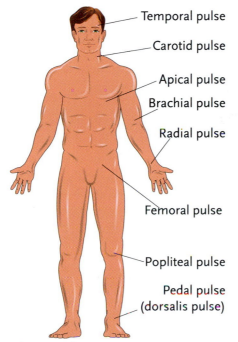

Temporal pulse
Carotid pulse
Apical pulse
Brachial pulse
Radial pulse

Femoral pulse

Popliteal pulse

Pedal pulse
(dorsalis pulse)

Fig. 14-12. Common pulse sites.

The **apical** (*AY-pi-kul*) pulse is heard by listening directly over the heart with a stethoscope. This is often the easiest method for measuring the pulse in infants and small children because their pulse points are harder to find. A **stethoscope** is an instrument designed to listen to sounds within the body, such as the heart beating or air moving through the lungs.

Taking and recording apical pulse

Equipment: stethoscope, watch with second hand

1. Wash your hands.

2. Explain procedure to client, speaking clearly, slowly, and directly, maintaining face-to-face contact whenever possible.

3. Provide privacy for the client.

4. Fit the earpieces of the stethoscope snugly in your ears. Place the flat metal diaphragm on the left side of the chest, just below the nipple (Fig. 14-13). Listen for the heartbeat.

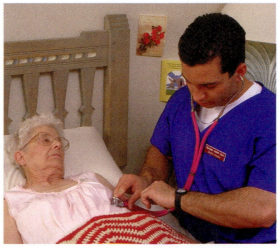

Fig. 14-13.

5. Use the second hand of your watch. Count the heartbeats for one minute. Each "lub-dub" that you hear is counted as one beat. A normal heartbeat is rhythmical. Leave the stethoscope in place to count respirations (see procedure later in chapter).

6. Document the pulse rate, date, time, and method used (apical). Note any irregularities in the rhythm.

7. Store stethoscope.

8. Wash your hands.

Respirations

Respiration is the process of breathing air into the lungs, or **inspiration**, and exhaling air out of the lungs, or **expiration**. Each respiration consists of an inspiration and an expiration. The chest rises during inspiration and falls during expiration.

The normal respiration rate for adults ranges from 12-20 breaths per minute. Infants and children have a faster respiratory rate. Infants normally breathe at a rate of 30-40 respirations per minute. People may breathe more quickly if they know they are being observed. Because of this, count respirations immediately after taking

14

Core Healthcare Skills

the pulse. Keep your fingers on a client's wrist or on the stethoscope over the heart. Do not make it obvious that you are observing the client's breathing.

If you find it difficult to remember the pulse rate after taking the respiratory rate, use a paper and pencil and jot down the pulse rate before counting respirations. Then document the pulse and respiration rates on the visit notes when you are finished.

Taking and recording radial pulse, and counting and recording respirations

Equipment: watch with a second hand

1. Wash your hands.

2. Explain procedure to client, speaking clearly, slowly, and directly, maintaining face-to-face contact whenever possible.

3. Provide privacy for the client.

4. Place fingertips on the thumb side of client's wrist to locate pulse (Fig. 14-14).

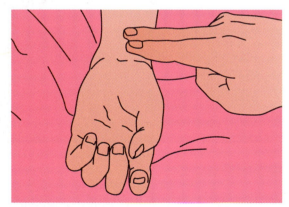

Fig. 14-14.

5. Count the beats for one full minute.

6. Keeping your fingertips on the client's wrist, count respirations for one full minute. Observe for the pattern and character of the client's breathing. Normal breathing is smooth and quiet. If you see signs of difficult breathing, shallow breathing, or noisy breathing, such as wheezing, report it to your supervisor.

7. Document the pulse rate, date, time, and method used (radial). Notify your supervisor if the pulse is less than 60 beats per minute, over 100 beats per minute, or if the rhythm is irregular. Document the respiratory rate and the pattern or character of breathing.

8. Wash your hands.

Blood Pressure

Blood pressure is an important indicator of a person's health. Blood pressure is measured in millimeters of mercury (mmHg). The measurement shows how well the heart is working. There are two parts of blood pressure, the systolic (*sis-TOL-ik*) measurement and diastolic (*DYE-a-stol-ik*) measurement.

In the **systolic** phase, the heart is at work, contracting and pushing the blood from the left ventricle of the heart. The reading you get shows the pressure on the walls of arteries as blood is pumped through the body. The normal range for systolic blood pressure is 100-139 mmHg.

The second measurement reflects the **diastolic** phase—when the heart relaxes. The diastolic measurement is always lower than the systolic measurement. It shows the pressure in the arteries when the heart is at rest. The normal range for adults is 60-89 mmHg.

People with high blood pressure, or **hypertension** (*high-per-TEN-shun*), have elevated systolic and/or diastolic blood pressures. A blood pressure level of 140/90 mmHg or higher is considered high.

However, if blood pressure is between 120/80 mmHg and 140/90 mmHg, it is called **prehypertension**. This means that the person does not have high blood pressure now but is likely to develop it in the future. Report to your supervisor if a client's blood pressure is over 140/90.

Many factors can cause increased blood pressure. These include aging, exercise, physical or emotional stress, pain, medications, and the volume of blood in the circulation. For example,

loss of blood will lead to abnormally low blood pressure, or **hypotension** (*high-poh-TEN-shun*). Hypotension can be life-threatening if it is not corrected.

Blood pressure is taken using a stethoscope and a blood pressure cuff, or **sphygmomanometer** (*sfig-moh-ma-NOM-e-ter*) (Fig. 14-15). Inside the cuff is an inflatable balloon that expands when air is pumped into the cuff. Two pieces of tubing are connected to the cuff. One leads to a rubber bulb that pumps air into the cuff. A pressure control button allows you to control the release of air from the cuff after it is inflated. The other piece of tubing is connected to a pressure gauge with numbers. The gauge is either a mercury column or a round dial.

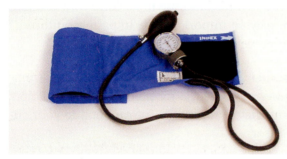

Fig. 14-15. A sphygmomanometer.

There may be an electronic sphygmomanometer in some homes. The systolic and diastolic pressure readings and pulse are displayed digitally. Some units have automatic inflation and deflation. You do not need a stethoscope with an electronic sphygmomanometer. Ask your supervisor for instructions on the proper use of the equipment.

When taking blood pressure, the first clear sound you will hear is the systolic pressure (top number). When the sound changes to a soft muffled thump or disappears, this is the diastolic pressure (bottom number). Blood pressure is recorded as a fraction. The systolic reading is on top and the diastolic reading is on the bottom (for example: 120/80).

Never measure blood pressure on an arm that has an IV, a dialysis shunt, or any medical equipment. Avoid a side that has a cast, recent trauma, or breast surgery (mastectomy).

Taking and recording blood pressure (two-step method)

Equipment: sphygmomanometer (blood pressure cuff), stethoscope, alcohol wipes, pen and paper

1. Wash your hands.

2. Explain procedure to client, speaking clearly, slowly, and directly, maintaining face-to-face contact whenever possible.

3. Provide privacy for the client.

4. Ask the client to roll up his or her sleeve. Do not measure blood pressure over clothing.

5. Position the client's arm with the palm up. The arm should be level with the heart.

6. With the valve open, squeeze the cuff to make sure it is completely deflated.

7. Place the blood pressure cuff snugly on client's upper arm, with the center of the cuff placed over the brachial artery (1-1½ inches above the elbow toward inside of elbow) (Fig. 14-16).

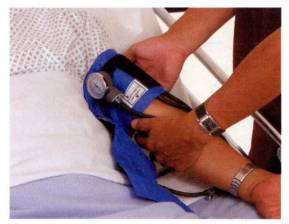

Fig. 14-16.

8. Locate the radial (wrist) pulse with your fingertips.

9. Close the valve (clockwise) until it stops. Inflate the cuff while watching the gauge.

10. Stop inflating when you can no longer feel the radial pulse. Note the reading. The number is an estimate of the systolic pressure. This estimate helps you not to inflate the cuff too high later in this procedure. Inflating the cuff too high is painful and may damage small blood vessels.

11. Open the valve to deflate cuff completely. An inflated cuff left on client's arm can cause numbness and tingling.

12. Write down the systolic reading.

13. Before using the stethoscope, wipe the diaphragm and earpieces of stethoscope with alcohol wipes.

14. Locate the brachial pulse with fingertips.

15. Place the earpieces of the stethoscope in your ears.

16. Place the diaphragm of the stethoscope over the brachial artery.

17. Close the valve (clockwise) until it stops. Do not tighten it (Fig. 14-17).

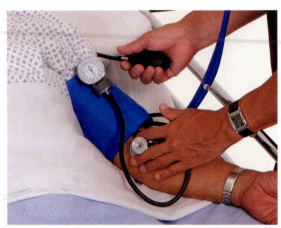

Fig. 14-17.

18. Inflate the cuff to 30 mmHg above your estimated systolic pressure.

19. Open the valve slightly with thumb and index finger. Deflate cuff slowly. Releasing the valve slowly allows you to hear beats accurately.

20. Watch the gauge and listen for sound of pulse.

21. Remember the reading at which the first clear pulse sound is heard. This is the systolic pressure.

22. Continue listening for a change or muffling of pulse sound. The point of a change or the point at which the sound disappears is the diastolic pressure. Remember this reading.

23. Open the valve to deflate cuff completely. Remove cuff.

24. Document both systolic and diastolic pressures. Write the numbers like a fraction, with the systolic reading on top and the diastolic reading on the bottom (for example: 120/80). Note which arm was used. Write "RA" for right arm and "LA" for left arm.

25. Wipe diaphragm and earpieces of stethoscope with alcohol. Store equipment.

26. Wash your hands.

Pain

It is important to observe and report on a client's pain. Pain is called the "fifth vital sign" because it is so important to monitor.

Because you spend the most time with clients, you play an important role in pain monitoring and prevention.

If a client complains of pain, ask the following questions to get the most accurate information. Immediately report the information to your supervisor.

- Where is the pain?

- When did the pain start?

- Is the pain mild, moderate or severe? To help assess this, ask the client to rate the pain on a scale of 1 to 10. Ten is the most severe.

- Ask the client to describe the pain. Make notes if you need to and use the client's words when reporting to your supervisor.

- Ask the client what he or she was doing before the pain started.

You may need to report the client's other vital signs when calling your supervisor. Be prepared to give this information.

Measures to reduce pain include the following:

- Report complaints of pain or unrelieved pain promptly to your supervisor.

- Gently position the body in good alignment. Use pillows for support. Assist in frequent changes of position if the client desires it.

- Give back rubs.

- Offer warm baths or showers.

- Assist the client to the bathroom or commode or offer the bedpan or urinal.

- Encourage slow, deep breaths when the client has difficulty breathing.

- Provide a calm and quiet environment. Use soft music to distract the client.

- If a client is taking pain medication, remind him or her when it is time to take it. See chapter 16 for information on medications.

- Be patient, caring, gentle, and sympathetic.

Height and Weight

You may be asked to check a client's weight and height as part of your care. Height is checked less frequently than weight. Weight changes can be signs of illness. They can also affect the medication doses a client needs. For these reasons, you must report any weight loss or gain, no matter how small.

Clients confined to bed can be weighed using a chair scale. Your agency will provide this equipment if it is needed. Ambulatory clients can be weighed on a bathroom scale or a standing scale. Keep the following in mind when weighing a client:

- Always explain what you will do before beginning any procedure. You will need your client's cooperation to measure weight properly.

- Provide for privacy, as some people are sensitive about their weight.

- Always weigh at the same time of day, with client wearing the same amount of clothing. Have the client void, or empty her bladder, before she is weighed.

Measuring and recording the weight of a client

Equipment: bathroom scale

1. Wash your hands.

2. Explain procedure to client, speaking clearly, slowly, and directly, maintaining face-to-face contact whenever possible.

3. Provide privacy for the client.

4. Set the scale on a hard surface in a place the client can get to easily.

5. Start with the scale balanced at zero before weighing the client. If it does not read zero, adjust the knob.

6. Help client to the scale as needed.

7. Have the client step on the scale. Assist as needed. Be sure she is not holding, touching, or leaning against anything. This interferes with weight measurement. Do not force someone to let go. If you are unable to obtain a weight, notify your supervisor.

8. When the dial has stopped moving, read the weight.

9. Have the client step off the scale and help her back into a comfortable position.

10. Document the weight.

11. Store the scale if it was moved.

12. Wash your hands.

Measuring and recording the height of a client

Some clients will be unable to get out of bed. If so, height can be measured using a tape measure (Fig. 14-18).

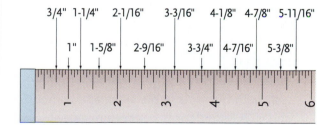

Fig. 14-18. A tape measure.

Equipment: tape measure and pencil

1. Wash your hands.

2. Explain procedure to client, speaking clearly, slowly, and directly, maintaining face-to-face contact whenever possible.

3. Provide privacy for the client.

4. Position the client lying straight in bed, flat

Core Healthcare Skills

14

Core Healthcare Skills

on his back with arms and legs at his sides. Be sure the bed sheet is smooth underneath the client.

5. Make a pencil mark on the sheet at the top of the head.

6. Make another mark at the client's heel (Fig. 14-19).

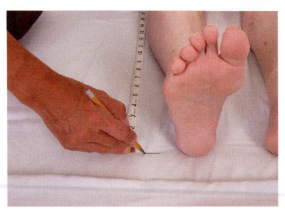

Fig. 14-19.

7. With the tape measure, measure the distance between the marks.

8. Document the height.

9. Store equipment.

10. Wash your hands.

For clients who can get out of bed, you will measure height while they stand against a wall.

Equipment: tape measure and pencil

1. Wash your hands.

2. Explain procedure to client, speaking clearly, slowly, and directly, maintaining face-to-face contact whenever possible.

3. Provide privacy for the client.

4. Have the client stand with his back to the wall, with his arms at his sides and without shoes. A hard floor is better than carpet.

5. Make a pencil mark on the wall at the top of the client's head.

6. Ask client to step away. Measure the distance between the pencil mark and the floor.

7. Document the height.

8. Store equipment.

9. Wash your hands.

2. List three types of specimens you may collect from a client

You may be asked to collect a specimen from a client. A **specimen** is a sample. Different types of specimens are used for different tests.

1. **Sputum** (*SPYOO-tum*) is mucus coughed up from the lungs. This may help diagnose illness or evaluate the effects of medication. Early morning is the best time to collect sputum.

2. **Stool** (feces) specimens are another type of sample collected. If the client uses a bedpan or portable commode for elimination, you will take the stool specimen from there. If the client uses the toilet, you will need a special container (often called a "**hat**"). A "hat" fits into the toilet bowl to collect the stool (Fig. 14-20).

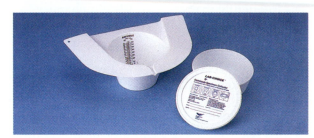

Fig. 14-20. A "hat" is a container that is placed under the toilet seat to collect specimens for clients who use the toilet.

3. Urine specimens may be routine, clean catch (mid-stream), or 24-hour. A **routine urine specimen** is collected anytime the client voids. The client will void into a bedpan, urinal, commode, or "hat." The **clean catch specimen** is called "mid-stream" because the first and last urine are not included in the sample. Its purpose is to determine the presence of bacteria in the urine. A **24-hour urine specimen** tests for certain chemicals and hormones. A 24-hour urine specimen collects all the urine voided by a client in a 24-hour period. Usually the collection begins at 7am and runs until 7am the next day. When beginning a 24-hour urine specimen collection, the client must void and discard the first urine so that the collection begins with an empty bladder. All urine must be collected and stored properly. If any is accidentally thrown away or improperly stored, the collection will have to be done over again another day.

Note: Different states have different rules about what home health aides are allowed to do. Be sure you understand your state's guidelines before performing any procedures. Check with your supervisor if you are uncertain.

Collecting a sputum specimen

Equipment: specimen container with cover (labeled with client's name, address, date and time), tissues, plastic bag, gloves, mask

1. Wash your hands.

2. Explain the procedure to the client, speaking clearly, slowly, and directly, maintaining face-to-face contact whenever possible.

3. Provide privacy for the client.

4. Put on mask and gloves. If the client has known or suspected tuberculosis or another infectious disease, you should wear a mask when collecting a sputum specimen. Coughing is one way TB germs can enter the air.

5. Ask the client to cough deeply, so that sputum comes up from the lungs. To prevent the spread of infectious material, give the client tissues to cover his or her mouth while coughing. Ask the client to spit the sputum into the specimen container.

6. When you have obtained a good sample (about two tablespoons of sputum), cover the container tightly. Wipe any sputum off the outside of the container with tissues. Discard the tissues. Put the specimen container in the plastic bag and seal.

7. Remove gloves and mask.

8. Wash your hands.

9. Document the procedure.

Collecting a stool specimen

Ask the client to let you know when he or she can have a bowel movement. Be ready to collect the specimen.

Equipment: specimen container and lid with label, 2 tongue blades, 2 pairs of gloves, bedpan, portable commode or toilet attachment (hat), 2 plastic bags, toilet tissue, washcloth or towel, supplies for perineal care

1. Wash your hands.

2. Explain procedure to client, speaking clearly, slowly, and directly, maintaining face-to-face contact whenever possible.

3. Provide privacy for the client.

4. Put on gloves.

5. When the client is ready to move bowels, ask him not to urinate at the same time and not to put toilet paper in with the sample. Provide a plastic bag to discard toilet paper separately.

6. Fit hat to toilet or commode, or provide client with bedpan. Leave the room and ask the client to call you when he is finished with the bowel movement.

7. After the bowel movement, assist as necessary with perineal care. Help client wash his or her hands at the sink or using the washcloth and towel. Make the client comfortable. Remove gloves.

8. Wash your hands again.

9. Put on clean gloves.

10. Using the two tongue blades, take about two tablespoons of stool and put it in the container. Without touching the inside of the container, cover it tightly.

11. Wrap the tongue blades in toilet paper and throw them away. Empty the bedpan or container into the toilet. Clean and store the equipment.

12. Store the specimen properly. It must be bagged and labeled.

13. Remove and dispose of gloves.

14. Wash your hands.

15. Document the procedure. Note amount and characteristics of stool.

Some clients will be able to collect their own urine specimens. Others will need your help. Be sure to explain exactly how the specimen must be collected.

14

Core Healthcare Skills

14

Core Healthcare Skills

Collecting a routine urine specimen

Equipment: urine specimen container and lid, label, gloves, bedpan or urinal (if client cannot use the bathroom), "hat" for toilet (if client can get to the bathroom), 2 plastic bags, washcloth, towel, paper towel, supplies for perineal care, PPE (if needed)

1. Wash your hands.

2. Explain procedure to client, speaking clearly, slowly, and directly, maintaining face-to-face contact whenever possible.

3. Provide privacy for the client.

4. Put on gloves.

5. Assist the client to the bathroom or commode, or offer the bedpan or urinal.

6. Have client void into "hat," urinal, or bedpan. Ask the client not to put toilet paper in with the sample. Provide a plastic bag to discard toilet paper separately.

7. After urination, assist as necessary with perineal care. Help client wash his or her hands at the sink or using the washcloth and towel. Make the client comfortable.

8. Take bedpan, urinal, or commode pail to the bathroom.

9. Pour urine from bedpan, urinal, or toilet attachment into the specimen container. Specimen container should be at least half full.

10. Cover the urine container with its lid. Wipe off the outside with a paper towel.

11. Place the container in a plastic bag.

12. If using a bedpan or urinal, discard extra urine. Rinse and clean equipment, and store.

13. Remove and dispose of gloves.

14. Complete the label for the container with the client's name, address, the date, and time.

15. Wash your hands.

16. Document the procedure. Note amount and characteristics of urine.

Collecting a clean catch (mid-stream) urine specimen

Equipment: specimen kit with container, label, cleansing solution, gauze or towelettes, gloves, bedpan or urinal (if client cannot use the bathroom), plastic bag, washcloth, paper towel, towel, supplies for perineal care, PPE (if needed)

1. Wash your hands.

2. Explain procedure to client, speaking clearly, slowly, and directly, maintaining face-to-face contact whenever possible.

3. Provide privacy for the client.

4. Put on gloves.

5. Open the specimen kit. Do not touch the inside of the container or the inside of the lid.

6. Using the towelettes or gauze and cleansing solution, clean the area around the urethra. **For females**, separate the labia and wipe from front to back along one side. Discard towelette/gauze. With a new towelette or gauze, wipe from front to back along the other labia. Using a new towelette or gauze, wipe down the middle.

   For males, clean the head of the penis using circular motions with the towelettes or gauze. Clean thoroughly, changing towelettes/gauze after each circular motion and discarding after use. If the man is uncircumcised, pull back the foreskin of the penis before cleaning and hold it back during urination. Make sure it is pulled back down after collecting the specimen.

7. Ask the client to urinate into the bedpan, urinal, or toilet, and to stop before urination is complete.

8. Place the container under the urine stream and have the client start urinating again. Fill the container at least half full. Have the client finish urinating in bedpan, urinal, or toilet.

9. Cover the urine container with its lid. Wipe off the outside with a paper towel.

10. Place the container in a plastic bag.

11. If using a bedpan or urinal, discard extra urine. Rinse and clean equipment, and store.

12. After urination, assist as necessary with perineal care. Remove and dispose of gloves. Wash your hands. Help client wash his hands at the sink or using the washcloth.

13. Complete the label for the container with the client's name and address, the date, and time.

14. Wash your hands again.

15. Document the procedure. Note amount and characteristics of urine.

Collecting a 24-hour urine specimen

Since you will probably not be present during all 24 hours of the test, it is important to explain the collection fully to the client and family members.

Equipment: container for urine: gallon bottle or a container from the lab, bedpan or urinal (for clients confined to bed), "hat" for toilet (if client can get to the bathroom), bucket of ice (if the urine must be kept cold) or a clearly-marked container can also be put in the refrigerator, funnel (if the container opening is small), gloves, washcloth or towel, supplies for perineal care, PPE (if needed)

1. Wash your hands.

2. Explain procedure to client, speaking clearly, slowly, and directly, maintaining face-to-face contact whenever possible.

3. Provide privacy for the client.

4. When beginning the collection, have the client completely empty the bladder. Discard the urine and note the exact time of this voiding. The collection will run until the same time tomorrow.

5. Label the container with client's name, address, dates and times the collection period began and ended (Fig. 14-21).

6. Put on gloves each time the client voids.

7. Pour urine from bedpan, urinal, or toilet attachment into the container, using the funnel as needed.

8. After each voiding, assist as necessary with perineal care. Help the client wash his or her

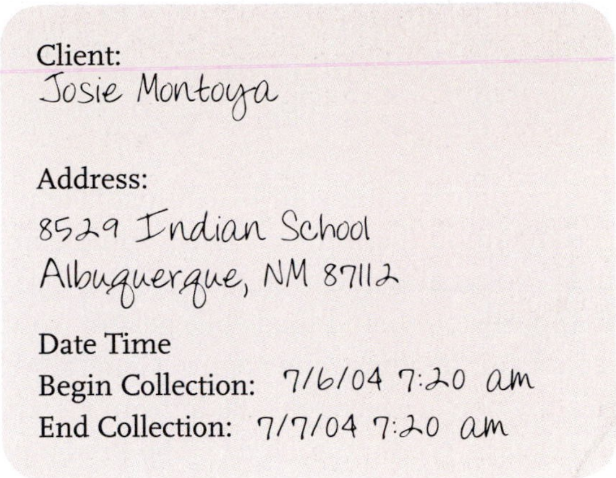

Client:
Josie Montoya

Address:
8529 Indian School
Albuquerque, NM 87112

Date Time
Begin Collection: *7/6/04 7:20 am*
End Collection: *7/7/04 7:20 am*

Fig. 14-21.

hands using the washcloth and towel after each voiding.

9. Be sure the client or a family member understands that all urine is to be saved, even when you are gone. Show them how to pour the urine into the container. Remind them to store the container in the bucket of ice or in the refrigerator if ordered.

10. Clean equipment after each voiding.

11. Remove gloves.

12. Wash your hands.

13. Document the time of the last void before the 24-hour collection period began, and the last void of the 24-hour collection period.

Urine is strained to discover the presence of **calculi**, or kidney stones, that can develop in the urinary tract. Urine straining is the process of pouring all urine through a fine filter to catch any particles that are present. Kidney stones can be as small as grains of sand or as large as golf balls. If any stones are found, they are saved and then sent to a laboratory for examination.

If you are going to strain urine, you will collect a routine urine specimen. After taking it to the bathroom, pour it through a disposable paper filter or a 4x4-inch piece of gauze into a specimen container. Any stones that are present are wrapped in the filter and placed in the specimen container to go to the laboratory.

14

Core Healthcare Skills

14

Core Healthcare Skills

3. Describe the importance of fluid balance and explain intake and output (I&O)

To maintain health, your body must take in a certain amount of fluid each day. Fluid comes in the form of liquids you drink and is also found in semi-liquid foods like gelatin, soup, ice cream, pudding, and yogurt. Generally, a healthy person needs to take in from 64 to 96 ounces (oz.) of fluid each day. The fluid a person consumes is called **intake**, or **input**. If a person's intake is not in a healthy range, he or she can become **dehydrated**. Dehydration is a serious medical condition that requires immediate attention. More information on dehydration is in chapter 22.

All fluid taken in each day cannot remain in the body. It must be eliminated as **output**. Output includes urine, feces, and vomitus. It also includes perspiration and moisture in the air we exhale. If a person's intake exceeds his or her output, the fluid is building up in body tissues. This fluid retention can cause medical problems and discomfort.

Fluid balance is maintaining equal input and output, or taking in and eliminating equal amounts of fluid. Most people regulate fluid balance automatically. But some clients must have their intake and output, or I&O, monitored and documented. To monitor this, you will need to measure and document all fluids the client takes by mouth, as well as all urine and vomitus the client produces.

To measure these amounts, use separate measuring containers for input and output. Be careful never to mix them up. Measuring cups can be used. If a client frequently drinks out of one type of cup, measure the amount that cup holds. You can even use masking tape on the outside of the cup to mark different quantities. This makes it easier to keep track of input.

To document intake and output, some agencies use a special form. This is called an Intake/Output (I&O) sheet (Fig. 14-22). Use this form if your employer provides it. Otherwise, make your own I&O sheet on regular paper.

Fig. 14-22. Many employers provide a form for documenting intake and output (I&O).

Conversions

A cubic centimeter (cc) is a unit of measure and is equal to one milliliter (ml.)

1 oz. = 30 cc or 30 ml.

2 oz. = 60 cc

3 oz. = 90 cc

4 oz. = 120 cc

5 oz. = 150 cc

6 oz. = 180 cc

7 oz. = 210 cc

8 oz. = 240 cc

¼ cup = 2 oz. = 60 cc

½ cup = 4 oz. = 120 cc

1 cup = 8 oz. = 240 cc

Measuring and recording input and output

Monitoring fluid balance begins with measuring intake.

Equipment: I&O sheet, graduate (Fig. 14-23), pen and paper

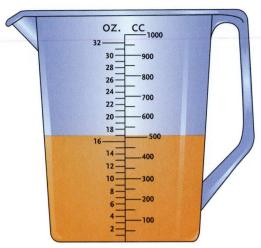

Fig. 14-23. A graduate is a measuring container.

1. Wash your hands.

2. Explain procedure to client, speaking clearly, slowly, and directly, maintaining face-to-face contact whenever possible.

3. Provide privacy for the client.

4. Using a measuring cup, measure the amount of fluid a client is served. Note the amount on paper, not in the visit notes.

5. When client has finished a meal or snack, measure any leftover fluids. Note this amount on paper.

6. Subtract the leftover amount from the amount served. If you have measured in ounces, convert to cubic centimeters (cc) by multiplying by 30.

7. Document the amount of fluid consumed (in cc) in the visit notes and/or I&O record, as well as the time and what fluid was taken.

Measuring output is the other half of monitoring fluid balance.

Equipment: I&O record, pen and paper, graduate, bedpan, urinal or toilet attachment, plastic bag for disposal of toilet paper, washcloth or towel, gloves

1. Wash your hands.

2. Explain procedure to client, speaking clearly, slowly, and directly, maintaining face-to-face contact whenever possible.

3. Provide privacy for the client.

4. Put on gloves.

5. Ask the client to put used toilet paper in the bag, not in the bedpan or toilet. Ask client not to move bowels at the same time as urinating, if possible.

6. Make client comfortable, assisting as necessary. Leave the room if your assistance is not needed.

7. Help the client wash his or her hands using the washcloth and towel.

8. Pour urine into measuring container. Note the amount on paper, converting to cc if necessary.

9. Discard urine. Wash and store equipment. Flush toilet paper down the toilet and discard plastic bag.

10. Remove gloves.

11. Wash your hands.

12. Document the time and amount of urine in output column on sheet. For example: 3:45pm 200 cc urine

    To measure vomitus, pour from basin into measuring container, then discard in the toilet. If client vomits on the bed or floor, estimate the amount. Document **emesis** (*EM-e-sis*, or vomiting) and amount in the visit notes and/or I&O sheet.

Emesis, or vomiting, must be documented. It may be a sign of illness or of a reaction to medication. Some clients, such as cancer patients undergoing chemotherapy, may vomit frequently as a result of treatment. Vomiting is unpleasant. Handle it calmly. Provide comfort to the client.

GUIDELINES
Vomiting

-   Treat vomitus as you treat urine and other potentially infectious wastes. Follow Standard Precautions. Always wear gloves when handling it. Flush vomitus down the toilet. Clean spills thoroughly with a disinfecting solution of bleach and water.

-   Provide comfort to a client who has vomited. Stay calm, and offer a basin if you think he or she may vomit more. Remove soiled

14

Core Healthcare Skills

198

sheets or clothing promptly. Provide a wet washcloth to wipe face, mouth or hands. Offer a drink of water or oral care to clean the mouth.

ⓖ Provide plenty of fluids to the client who has vomited. Water, diluted juices, or sports drinks may help prevent dehydration. Discontinue solid foods when vomiting occurs. Check with your supervisor for what you can serve. Clear liquids or a bland diet may be recommended.

Observing, reporting, and documenting emesis

Because you may not know when a client is going to vomit, you may not have time to explain what you will do and assemble supplies ahead of time. Talk to the client soothingly as you help him clean up. Tell him what you are doing to help him.

1. Put on gloves when client has vomited.

2. Provide a basin and remove it when vomiting has stopped.

3. Remove soiled linens or clothes. Set aside for laundering. Replace with fresh linens or clothes.

4. If client's I&O is being monitored, measure and note amount of vomitus.

5. Flush vomit down the toilet. Wash and store basin.

6. Remove gloves.

7. Wash your hands.

8. Put on fresh gloves.

9. Provide comfort to client: wipe face and mouth, position comfortably, offer a drink of water or oral care (Fig. 14-24).

10. Launder soiled linens and clothes promptly in hot water.

11. Remove gloves.

12. Wash your hands again.

13. Document time, amount, color, and consistency of vomitus. Look for blood in vomitus or blood-tinged vomitus.

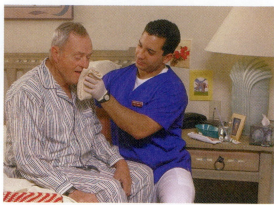
Fig. 14-24.

14. Report to your supervisor immediately and get instructions for diet.

4. Describe the guidelines for catheter care

A **catheter** (*KATH-et-er*) is a tube used to drain urine from the bladder. A **straight catheter** does not remain inside the person. It is removed immediately after urine is drained. An **indwelling catheter** remains inside the bladder for a period of time (Fig. 14-25). The urine drains into a bag. Home health aides never insert, remove, or irrigate catheters. However, you may be asked to provide daily care for the catheter, cleaning the area around the urethral opening and emptying the drainage bag.

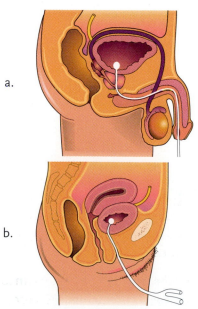
Fig. 14-25. a) An indwelling catheter (male). b) An indwelling catheter (female).

An **external**, or **condom catheter**, has an attachment on the end that fits onto the penis (Fig. 14-26). The attachment is fastened with a Velcro strap or self-adhesive strip. The external catheter is changed daily. In some states home health aides are allowed to change an external catheter. However, in other states nurses must perform this procedure. As always, provide only the care you are assigned to provide.

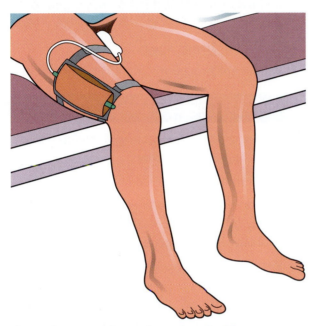

Fig. 14-26. An external or condom catheter (male).

You may be asked to collect a urine specimen from a client who uses a catheter. Be aware of what to report to your supervisors about clients with catheters.

GUIDELINES
Working with Clients who have Catheters

- The drainage bag must always be kept lower than the hips or bladder. Urine must never flow from the bag or tubing back into the bladder. This can cause infection.

- Tubing should be kept as straight as possible and should not be kinked. Kinks, twists, or pressure on the tubing (such as from the client sitting or lying on the tubing) can prevent urine from draining.

- The genital area must be kept clean to prevent infection. Because the catheter goes all the way into the bladder, germs can enter

the bladder more easily. Daily care of the genital area is especially important.

OBSERVING AND REPORTING
Catheter Care

Report any of the following to your supervisor:

- blood in the urine or any other unusual appearance
- catheter bag does not fill after several hours
- catheter bag fills suddenly
- catheter is not in place
- urine leaks from the catheter
- client reports pain
- odor

You may be asked to collect a urine specimen from a client who is wearing a catheter. If so, you will disconnect the tubing from the drainage bag. Allow the specimen to drip directly into the specimen container. If the client's input and output is being monitored, measure the amount of urine collected. Collecting a specimen this way may take some time. Do not collect a urine sample from the drainage bag unless ordered to do so.

Providing catheter care

Many clients can clean the catheter site themselves. If you need to provide this care for a client, follow the steps below.

Equipment: bath blanket, protective pad, bath basin, bath thermometer, soap, 2-4 washcloths, 1 towel, gloves

1. Wash your hands.
2. Explain procedure to client, speaking clearly, slowly, and directly, maintaining face-to-face contact whenever possible.
3. Provide privacy for the client.
4. If the bed is adjustable, adjust bed to a safe working level, usually waist high.
5. Lower head of bed. Position client lying flat on her back. Raise the side rail farthest from you.

14

Core Healthcare Skills

6. Remove or fold back top bedding, keeping client covered with bath blanket.

7. Test water temperature with thermometer or your wrist and ensure it is safe. Water temperature should be 105° to 109°F. Have client check water temperature. Adjust if necessary.

8. Put on gloves.

9. Ask the client to flex her knees and raise the buttocks off the bed by pushing against the mattress with her feet. Place clean protective pad under her buttocks.

10. Expose only the area necessary to clean the catheter.

11. Place towel or pad under catheter tubing before washing.

12. Apply soap to wet washcloth.

13. Hold catheter near meatus to avoid tugging the catheter.

14. Clean at least four inches of catheter nearest meatus. Move in only one direction, away from meatus. Use a clean area of the cloth for each stroke.

15. Dip a clean washcloth in the water. Rinse at least four inches of catheter nearest meatus. Move in only one direction, away from meatus (Fig. 14-27). Use a clean area of the cloth for each stroke.

16. Empty the water into the toilet. Dispose of linen in proper containers.

17. Remove and dispose of gloves.

18. If you raised an adjustable bed, be sure to return it to its lowest position.

19. Wash your hands.

20. Help the client dress. Arrange covers. Check that the catheter tubing is free from kinks and twists and that it is securely taped to the leg.

21. Wash your hands again.

22. Document procedure and any observations.

Emptying the catheter drainage bag

Equipment: graduate (measuring container), alcohol wipes, paper towels, gloves

1. Wash your hands.

2. Explain procedure to client, speaking clearly, slowly, and directly, maintaining face-to-face contact whenever possible.

3. Put on gloves.

4. Place paper towel on the floor under the drainage bag. Place measuring container on the paper towel.

5. Open the drain or spout on the bag so that urine flows out of the bag into the measuring container (Fig. 14-28).

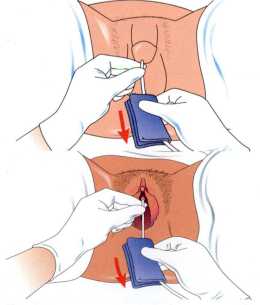

Fig. 14-27.

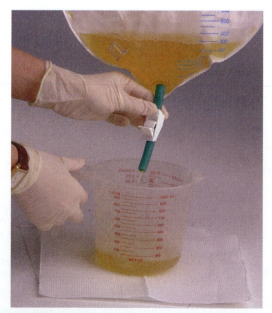

Fig. 14-28.

6. When urine has drained, close spout. Using alcohol wipe, clean the drain spout. Replace the drain in its holder on the bag.

7. Mentally note the amount and the appearance of the urine. Empty into toilet.

8. Clean and store measuring container.

9. Remove gloves.

10. Wash your hands.

11. Document procedure and amount of urine.

Applying a condom catheter

Equipment: condom catheter and collection bag, Velcro band or tape, gloves, plastic bag, bath blanket, supplies for perineal care

1. Wash your hands.

2. Explain procedure to client, speaking clearly, slowly, and directly, maintaining face-to-face contact whenever possible.

3. Provide privacy for the client.

4. If the bed is adjustable, adjust bed to a safe working level, usually waist high.

5. Lower head of bed. Position client lying flat on his back. Raise the side rail farthest from you.

6. Remove or fold back top bedding, keeping client covered with bath blanket.

7. Put on gloves.

8. Adjust bath blanket to only expose genital area.

9. If condom catheter is present, gently remove it. Place it in the plastic bag.

10. Assist as necessary with perineal care.

11. Attach collection bag to leg.

12. Hold penis firmly. Place condom at tip of penis and roll towards base of penis. Leave space between the drainage tip and glans of penis to prevent irritation. If client is not circumcised, be sure that foreskin is in normal position.

13. Secure condom to penis with Velcro band or tape provided (Fig. 14-29).

14. Connect catheter tip to drainage tubing. Make sure tubing is not twisted or kinked.

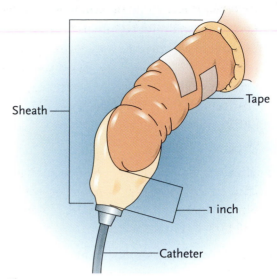

Sheath — Tape — 1 inch — Catheter

Fig. 14-29.

15. Discard used supplies in plastic bag. Remove and dispose of your gloves.

16. If you raised an adjustable bed, be sure to return it to its lowest position.

17. Wash your hands.

18. Remove bath blanket and store it. Make sure client is comfortable.

19. Document procedure and any observations.

5. Explain the benefits of warm and cold applications

Applying heat or cold to injured areas can have several good effects. Heat tends to relieve pain and muscular tension. It reduces swelling, elevates the temperature in the tissues, and increases blood flow. Increased blood flow brings more oxygen and nutrients to the tissues for healing.

Cold applications can help stop bleeding. They reduce swelling and pain, and bring down high fevers. Applying ice bags or cold compresses immediately after an injury can stop bleeding and reduce swelling.

Home health aides may be allowed to prepare and apply warm water bottles, heating pads, warm compresses or soaks, ice packs, and cold compresses. If your agency and state allow you to use other methods, your supervisor will train

14

Core Healthcare Skills

you. Never perform a procedure you are not trained or allowed to do. Only perform procedures that are assigned to you.

Warm and Cold Applications

Report the following to your supervisor:

- **O&R** excessive redness
- **O&R** pain
- **O&R** blisters
- **O&R** numbness

If you observe these signs, the application may be causing tissue damage.

Electric heating pads can also be used as heat applications. Follow the care plan. Do not use a heating pad unless it has been ordered in the care plan or by your supervisor.

Electric Heating Pad

- **g** Check the skin frequently for redness or pain. Electric heating pads do not cool down. Having it just a little too hot can be very dangerous for the client.

- **g** Make sure any electric heating pad you use is in good shape. Do not use it if the cord is frayed or if wires are exposed.

- **g** Do not use a pin to fasten the pad. The pin could contact a wire inside the pad and cause a shock.

- **g** Do not allow the client to lie on top of an electric heating pad.

- **g** Do not allow the client to use an electric heating pad near a source of water.

Another type of heat application is a **sitz bath**, or a warm soak of the perineal area. Sitz baths clean perineal wounds and reduce inflammation and pain. Circulation in the perineal area is increased. Voiding may be stimulated by a sitz bath. Clients with perineal swelling (such as hemorrhoids), or perineal wounds (such as those that occur during childbirth), may be ordered to take sitz baths. Because the sitz bath

causes increased blood flow to the pelvic area, blood flow to other parts of the body is decreased. Clients may feel weak, faint, or dizzy after taking a sitz bath.

Preparing and applying warm compresses

Equipment: washcloth, plastic wrap, towel, basin, bath thermometer

1. Wash your hands.

2. Explain procedure to client, speaking clearly, slowly, and directly, maintaining face-to-face contact whenever possible.

3. Provide privacy for the client.

4. Fill basin one-half to two-thirds full with hot water. Test water temperature with thermometer or your wrist and ensure it is safe. Water temperature should be 105° to 115°F. Have client check water temperature. Adjust if necessary.

5. Soak the washcloth in the water and wring it out. Immediately apply it to the area needing a warm compress. Note the time. Quickly cover the washcloth with plastic wrap and the towel to keep it warm (Fig. 14-30).

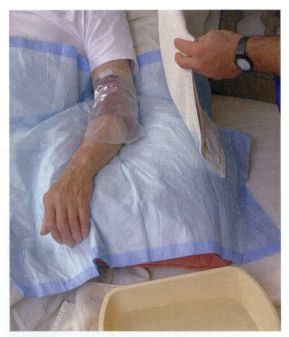

Fig. 14-30.

6. Check the area every five minutes. Remove the compress if the area is red or numb or if

14

Core Healthcare Skills

the client complains of pain or discomfort. Change the compress if cooling occurs. Remove the compress after 20 minutes.

7. Commercial warm compresses are also available. If these are provided, follow the package directions and your supervisor's instructions.

8. Discard water in the toilet. Clean and store basin and other supplies. Put laundry in hamper. Discard plastic wrap.

9. Wash your hands.

10. Document the time, length, and site of procedure, and any observations.

Administering warm soaks

Equipment: basin or bathtub (depending on the area to be soaked) bath thermometer, bath blanket, towel

1. Wash your hands.

2. Explain procedure to client, speaking clearly, slowly, and directly, maintaining face-to-face contact whenever possible.

3. Provide privacy for the client.

4. Fill the basin or tub half full of warm water. Test water temperature with thermometer or your wrist and ensure it is safe. Water temperature should be 105° to 110°F. Have client check water temperature. Adjust if necessary.

5. Immerse the body part in the basin, or help the client into the tub. Pad the edge of the basin with a towel if needed (Fig. 14-31). Use a bath blanket to cover the rest of the client if needed for extra warmth.

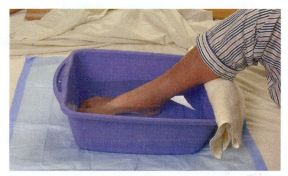

Fig. 14-31.

6. Check water temperature every five minutes.

Add hot water as needed to maintain the temperature. Never add water hotter than 110°F to avoid burns. To prevent burns, tell the client not to add hot water him- or herself. Observe the area for redness. Discontinue the soak if the client complains of pain or discomfort.

7. Soak for 15–20 minutes, or as ordered in the care plan.

8. Remove basin or help the client out of the tub. Use the towel to dry client.

9. Drain the tub or discard water. Clean and store basin and other supplies. Put laundry in hamper.

10. Wash your hands.

11. Document the time, length, and site of procedure. Report the client's response and any of your observations about the skin.

Using a hot water bottle

Equipment: hot water bottle, cloth cover or towel, bath thermometer

1. Wash your hands.

2. Explain procedure to client, speaking clearly, slowly, and directly, maintaining face-to-face contact whenever possible.

3. Provide privacy for the client.

4. Fill the bottle half full with warm water (105°F-115°F, or 98°F-110°F for infants and small children or older adults).

5. Press out excess air and seal the bottle.

6. Dry the bottle and check for leaks. Cover with a cloth cover or towel.

7. Apply the bottle to the area ordered. Check skin every five minutes for redness or pain. If redness or pain are present, add cold water to the bottle to reduce the temperature.

8. Remove the bottle after 20 minutes or as ordered in the care plan.

9. Empty the hot water bottle. Wash and store supplies.

10. Wash your hands.

14

Core Healthcare Skills

11. Document the time, length, and site of procedure. Document the client's response and any of your observations about the skin.

Assisting with a sitz bath

A disposable sitz bath fits on the toilet seat and is attached to a rubber bag containing warm water (Fig. 14-32).

Equipment: disposable sitz bath, bath thermometer, towels, gloves

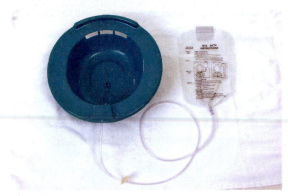

Fig. 14-32.

1. Wash your hands.
2. Explain procedure to client, speaking clearly, slowly, and directly, maintaining face-to-face contact whenever possible.
3. Provide privacy for the client.
4. Put on gloves.
5. Fill the sitz bath two-thirds full with hot water. Place the disposable sitz bath on the toilet seat. If the sitz bath is prescribed for cleaning the perineal area, the temperature should be 100°F-104°F. For a sitz bath given for pain and to stimulate circulation, the water temperature should be 105°F-110°F. Check the water temperature using the bath thermometer.
6. Help the client undress and be seated on the sitz bath. A valve on the tubing connected to the bag allows the client or you to replenish the water in the sitz bath with hot water.
7. Leave the room, but check on the client every five minutes to make sure he or she is not dizzy or weak. Stay with a client who seems unsteady.
8. Assist the client out of the sitz bath in 20 minutes. Provide towels and help with dressing if needed.
9. Clean and store supplies.
10. Remove gloves.
11. Wash your hands.
12. Document the procedure, including the time started and ended, the client's response, and the water temperature.

Applying ice packs

Equipment: ice pack or sealable plastic bag and crushed ice, towel to cover pack or bag

1. Wash your hands.
2. Explain procedure to client, speaking clearly, slowly, and directly, maintaining face-to-face contact whenever possible.
3. Provide privacy for the client.
4. Fill plastic bag or ice pack one-half to two-thirds full with crushed ice. Remove excess air. Cover bag or ice pack with towel.
5. Apply bag to the area as ordered (Fig. 14-33). Note the time. Use another towel to cover bag if it is too cold.

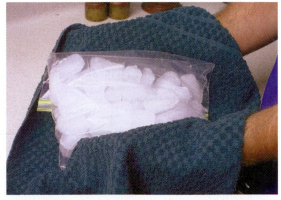

Fig. 14-33.

6. Check the area after ten minutes for blisters, pale, white, or gray skin. Stop treatment if client complains of numbness or pain.
7. Remove ice after 20 minutes or as ordered in the care plan.
8. Return ice bag or pack to freezer.
9. Wash your hands.

10. Document the time, length, and site of procedure. Report the client's response and any of your observations about the skin.

Applying cold compresses

Equipment: basin filled with water and ice, two washcloths, plastic or rubber sheet, towels

1. Wash your hands.

2. Explain procedure to client, speaking clearly, slowly, and directly, maintaining face-to-face contact whenever possible.

3. Provide privacy for the client.

4. Position client on plastic sheet. Rinse washcloth in basin and wring out. Cover the area to be treated with a cloth sheet or towel. Apply cold washcloth to the area as directed (Fig. 14-34). Change washcloths often to keep area cold.

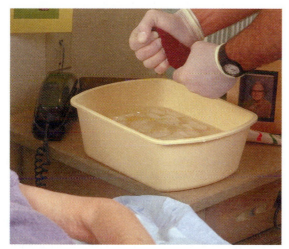

Fig. 14-34.

5. Check the area after five minutes for blisters, pale, white, or gray skin. Stop treatment if client complains of numbness or pain.

6. Remove compresses after 20 minutes or as ordered in the care plan. Give client towels as needed to dry the area.

7. Clean and store basin.

8. Wash your hands.

9. Document the time, length, and site of procedure. Report the client's response and any observations about the skin.

6. Explain how to apply non-sterile dressings

Sterile dressings are those that cover open or draining wounds. A nurse changes these dressings. Non-sterile dressings are applied to dry wounds that have less chance of infection. Home health aides may assist with non-sterile dressing changes.

Changing a dry dressing using non-sterile technique

Equipment: package of square gauze dressings, adhesive tape, scissors, 2 pairs of gloves, waste bag

1. Wash your hands.

2. Explain procedure to client, speaking clearly, slowly, and directly, maintaining face-to-face contact whenever possible.

3. Provide privacy for the client.

4. Cut pieces of tape long enough to secure the dressing. Hang tape on the edge of a table within reach. Open the four-inch gauze square package without touching the gauze. Place the opened package on a flat surface.

5. Put on gloves.

6. Remove soiled dressing by gently peeling tape toward the wound. Lift dressing off the wound. Do not drag it over the wound. Observe the dressing for odor or drainage. Notice the color of the wound. Dispose of used dressing in the waste bag. Remove your gloves. Place them in the waste bag.

7. Put on new gloves. Touching only outer edges of new four-inch gauze, remove it from package. Apply it to the wound. Tape gauze in place. Secure it firmly (Fig. 14-35).

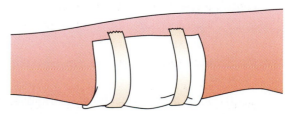

Fig. 14-35.

8. Remove gloves. Discard in the waste bag.

9. Wash your hands.

10. Document the procedure and your observations.

7. Describe the purpose of anti-embolic hose

For some cases of poor circulation to legs and feet, elastic stockings are ordered. These special stockings help prevent swelling and blood clots. They promote circulation. These stockings are called anti-embolic hose, or TED hose. Follow the manufacturer's instructions and illustrations on how to put on stockings.

Applying anti-embolic hose

Equipment: anti-embolic hose

1. Wash your hands.

2. Explain procedure to client, speaking clearly, slowly, and directly, maintaining face-to-face contact whenever possible.

3. Provide privacy for the client.

4. With client lying down, remove his or her socks, shoes, or slippers, and expose one leg.

5. Turn stocking inside-out at least to heel area (Fig. 14-36).

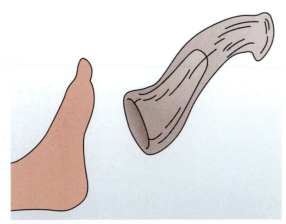

Fig. 14-36.

6. Gently place the foot of the stocking over toes, foot, and heel. Make sure the heel is in the right place (Fig. 14-37).

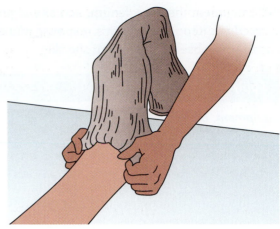

Fig. 14-37.

7. Gently pull the top of stocking over foot, heel, and leg (Fig. 14-38).

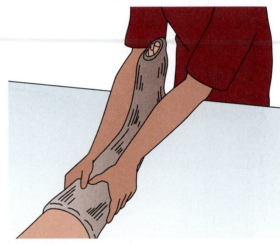

Fig. 14-38.

8. Make sure that there are no twists and wrinkles in the stocking after it is applied. It must fit smoothly. If you have trouble putting the stocking on, try applying powder to the client's leg before pulling the stocking up.

9. Repeat for the other leg.

10. Wash your hands.

11. Document the procedure.

8. Define the term ostomy and list care guidelines

An **ostomy** (*OS-toh-mee*) is the surgical removal of a portion of the intestines. It may be necessary due to bowel disease, cancer, or trauma. In

a client with an ostomy, the end of the intestine is brought out of the body through an artificial opening in the abdomen. This opening is called a **stoma** (*STOH-ma*). Stool, or feces, are eliminated through the ostomy rather than through the anus.

The terms "**colostomy**" (*koh-LOS-toh-mee*) and "**ileostomy**" (*il-ee-OS-toh-mee*) indicate what section of the intestine was removed and the type of stool that will be eliminated. In a colostomy, stool will generally be semi-solid. With an ileostomy, stool may be liquid and irritating to the client's skin.

Clients who have had an ostomy wear a disposable bag that fits over the stoma to collect the feces (Fig. 14-39). The bag is attached to the skin by adhesive. A belt may also be used to secure it.

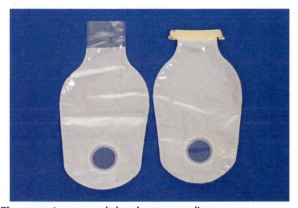

Fig. 14-39. An open and closed ostomy appliance.

Many people manage the ostomy appliance by themselves. Your employer should provide training before you provide this care. If you are providing ostomy care, make certain the client receives good skin care and hygiene. The ostomy bag should be emptied and cleaned or replaced whenever a stool is eliminated. Always wear gloves and wash hands carefully when providing ostomy care. Teach proper handwashing techniques to clients with ostomies.

Many clients with ostomies feel they have lost control of a basic bodily function. They may be embarrassed or angry about the ostomy. Be sensitive and supportive when working with these clients. Always provide privacy for ostomy care.

Caring for an ostomy

Equipment: bedpan, disposable bed protector, bath blanket, clean ostomy bag and belt/appliance, toilet paper, basin of warm water, soap or cleanser, washcloth, skin cream as ordered, two towels, plastic disposable bag, 3 pairs of gloves

1. Wash your hands.

2. Explain procedure to client, speaking clearly, slowly, and directly, maintaining face-to-face contact whenever possible.

3. Provide privacy for the client.

4. If the bed is adjustable, adjust bed to a safe working level, usually waist high.

5. Place bed protector under client. Cover client with a bath blanket. Pull down the top sheet and blankets. Only expose the ostomy site. Offer client a towel to keep clothing dry.

6. Put on gloves.

7. Remove ostomy bag carefully. If it will be washed and reused, place it in the bedpan. If it will be discarded, place it in the plastic bag. Note the color, odor, consistency, and amount of stool in the bag.

8. Wipe the area around the stoma with toilet paper. Discard paper in plastic bag.

9. Using a washcloth and warm soapy water, wash the area around the stoma (Fig. 14-40). Pat dry with another towel. Apply cream as ordered.

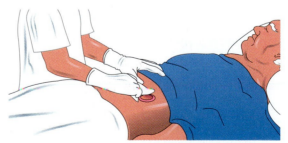

Fig. 14-40.

10. Place the clean ostomy appliance on client, following your supervisor's instructions. Make sure the bottom of the bag is clamped.

11. Remove disposable bed protector and discard.

12. Remove gloves. Make the client comfortable. Put on fresh gloves and change linens if necessary. Cover the client and remove bath blanket and towel. Place soiled linens in appropriate containers. Remove gloves.

13. Put on new gloves. Take bedpan and other supplies to bathroom. Empty bag into toilet and flush, along with used toilet paper. Wash out bag. Use a deodorant in the bag as directed.

14. Clean bedpan, pouring rinse water into toilet. Return to proper storage.

15. Remove and dispose of gloves properly.

16. Return bed to appropriate level if previously adjusted.

17. Wash your hands.

18. Document procedure and any observations.

Note: Call your supervisor if stoma appears very red or blue, or if swelling or bleeding is present.

Chapter Review

1. List five vital signs that must be monitored.

2. What temperature site is considered to be the most accurate?

3. What are the two parts of measuring blood pressure?

4. What other measurements may you be asked to check besides vital signs?

5. What is a specimen?

6. List the types of specimens you may have to collect.

7. You serve Mrs. Wyant a glass of milk. You know the glass holds 180 cc. She finishes most, but not all, of the milk. You measure the leftover milk, and it measures ¼ cup.

   How many cc of milk were left?

8. Miss Cahill drinks tea in the morning. Her mug holds 10 oz., and 3 oz. are left in the mug. What was her input in cc?

9. Why should the catheter drainage bag always be kept lower than the hips or the bladder?

10. Why should catheter tubing be kept as straight as possible?

11. What signs should you watch for at the site of a heat or cold application?

12. When are non-sterile dressings usually used?

13. Why may elastic stockings be ordered?

14. What type of client might have had an ostomy?

15. How often should an ostomy bag be emptied?

15

Rehabilitation and Restorative Care

1. List goals of restorative home care

Restorative care or **rehabilitation** involves helping clients move from illness, disability, and dependence, toward health, ability, and independence. Goals of a restorative or rehabilitative program include the following:

- To help a client regain abilities or recover from illness

- To develop and promote a client's independence

- To allow a client to feel in control of his or her life

- To help a client accept or adapt to the limitations of a disability

Rehabilitation will be used for many of your clients, particularly those who have suffered a stroke, accident, or trauma. Because you spend many hours with these clients, you play a critical role in helping them recover and regain independence. Rehabilitation is one of the great joys of working as a caregiver. Enjoy seeing clients progress toward independence or recovery. Take pride in your contributions to their improving health.

2. Explain the home care rehabilitation model

When you work with clients who need restorative care you will be working as part of a team. Some different members of the team and their roles are listed below.

The physician and nurses will establish goals of care. This includes promoting independence in activities of daily living (ADLs) and restoring health to optimal condition (Fig. 15-1).

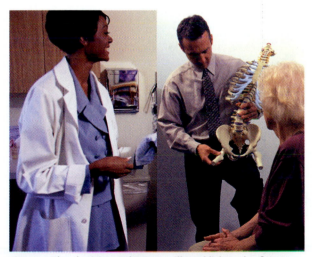

Fig. 15-1. The physician and nurses will establish goals of care.

The physical therapist, occupational therapist, or speech therapist will work with the client to help restore or adapt specific abilities (Fig. 15-2). Social workers or other counselors may see the client to help promote attitudes of independence and acceptance.

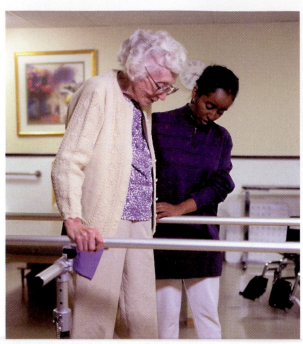

Fig. 15-2. A physical therapist will help restore specific abilities.

You, the home health aide, will be in the home, carrying out instructions of the other care team members. You will assist in achieving the client's goals. You will also observe and report the client's progress (Fig. 15-3).

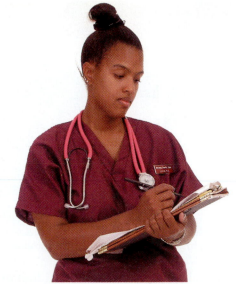

Fig. 15-3. Observing and documenting a client's progress are some of the most important duties you'll have.

3. Describe guidelines for assisting with restorative care

When assisting with restorative care, these guidelines are critical to your clients' progress:

- **Patience**. Progress may be slow, and it will seem slower to you and your client if you are impatient. Your clients must do as much as possible for themselves. Encourage self-care, regardless of how long it takes or how poorly they are able to do it. The more patient you are, the easier it will be for them to regain abilities and confidence.

- **Positive attitude**. Your attitude can set the tone. Family members and clients will take cues from you as to how they should behave. If you are encouraging and positive, you help create a supportive atmosphere for rehabilitation.

In addition, your expectations and reactions contribute to rehabilitation. Keep the following tips in mind:

- **Focus on small tasks and small accomplishments**. For example, dressing themselves may seem like an overwhelming task to some clients. Break the task down into smaller steps. For example, today the goal might be putting on a shirt without buttoning it. Next week the goal could be buttoning the shirt if that seems manageable. When the client is able to put the shirt on without assistance, congratulate him on this. Take everything one step at a time.

- **Recognize that setbacks occur**. Progress occurs at different rates. Sometimes a client can do something one day that he or she cannot do the next. Reassure clients that setbacks are normal. However, document in your notes any decline in a client's abilities.

- **Be sensitive to the client's needs**. Some clients may need more encouragement than others. Some may feel embarrassed by certain kinds of encouragement. Get to know your clients and understand what motivates them. Adapt your encouragement to fit an individual's personality.

OBSERVING AND REPORTING
Restorative Care

O&R any increase or decrease in abilities

O&R any change in attitude or motivation, positive or negative

- any decline in ability (for example "Yesterday Mr. Hogan used the portable commode without assistance. Today he asked for the bedpan.")
- any change in general health, including changes in skin condition, appetite, energy level, or general appearance
- signs of depression or mood changes

4. Describe how to assist with range of motion exercises

Exercise helps people regain strength and mobility. It prevents disabilities from developing. People who are in bed for long periods of time are more likely to develop contractures (*kon-TRAK-churs*). A **contracture** is the permanent and often very painful stiffening of a joint and muscle. They are generally caused by immobility. Contractures can result in the loss of ability. **Range of motion** (ROM) exercises are exercises that put a particular joint through its full arc of motion. The purpose of range of motion exercises is to decrease or prevent contractures, improve strength, and increase circulation.

Passive range of motion (PROM) exercises are used when clients are not able to move on their own. When assisting with PROM exercises, support the client's joints and move them through the range of motion. **Active range of motion** (AROM) exercises are performed by a client himself. Your role in AROM exercises is to encourage the client. **Active assisted range of motion** (AAROM) exercises are performed by the client with some assistance and support from you.

You will not perform ROM exercises without a specific order from a doctor, nurse, or physical therapist. Depending on the care plan, you will repeat each exercise two to five times, once or twice a day, working on both sides of the body. When performing ROM exercises, begin at the client's head and work down the body. Exercise the upper extremities (arms) before the lower extremities (legs). Give support above and below the joint. Stop the motion if the client complains of pain. These exercises are specific for each body area. They include the following movements (Fig. 15-4):

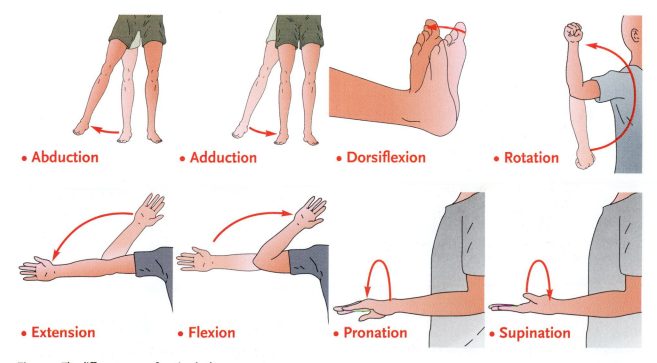

- **Abduction**
- **Adduction**
- **Dorsiflexion**
- **Rotation**
- **Extension**
- **Flexion**
- **Pronation**
- **Supination**

Fig. 15-4. The different range of motion body movements.

- **Abduction**: moving a body part away from the body

- **Adduction**: moving a body part toward the body

- **Dorsiflexion**: bending backward

- **Rotation**: turning a joint

- **Extension**: straightening a body part

- **Flexion**: bending a body part

- **Pronation**: turning downward

- **Supination**: turning upward

Assisting with passive range of motion (PROM) exercises

1. Wash your hands.

2. Explain the procedure to the client, speaking clearly, slowly, and directly, maintaining face-to-face contact whenever possible.

3. Provide privacy if the client desires it.

4. If the bed is adjustable, adjust bed to a safe working level, usually waist high. If the bed is movable, lock bed wheels.

5. Position the client supine—lying flat on his or her back—on the bed. Position the body in good alignment.

6. **Shoulder**. Support the client's arm at the elbow and wrist while performing ROM for the shoulder. Place one hand above the elbow and the other hand around the wrist. Move the arm upward so that the upper arm is aligned with the side of the head (forward flexion) (Fig. 15-5).

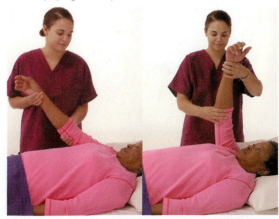

Fig. 15-5.

Move the arm downward to the side (extension) (Fig. 15-6). Return arm to side.

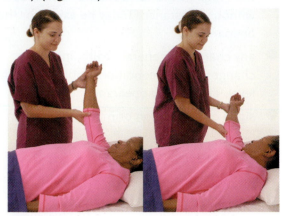

Fig. 15-6.

Bring the arm sideways away from the body to above the head (abduction) and back down to midline (adduction) (Fig. 15-7).

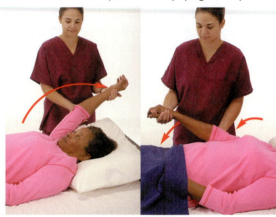

Fig. 15-7.

Bend the elbow and position it at the same level as the shoulder. Move the forearm down toward the midline of the body (internal rotation). Now move the forearm toward the head (external rotation) (Fig. 15-8).

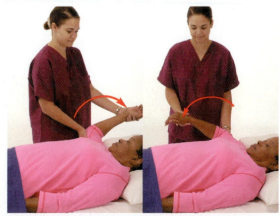

Fig. 15-8.

7. **Elbow**. Hold the client's wrist with one hand, the elbow with the other hand. Bend the elbow so that the hand touches the shoulder on that same side (flexion). Straighten the arm (extension) (Fig. 15-9).

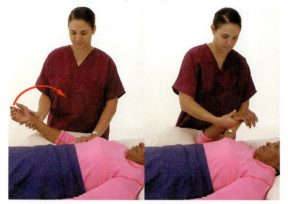

Fig. 15-9.

Exercise the forearm by moving it so the palm is facing downward (pronation) and then the palm is facing upward (supination) (Fig. 15-10).

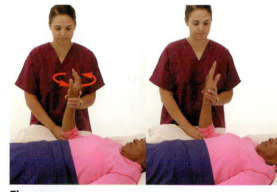

Fig. 15-10.

8. **Wrist**. Hold the wrist with one hand and use the fingers of the other hand to help the joint through the motions. Bend the hand down (flexion); bend the hand backwards (extension) (Fig. 15-11).

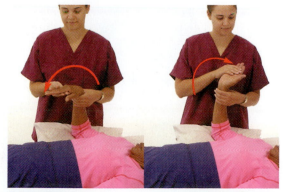

Fig. 15-11.

Turn the hand in the direction of the thumb (radial flexion). Then turn the hand in the direction of the little finger (ulnar flexion) (Fig. 15-12).

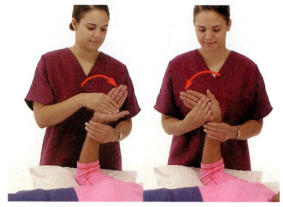

Fig. 15-12.

9. **Thumb**. Move the thumb away from the index finger (abduction). Move the thumb back next to the index finger (adduction) (Fig. 15-13).

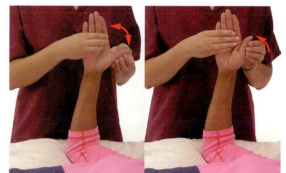

Fig. 15-13.

Touch each fingertip with the thumb (opposition) (Fig. 15-14).

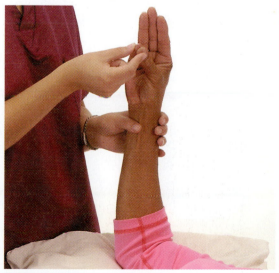

Fig 15-14

Bend thumb into the palm (flexion) and out to the side (extension) (Fig. 15-15).

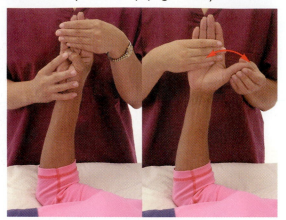

Fig. 15-15.

10. **Fingers**. Make the hand into a fist (flexion). Gently straighten out the fist (extension) (Fig. 15-16).

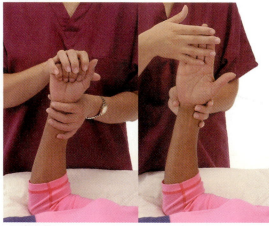

Fig. 15-16.

Spread the fingers and the thumb far apart from each other (abduction). Bring the fingers next to each other (adduction) (Fig. 15-17).

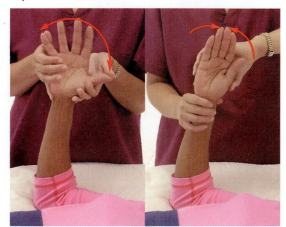

Fig. 15-17.

11. **Hip**. Support the leg by placing one hand under the knee and one under the ankle. Straighten the leg and raise it gently upward. Move the leg away from the other leg (abduction). Move the leg toward the other leg (adduction) (Fig. 15-18).

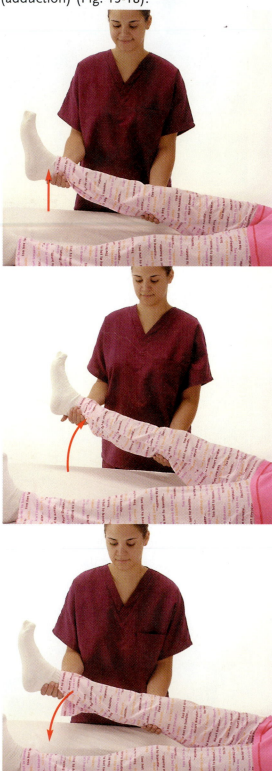

Fig. 15-18.

15

Rehabilitation and Restorative Care

Gently turn the leg inward (internal rotation), then turn the leg outward (external rotation) (Fig. 15-19).

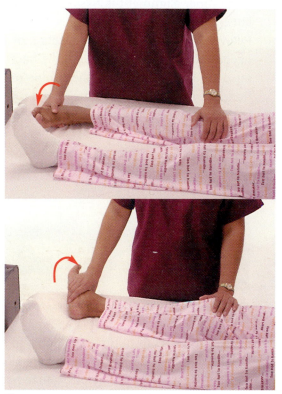

Fig. 15-19.

12. **Knees**. Bend the leg at the knee (flexion). Straighten the leg (extension) (Fig. 15-20).

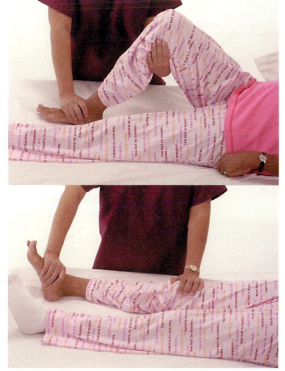

Fig. 15-20.

13. **Ankles**. Bend the foot up toward the leg (dorsiflexion). Turn the foot down away from the leg (plantar flexion) (Fig. 15-21).

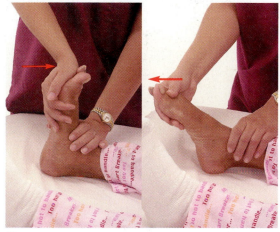

Fig. 15-21.

Turn the inside of the foot inward toward the body (supination) and the sole of the foot so that it faces away from the body (pronation) (Fig. 15-22).

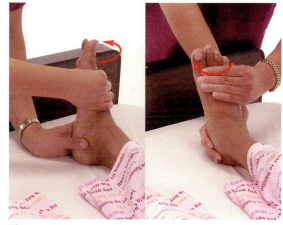

Fig. 15-22.

14. **Toes**. Curl and straighten the toes (flexion and extension) (Fig. 15-23).

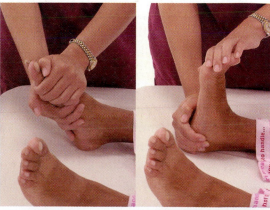

Fig. 15-23.

6. List five important observations about changes in a client's skin

Gently spread the toes apart (abduction) (Fig. 15-24).

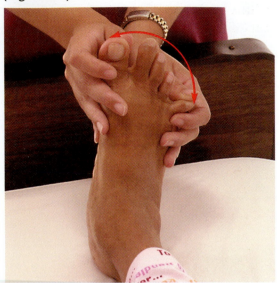

Fig. 15-24.

15. Return the client to a comfortable resting position and cover as appropriate. If you raised an adjustable bed, be sure to return it to its lowest position.

16. Wash your hands.

17. Document the procedure. Note any decrease in range of motion or any pain experienced by the client. Notify the supervisor or the physical therapist if you find increased stiffness or physical resistance. Resistance may be a sign that a contracture is developing.

Note any decrease in range of motion or any pain experienced by the client. Notify the supervisor or the physical therapist if you find increased stiffness or physical resistance. Resistance may be a sign that a contracture is developing.

5. Explain guidelines for maintaining proper body alignment

Clients who are confined to bed need to maintain good body alignment. This promotes recovery and prevents injury to muscles and joints. Chapter 12 includes specific instructions for positioning clients. The following guidelines help clients maintain good alignment and make progress when they can get out of bed.

GUIDELINES
Alignment and Positioning

⑧ Observe principles of alignment. Remember that proper alignment is based on straight lines. The spine should lie in a straight line. Pillows or rolled or folded blankets may be needed to support the small of the back and raise the knees or head in the supine position. They can support the head and one leg in the lateral position (Fig. 15-25).

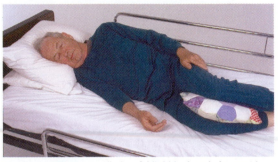

Fig. 15-25. Pillows or rolled or folded blankets help provide extra support.

⑧ Keep body parts in natural positions. In a natural hand position, the fingers are slightly curled. Use a rolled washcloth, gauze bandage, or a rubber ball inside the palm to support the fingers in this position. Use footboards to keep covers from resting on feet in the supine position.

⑧ Prevent external rotation of hips. When legs and hips are allowed to turn outward during long periods of bedrest, hip contractures can result. A rolled blanket or towel that is tucked alongside the hip and thigh can prevent the leg from turning outward.

⑧ Change positions frequently to prevent muscle stiffness and pressure ulcers. Every two hours is usually adequate. Which position the client uses will depend on the client's condition and preference. Check the skin every time you reposition the client.

6. List important observations to make about changes in a client's skin

Immobility reduces the amount of blood that circulates to the skin. Clients who have restricted mobility have increased risk of skin

deterioration at **pressure points**. Pressure points are areas of the body that bear much of the body weight. Pressure points are mainly located at bony prominences. **Bony prominences** are areas of the body where the bone lies close to the skin. These areas include elbows, shoulder blades, tailbone, hip bones, ankles, heels, and the back of the neck and head.

Other areas at risk are the ears, the area under the breasts, and the scrotum. The pressure on these areas reduces circulation, decreasing the amount of oxygen the cells receive. Warmth and moisture also contribute to skin breakdown. Once the surface of the skin is weakened, pathogens can invade and cause infection. When infection occurs, the healing process slows down.

When the skin begins to break down, it becomes pale, white or a reddened color. Darker skin may appear purple. The client may also complain of tingling or burning in the area. This discoloration does not go away, even when the client's position is changed. If pressure is allowed to continue, the area will further deteriorate, or break down. The resulting wound is called a **pressure sore**, **bed sore**, or **decubitus** (*dee-KYOO-bi-tus*) **ulcer** (Fig. 15-26). Once a

pressure sore forms, it can get bigger, deeper, and infected. Pressure sores are painful and are difficult to heal. They can lead to life-threatening infections. Prevention is very important.

OBSERVING AND REPORTING
Client's Skin

Report any of the following to your supervisor:

- pale, white, reddened, or purple areas, or blistered or bruised areas on the skin
- complaints of tingling, warmth, or burning of the skin
- dry or flaking skin
- itching or scratching
- rash or any skin discoloration
- swelling
- blisters
- fluid or blood draining from skin
- broken skin
- wounds or ulcers on the skin
- changes in an existing wound or ulcer (size, depth, drainage, color, odor)
- redness or broken skin between toes or around toenails

7. List guidelines for providing basic skin care and preventing pressure sores

The following are guidelines for basic skin care. It is important that family caregivers also understand and follow these guidelines.

GUIDELINES
Basic Skin Care

- Report changes you observe in a client's skin.

- Provide regular care for skin to keep it clean and dry. When complete baths are not given or taken every day, check the client's skin and provide skin care daily.

- Reposition immobile clients frequently (at least every two hours).

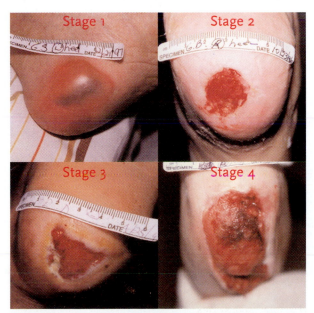

Fig. 15-26. Pressure sores are categorized by four stages. (Photos courtesy of Dr. Tamara D. Fishman and The Wound Care Institute, Inc.)

ⓖ Provide frequent and thorough skin care as often as needed for incontinent clients. Change clothing and linens often as well.

ⓖ Avoid scratching or irritating the skin in any way. Report to your supervisor if a client wears shoes or slippers that cause blisters or sores.

ⓖ Massage the skin frequently, using light, circular strokes to increase circulation. Use little or no pressure on bony areas. Do not massage a white, red, or purple area or put any pressure on it. Massage the healthy skin and tissue surrounding the area.

For clients who are confined to bed or who cannot change positions easily, remember the following points:

• Keep the bottom sheet tight and free from wrinkles and the bed free from crumbs.

• Avoid pulling the client across sheets during transfers or repositioning. This causes shearing, or pressure, when the surfaces rub against each other. Shearing can lead to skin breakdown, as explained in chapter 12.

• Place a sheepskin, chamois skin, or bed pad under the back and buttocks to absorb moisture. This also protects the skin from irritating bed linens (Fig. 15-27).

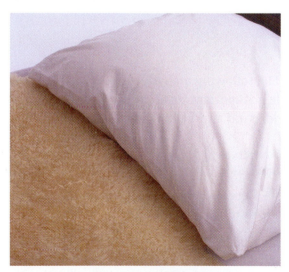

Fig. 15-27. A sheepskin or chamois skin may be placed to absorb moisture. (Photo courtesy of Briggs Corporation)

• Relieve pressure under bony prominences. Place foam rubber or sheepskin pads under

them. Heel and elbow protectors that are made of foam and sheepskin are available (Fig. 15-28).

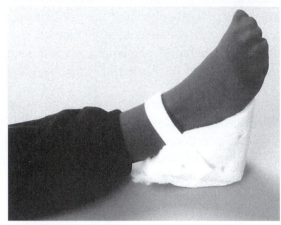

Fig. 15-28. Heel and elbow protectors can help relieve pressure under bony prominences. (Photo courtesy of Briggs Corporation)

• A bed or chair can be made softer with flotation pads or an egg crate mattress (Fig. 15-29).

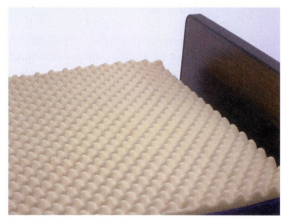

Fig. 15-29. An egg crate mattress is made of foam and is placed on top of a regular mattress.

• Use a bed cradle to keep top sheets from rubbing the client's skin. A bed cradle is made of metal or from a cardboard box (see chapter 12).

• Clients seated in chairs or wheelchairs need to be repositioned frequently, too.

8. Describe the guidelines for caring for clients who have fractures or casts

Fractures are broken bones caused by accidents or by **osteoporosis** (*os-tee-oh-poh-ROH-sis*).

Osteoporosis causes brittle bones that easily crack or break. Osteoporosis occurs more frequently in elderly people, particularly women. It may due to age, lack of hormones, a loss of calcium from the bones, alcohol consumption, or lack of exercise. Signs and symptoms of a fracture are pain, swelling, bruising, changes in skin color at the site of the fracture, and limited movement.

When bones are fractured, the sections of broken bone must be placed in alignment so the body can heal. The body can grow new bone tissue and fuse the sections of fractured bone together. The bone must be immobilized to allow this healing to occur. Immobilization is often accomplished by the use of a **cast**.

Some casts will allow the client to bear weight, and some will not. A client who has had a cast applied must wait until the cast is completely dry before bearing weight on it. A wet cast is grey, dull, cool, and smells musty. A dry cast is white, shiny, and odorless. As a cast dries, it gives off heat. This heat must be allowed to escape or it will burn the skin. Never cover a cast with any material until it has completely dried.

GUIDELINES
Caring for a Client who has a Cast

ⓖ If caring for a client who has a wet cast, do not cover the cast until it is dry. Assist the client in changing positions to allow the cast to dry evenly. Do not place the cast on a hard surface. Place it on pillows. A hard surface alters the shape of the cast. Use the palms of the hands to lift the cast. Fingers will dent it and dents will cause pressure on the client's skin.

ⓖ Elevate the extremity that is in a cast. This helps stop swelling in the injured tissue (Fig. 15-30).

ⓖ Observe the affected extremity for swelling, skin discoloration, odor, and loss of sensation or feeling cold. Compare to the extremity that does not have a cast. Report any one of these to a supervisor.

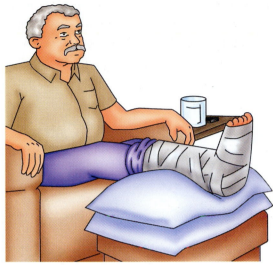
Fig. 15-30. To stop swelling, elevate the extremity that is in a cast.

ⓖ Protect the client's skin from the rough edges of the cast. The stocking that lines the inside of the cast can be pulled up and over the edges and secured with tape. Inform your supervisor if cast edges are irritating the client's skin.

ⓖ Keep the cast dry at all times. Wet casts lose their shape.

ⓖ Do not insert or allow the client to insert anything inside the cast, even when skin itches. Pointed or blunt objects may injure the skin, which is already dry and fragile. Skin can become infected under the cast.

9. List the guidelines for caring for a client who has a hip fracture

Weakened bones make hip fractures more common (Fig. 15-31). A sudden fall can result in a fractured hip that takes months to heal. Preventing falls is very important. Hip fractures can also occur because of weakened bones that fracture and then cause a fall. A hip fracture is a serious condition. The elderly heal slowly, and they are at risk for secondary illnesses and disabilities.

Most fractured hips require surgery. Total hip replacement is surgery that replaces the head of the long bone of the leg (femur) where it joins

the hip. After the surgery, the client is not able to stand on that leg while the hip heals. A physical therapist will assist after surgery. The goals of care include slowly strengthening the hip muscles and getting the client walking on that leg.

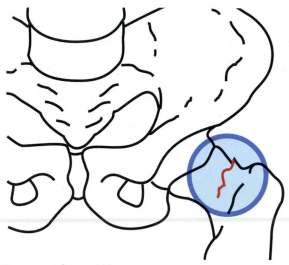

Fig. 15-31. A fractured hip.

GUIDELINES
Caring for Clients Recovering from Hip Replacements

ⓖ Keep often-used items, such as medications, telephone, tissues, call signal, and water within easy reach. Avoid placing items in high places.

ⓖ Dress starting with the affected side first.

ⓖ Never rush the client. Use praise and encouragement often. Do this even for small accomplishments.

ⓖ Have the client sit to do tasks and save his or her energy.

ⓖ Follow the care plan exactly, even if the client wants to do more than is ordered.

ⓖ Never perform ROM exercises on a leg on the side of a hip replacement unless directed by your supervisor.

ⓖ Caution the client not to sit with his or her legs crossed. The hip cannot be at less than a 90-degree angle. It cannot be turned outward (Fig. 15-32).

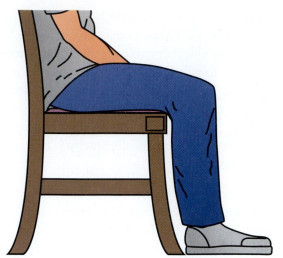

Fig. 15-32. The hip must maintain a 90-degree angle in the sitting position.

OBSERVING AND REPORTING
Hip Replacement

Report any of the following to your supervisor:

O&R if the incision is red, draining, or warm to the touch

O&R an increase in pain

O&R abnormal vital signs, especially elevated temperature

O&R if the client is unable to use equipment properly and safely

O&R if the client is not following doctor's orders for activity and exercise

O&R any problems with appetite

O&R increasing strength and improving ability to walk

A cast or traction may also be used to immobilize the hip. A client in traction will require special care that will be in the care plan. Traction assembly must never be disconnected. Good skin care and repositioning according to the care plan are essential for all clients who are immobilized. Skin will rapidly deteriorate over pressure points.

The assignment sheet and your supervisor will explain the type of care to be provided. Only provide the care that is in the client's care plan.

15

Rehabilitation and Restorative Care

10. List ways to adapt the environment for people with physical limitations

Many devices are available to assist people who are recovering from or adapting to a physical condition. Always check for hazards that could cause weak or confused clients to trip or otherwise injure themselves. For example, raised seating makes it simpler for a client with weak legs to stand. Armchairs allow a client to push with his arms to stand. Keeping frequently-used objects on low shelves may help a client avoid reaching. The items shown in Fig. 15-33 can be useful as clients relearn old skills or adapt to new limitations.

11. Identify reasons clients lose bowel or bladder control

When people cannot control the muscles of the bowels or bladder, they are said to be **incontinent** (*in-KON-ti-nent*). Incontinence can occur in clients who are confined to bed, ill, elderly,

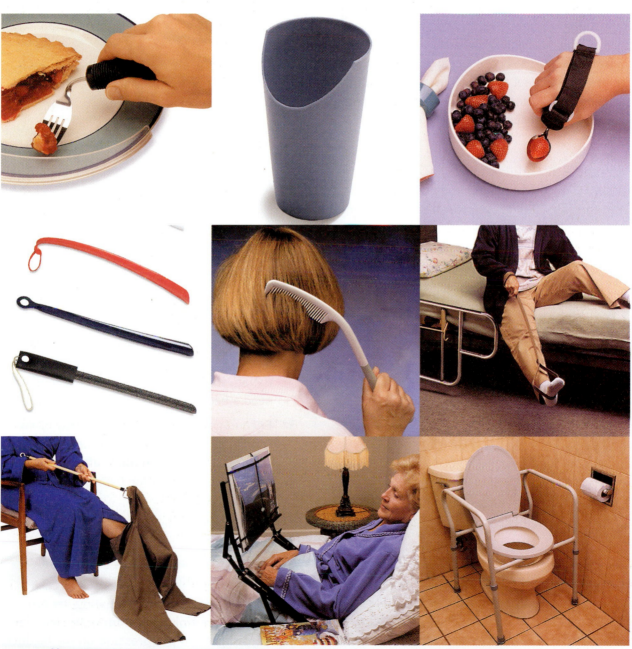

Fig. 15-33. Many adaptive items are available to help clients. (Photos courtesy of North Coast Medical, Inc. 800-821-9319)

15

Rehabilitation and Restorative Care

paralyzed, or who have circulatory or nervous system diseases or injuries. Diarrhea can also cause temporary incontinence. Incontinence is not a normal part of aging.

Clients who are incontinent need reassurance and understanding. Offer them a bedpan or take them to the bathroom more frequently. Keep them clean, dry, and free from odor. They will need good skin care as well. Urine and feces are very irritating to the skin. They should be washed off completely by bathing and good perineal care.

Clients who are confined to bed should have a plastic, latex, or disposable sheet placed under them to protect the bed. Place a draw sheet over the protective sheet to absorb moisture and protect the client's skin from the rubber or plastic. Double a regular flat sheet to make a draw sheet.

Disposable incontinence pads or briefs for adults are available to keep body wastes away from the skin (Fig. 15-34). Never refer to an incontinence brief or pad as a "diaper." Clients are not children and this is disrespectful.

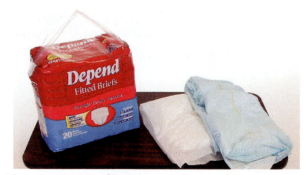

Fig. 15-34. One type of incontinence pad.

12. Explain the guidelines for assisting with bowel or bladder retraining

Clients who have had a disruption in their bowel and bladder routines from illness, injury, or inactivity may need assistance in re-establishing a regular routine and normal function. The physician may order suppositories, laxatives, stool softeners, or enemas to assist the client.

Always be professional and matter-of-fact when handling incontinence or working to re-establish routines. It is hard enough for clients to handle incontinence without having to worry about your reactions. Offer a trip to the commode or a bedpan before beginning long procedures or bathing (Fig. 15-35).

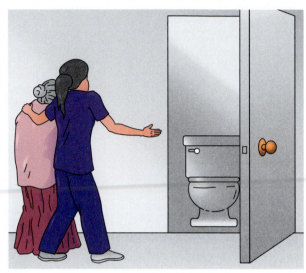

Fig. 15-35. Offer regular trips to the bathroom.

GUIDELINES
Bowel or Bladder Retraining

- Follow Standard Precautions. Wear gloves when handling body wastes.

- Explain the bowel or bladder training schedule to the client.

- Keep a record of the client's bowel and bladder habits. When you see a pattern of elimination, you can predict when the client will need a bedpan or a trip to the bathroom.

- Encourage the client to drink plenty of fluids. Do this even if urinary incontinence is a problem. About 30 minutes after fluids are taken, offer a trip to the bathroom, or a bedpan or urinal.

- Encourage the client to eat foods that are high in fiber, as appropriate or assigned. Chapter 22 provides more information on diet and nutrition.

- If a client has difficulty urinating, try running water in the sink. Have him or her lean forward slightly to put pressure on the bladder.

- ⓖ Do not rush the client.
- ⓖ Assist your client with good perineal care. This prevents skin breakdown and promotes proper hygiene. Carefully observe for skin changes.
- ⓖ Discard wastes properly according to your agency's policies.
- ⓖ Offer positive words for successes or even attempts to control bladder and bowels.
- ⓖ Never show frustration or anger toward clients who are incontinent. The problem is out of their control. Your negative reactions will only make things worse.

13. Describe the benefits of deep breathing exercises

Deep breathing exercises help expand the lungs, clearing them of mucus and preventing infections (such as pneumonia). Clients who are paralyzed or who have had abdominal surgery are often told to do deep breathing exercises regularly to expand the lungs.

The care plan may include using a deep breathing device called an **incentive spirometer** (Fig. 15-36). Do not assist with these exercises if you have not been trained. Ask your supervisor for instruction. The following procedure is intended as general instruction only.

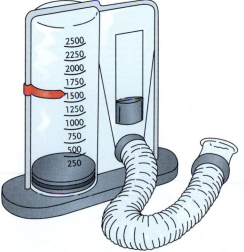

Fig. 15-36. Incentive spirometers are used for deep breathing exercises.

1. Wash your hands.
2. Explain the procedure to the client, speaking clearly, slowly, and directly, maintaining face-to-face contact whenever possible.
3. Provide privacy if the client desires it.
4. Put on a mask, eye shield, and gown as indicated by Standard Precautions. Be sure to put on a HEPA (high efficiency particulate air) or N-95 mask if the client has known or suspected tuberculosis. Deep breathing exercises may stimulate the client to cough and produce mucous.
5. Put on gloves.
6. With client sitting up, if possible, have him or her breathe in as deeply as possible through the nose. You should see the chest and then the abdomen expand and fill with air.
7. Have the client exhale through the mouth until all air is expelled.
8. Repeat this exercise five to ten times, as specified in the care plan.
9. If the client coughs or brings up mucous from the lungs during the exercise, offer the client tissues or the basin to catch the mucous.
10. Dispose of the used tissues and clean the basin.
11. Remove gloves, eye shield, mask, and gown.
12. Wash your hands.
13. Put on fresh gloves.
14. Provide mouth care as desired, and help the client return to a comfortable position.
15. Remove gloves.
16. Wash your hands again.
17. Document the procedure and any reactions you observe, including pain, prolonged coughing, and color or amount of mucous.

15

Rehabilitation and Restorative Care

Chapter Review

1. What does restorative care or rehabilitation involve?

2. In the home care rehabilitation model, who establishes the goals of care?

3. What attitudes can you adopt to assist in your clients' restorative care? Give an example of each.

4. What is the purpose of range of motion exercises?

5. Describe the difference between passive, active, and active assisted range of motion.

6. List guidelines you should follow to help clients maintain good alignment.

7. Why should you change a client's position frequently?

8. Why is prevention of pressure sores so important?

True or False. Mark each statement with either a "T" for true or "F" for false.

9. ___ You should check a client's skin only on bath days.

10. ___ It can be helpful to massage pale, white, or reddened areas of the skin.

11. ___ You should report to your supervisor if a client wears shoes or slippers that cause blisters.

12. ___ Linens should be changed no more than once a day.

13. ___ Immobile clients should be repositioned every two hours.

14. What guidelines should you follow for a client who has a cast?

15. Why is a hip fracture a serious condition for an elderly person?

16. A person recovering from a hip replacement should not sit at an angle less than how many degrees?

17. Look at the adaptive devices in Figure 15-33. Choose one and describe how it might help a client who is recovering from or adapting to a physical condition.

18. Why do incontinent clients need good skin care?

19. Why should you never refer to an incontinence brief as a "diaper?"

20. About how long after fluids are taken should you offer to take a client to the bathroom?

21. Why can it be helpful to keep track of your client's bowel or bladder habits?

22. What type of client might have been instructed to do deep breathing exercises?

16

Medications and Technology in Home Care

1. List four guidelines for safe and proper use of medications

People who need home care often need medications. Clients who have problems such as coronary artery disease, high blood pressure, and diabetes may take many drugs, all with different effects. Home health aides do not usually handle or give medications. However, you need to understand the kinds of medicine your clients may be taking. You also need to know what to do if a client experiences side effects or refuses to take medication.

GUIDELINES
Safe and Proper Use of Medications

Ⓖ Never handle or give medications unless you are specifically trained and assigned to do so. Do not touch the inside of a medicine bottle or the pills or other medicines themselves. Do not put any medication in a client's mouth. Handling or giving medication can have serious consequences. You are not trained to give medications.

Ⓖ Observe clients taking their medication. Although you cannot handle or give medication, you can remind clients to take their medications. You can also bring medication containers to clients, and provide water or food as needed to take with the medication. Always observe, report, and document as appropriate.

Ⓖ Know the difference between prescription drugs and over-the-counter drugs. Antibiotics (such as penicillin), heart drugs (such as nitroglycerin), and potent pain medication (such as codeine) are examples of prescription drugs. Aspirin or cold medications, such as decongestants, are over-the-counter drugs (Fig. 16-1).

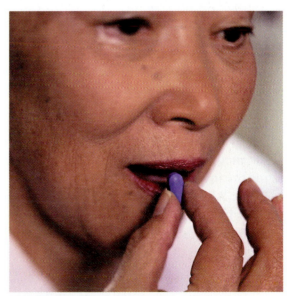

Fig. 16-1. Be aware of all medications a client is taking. Know the difference between prescription and over-the-counter medications.

Ⓖ Be aware of all medications a client is taking. There are many possible side effects and interactions among medications. Watch for symptoms such as itching, trembling or shaking, anxiety, stomachache, diarrhea, confusion, vomiting, rash, hives, or

headache. Any of these symptoms could indicate a side effect or interaction. Report any of these symptoms to your supervisor.

2. Identify the five "rights" of medications

Knowing and remembering the five "rights" of medications will help prevent mistakes.

1. **The Right Client.** Always check the label on the medication container to make sure the client's name is on it.

2. **The Right Medication.** Check the expiration date and the name of the medication before giving the container to the client. Make sure the medication name on the container matches the name listed in the care plan.

3. **The Right Time.** Make sure the instructions on the container label for what time or how often to take the medication match the instructions in the care plan.

4. **The Right Route.** Check the label for instructions on how the medication is to be taken. Make sure the instructions on the label match those in the care plan.

5. **The Right Amount.** Make sure the instructions on the container label for how much medication to take match the instructions in the care plan.

If the medication label and the care plan do not agree on any of the five "rights," call your supervisor. Also, if there is not enough information, or if you have noticed another problem with the medication (for example, the client's name is not on the container), call your supervisor.

3. Explain how to assist a client with self-administered medications

Some elderly people have a hard time remembering to take all their medications. In addition, there may be instructions to remember. Examples of instructions include taking pills with food or on an empty stomach, or drinking

plenty of fluids. Pay close attention to the medication schedule. The nurse usually sets this schedule. Become familiar with all doctors' instructions on how and when to take medications. If the specified time for a dose passes, remind the client to take the medicine. Report to your supervisor if the client does not take a medication that has been ordered.

If specified, you may be instructed to help the client with self-medication by doing any of the following:

*   Remind the client when it is time for medication.

*   Bring the bottle or container of medication to the client.

*   Provide food or water to take with the medication, as directed.

*   Observe the client taking the medication.

*   Document that the client took the medication, the time, and any other medications or food taken at the same time (Fig. 16-2).

*   Report any possible reactions to your supervisor.

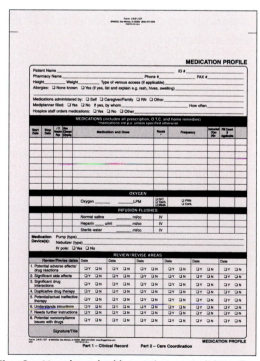

Fig. 16-2. **Many home health agencies use medication forms to help the client or aide document the client's self-medication. (Reprinted with permission of Briggs Corporation, Des Moines, Iowa, 800-247-2343)**

Some clients have reactions to certain medications, or some medications will interact with others, causing problems. To avoid these problems, document all medication that is taken. Report drugs, prescription or nonprescription, that the client takes that are not part of the care plan. Even a pill as innocent as aspirin should be noted. It is very important to report to your supervisor and document any reactions the client may have to medications.

Avoiding certain foods or substances can be important when taking certain medications. For example, drugs that have sedative or calming effects should never be mixed with alcohol. If the client does not follow these restrictions, notify your supervisor immediately. The doctor and pharmacist will inform the client and the family of any possible side effects from the medication. Be aware of what side effects to watch for. Common side effects include dizziness, drowsiness, headache, nausea and vomiting, or confusion. More serious side effects occur when there is an allergic reaction to the medication. Allergic reactions with symptoms like hives, fever, rash, or difficulty breathing, can be life-threatening. They may require emergency help.

4. Identify observations about medications that should be reported right away

If a client shows signs of a reaction to a medication, or complains of side effects, report it right away. Your supervisor can assess whether the symptom is caused by the medication. Your responsibility is to report your observations.

OBSERVING AND REPORTING
Medications

- dizziness, fainting
- nausea, vomiting
- rash, hives, itching
- difficulty breathing, swelling of throat or eyes
- drowsiness
- headache, blurred vision
- abdominal pain
- diarrhea
- any other unusual sign

In addition, report any of the following problems immediately:

- Client refuses to take medication as directed.
- Client takes the wrong dose (amount) of medication.
- Client takes medication at the wrong time.
- Client takes the wrong medication.
- A medication container is missing or empty.

5. Describe what to do in an emergency involving medications

If a client has a severe allergic reaction to a medication, takes the wrong dose, or takes medications together that cause complications, emergency medical treatment is necessary. Treat an overdose, whether it was accidental or intentional, as a poisoning. Call the local poison control number immediately. Follow their instructions. Poison control will send paramedics or an ambulance if needed.

For severe drug reactions or interactions, call 911 or 0 for emergency help. Stay with the client. Do not give any liquids, food, or other medications unless instructed to do so by emergency personnel. Notify your supervisor as soon as possible.

6. Identify methods of medication storage

You may be required to assist with the proper storage of medications. Keep the following in mind:

- Keep the client's medications in one place, separate from medicine used by other members of the household.

- If there are young children or a disoriented elderly person in the home, recommend to the family that medications be locked away.

16

Medications and Technology in Home Care

- All medications should be kept in child-proof containers if children are in the home. To avoid an accidental overdose, keep medications out of reach of children.

- If medicine requires refrigeration, make sure the bottle is on an upper shelf in the back, out of a child's reach (Fig. 16-3).

- All medications should be stored away from heat and light, as appropriate.

- The client or a family member should discard medications that have expired, are not labeled, or are discolored. Make sure these medications are not discarded in the trash. Children or animals may have access to them. Ask your supervisor for specific disposal instructions or if the client or family will not dispose of expired medications. Do not dispose of them yourself.

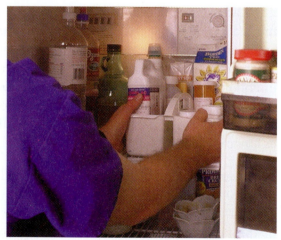

Fig. 16-3. Keep medications out of the reach of children.

7. Identify signs of drug misuse and abuse and know how to report these

Drug misuse and abuse may be accidental or deliberate. It includes the following:

- refusing to take medications

- taking the wrong dose or taking it at the wrong time

- mixing medication with alcohol

- taking drugs that have not been prescribed for the client

- taking illegal drugs

Misuse and abuse of drugs is extremely dangerous. It can even be fatal.

If your client refuses to take certain medications, explain that recovery often depends on taking the right medication. If the client still refuses, notify your supervisor. Do not push the client to take the medication. However, try to find out what is making him or her reluctant to take it. Getting the client to express uncertainties may help you get information to members of the healthcare team. A doctor or nurse can then either persuade the client to take the medication or adjust the treatment.

People may avoid taking prescribed medication because they cannot afford it or because they have difficulty getting it. Sometimes the client is confused about which drugs to take, at what hour, and in what quantities. You can help. If the client wants to know why he needs to be taking certain medications, ask the nurse or doctor to provide an explanation. People who have conditions, such as Alzheimer's disease, that affect mental function, will greatly benefit from your friendly reminders. Other reasons people do not take medicine are the dislike of side effects and difficulty swallowing the pills. These problems can be overcome once you have informed your supervisor.

Be alert to the signs of misuse or abuse and report them to your supervisor immediately.

OBSERVING AND REPORTING
Drug Misuse and Abuse

- O&R depression
- O&R anorexia
- O&R change in sleep patterns
- O&R withdrawn behavior or moodiness
- O&R secrecy
- O&R verbal abusiveness
- O&R poor relationships with family members

The drugs that pose the highest risk for causing drug dependency are pain medications and tranquilizers.

8. Demonstrate an understanding of oxygen equipment

Some clients with breathing difficulties may receive oxygen. It is more concentrated than what we breathe in the air. A doctor prescribes oxygen. You should never stop, adjust, or administer oxygen for a client. Oxygen will be delivered to the home in tanks or produced by an oxygen concentrator. An oxygen concentrator changes air in the room into air with more oxygen. The agency that supplies the oxygen will service the equipment and will provide training in its use.

Some clients receive oxygen through a **nasal cannula** (*KAN-ye-la*). A nasal cannula is a piece of plastic tubing that fits around the face and is secured by a strap that goes over the ears and around the back of the head (Fig. 16-4). The face piece has two short prongs made of tubing. These prongs fit inside the nose, and oxygen is delivered through them. A respiratory therapist fits the cannula. The length of the prongs (usually no more than half an inch) is adjusted for the client's comfort. The client can talk and eat while wearing the cannula.

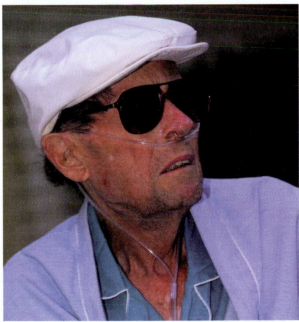

Fig. 16-4. A client with a nasal cannula.

Clients who do not need concentrated oxygen all the time may use a face mask when they need oxygen. The face mask fits over the nose and mouth. It is secured by a strap that goes over the ears and around the back of the head. It is difficult for a client to talk when wearing an oxygen face mask. The mask must be removed for the client to eat or drink anything.

Oxygen can be irritating to the nose and mouth. The strap of a nasal cannula or face mask can also cause irritation around the ears. Wash and dry skin carefully, and provide frequent mouth care. Offer the client plenty of fluids. Report and document any irritation you observe.

Oxygen is a highly **combustible** (*kom-BUS-ti-bel*) gas. This means it can very easily explode or catch fire. Working around oxygen requires special safety precautions.

GUIDELINES
Working Safely Around Oxygen

- Remove all fire hazards from the area. Fire hazards include electrical appliances, cigarettes, matches, and fluids that may catch fire easily (Fig. 16-5). Notify your supervisor if a fire hazard is present and the client does not want it removed.

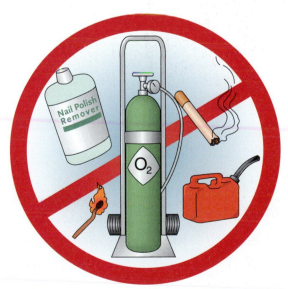

Fig. 16-5.

- Post "No Smoking" and "Oxygen in Use" signs. Never allow smoking in the room or area where oxygen is used or stored.

🅖 Never allow candles or other open flames around oxygen.

🅖 Learn how to turn oxygen off in case of fire. Never adjust oxygen level.

🅖 Report if the nasal cannula or face mask is causing skin irritation. Check behind the ears for irritation from the nasal cannula.

9. Explain guidelines for the care of a client with an IV

IV stands for **intravenous** (*in-tra-VEE-nus*), or into a vein. A client with an IV is receiving medication, nutrition, or fluids through a vein. When a physician prescribes an IV, a nurse inserts a needle into a vein. This allows direct access to the bloodstream. Medication, nutrition, or fluids either drip from a bag suspended on a pole or are pumped by a portable pump through a tube and into the vein (Fig. 16-6). Some clients with chronic conditions may have a permanent opening for IVs. This opening has been surgically created to allow easy access for IV fluids.

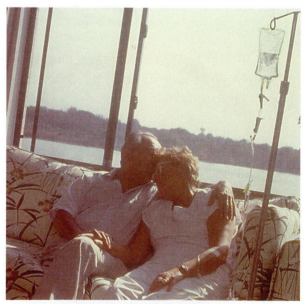

Fig. 16-6. A client receiving intravenous medication.

Home health aides never insert or remove IV lines. You will not be responsible for care of the IV site. Your only responsibility for IV care is to report and document any observations of changes or problems with the IV.

IVs

O&R The needle falls out or is removed.

O&R The dressing around the IV site is loose or not intact.

O&R Blood is in the tubing or around the site of the IV.

O&R The site is swollen or discolored.

O&R The client complains of pain.

O&R The bag is broken, or the level of fluid does not seem to decrease.

O&R The IV fluid is not dripping.

O&R The IV fluid is nearly gone.

O&R The pump beeps, indicating a problem.

O&R The pump is dropped.

As always, document your observations, your call, instructions received, and care provided.

Having an IV in place makes some basic care procedures more difficult. Always be careful not to pull or catch on IV tubing when performing or assisting with routine care of clients with IVs.

Assisting in changing clothes for a client who has an IV

Equipment: clean clothes

1. Wash your hands.

2. Explain the procedure to the client, speaking clearly, slowly, and directly, maintaining face-to-face contact whenever possible.

3. Provide privacy if the client desires it.

4. Wash your hands.

5. If the bed is adjustable, lower it as far as possible. Adjust so that client may sit with feet flat on the floor.

6. Help the client sit up at the edge of the bed, if possible.

7. Have the client remove the arm without the IV from clothing. Assist as necessary.

8. Help the client gather the clothing on the arm with the IV. Carefully lift the clothing over the IV site and move it up the tubing

toward the IV bag (Fig. 16-7).

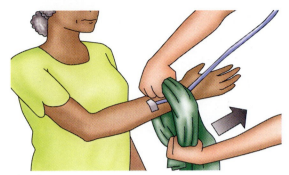

Fig. 16-7.

9. Lift the IV bag off its pole. Keep it higher than the IV site. Carefully slide the clothing over the bag. Place the IV bag back on the pole.

10. Set the used clothing aside to be placed with the soiled laundry when the client is finished changing clothes.

11. Gather the sleeve of the clean clothing.

12. Lift the IV bag off its pole and, keeping it higher than the IV site, carefully slide the clothing over the bag (Fig. 16-8). Place the IV bag back on the pole.

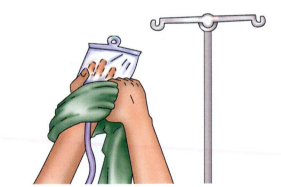

Fig. 16-8.

13. Carefully move the clean clothing down the IV tubing, over the IV site, and onto the client's arm.

14. Have the client put his other arm in the clothing. Assist as necessary.

15. Check that the IV is dripping properly. Make sure none of the tubing is dislodged and the IV site dressing is in place.

16. Assist the client with changing the rest of his clothing, as necessary.

17. Place soiled clothes in the laundry basket.

18. Adjust bed if necessary.

19. Wash your hands.

20. Document the procedure and any observations.

Chapter Review

1. What are the four guidelines for promoting the safe and proper use of medications? Briefly describe in your own words why each guideline is important.

2. List the five "rights" of medications and explain what they mean.

3. What should you do if you have noticed any problem with a patient's medication?

4. What are your duties if you are instructed to help the client with self-medication?

5. What are some signs of an allergic reaction to a medication?

6. Name some common side effects of medications.

7. List six signs you should report immediately to your supervisor that might indicate a reaction to medication.

8. How should you treat an overdose? Whom should you call?

9. What is the best place to keep medications if there are young children in the home?

10. What does drug abuse and misuse include?

11. What are two common reasons people avoid taking prescribed medication?

12. List four guidelines for working safely around oxygen equipment.

13. List seven things to observe and report about an IV.

17
Clients with Disabilities

A **disability** is the impairment of a physical or mental function. Disability may result from a disease, a complication of pregnancy, or an injury. A disability can be temporary or permanent.

Depending on the disability, a person may not be able to perform activities of daily living (ADLs). Work and social activities may be limited. People with disabilities may be more susceptible to illness. By strictly following the care plan and carefully observing and reporting, you can help your clients with disabilities avoid illness. Your efforts may also help clients lead more independent lives.

Families of people with disabilities may find it difficult to cope with the stress a disability can cause. They may feel resentment, disappointment, guilt or shame, and anger or frustration. Caring for someone with a disability can be a big responsibility. It affects a family's time, energy, patience, and financial resources. Home health aides can give family members a much-needed break (Fig. 17-1).

Clients and their families may need additional support, including counseling, to help deal with the disability. Tell your supervisor if you think a client or family member needs additional support.

Many clients with disabilities develop strong emotional attachments to their caregivers.

Clients may also become angry with caregivers.

Clients may resent being dependent or afraid of efforts to encourage independence. Be patient with clients. If a client's emotions are more than you can handle, speak to your supervisor.

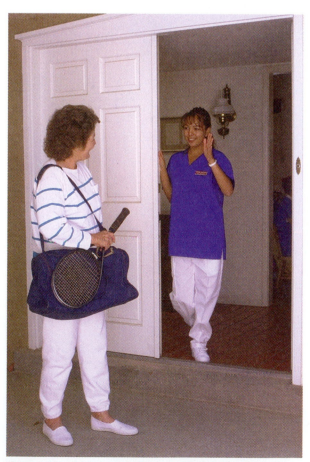

Fig. 17-1. The time a home health aide spends with a client with disabilities may be the only break a family member receives.

1. Identify common causes of disabilities

There are hundreds of diseases and disorders that may cause disability. Among them are diabetes, stroke (CVA), muscular dystrophy (*DIS-troh-fee*) or MD, congestive heart failure, AIDS, chronic obstructive pulmonary disease (COPD), Parkinson's disease, rheumatoid (*ROOM-a-toyd*) arthritis, osteoarthritis (*ah-stee-oh-ar-THRYE-tis*), and multiple sclerosis (*skler-OH-sis*, or MS).

Disabilities are also frequently caused by accidents. Head or spinal cord injuries can cause severe disabilities, including paralysis and brain damage. Accidents can also cause vision loss, hearing loss, or a number of other disabilities.

A person may be born with a disability due to a complication of pregnancy or childbirth, or because of an inherited gene. Cerebral palsy, which can cause mild to severe physical disability, can result from premature birth. Malnutrition or drug or alcohol abuse during pregnancy can cause lasting disability in babies. Down syndrome is a genetic abnormality that causes physical and mental disability.

2. Describe daily challenges a person with a disability may face

Which activities are challenging for a person with a disability depends on the disability. A person who is mentally retarded will face different challenges than a person who is confined to a wheelchair. However, any of the following activities may pose a challenge for a person with a disability:

- getting out of bed (Fig. 17-2)
- preparing or eating meals
- washing, dressing, or grooming him- or herself
- getting to the bathroom
- communicating with family, friends, or caregivers
- meeting basic human needs for acceptance, belonging, and community

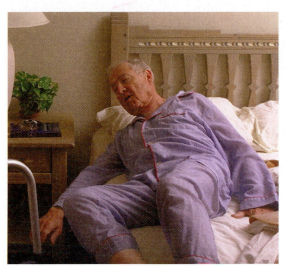

Fig. 17-2. Even getting out of bed in the morning may pose a challenge for a person with a disability.

- getting from one place to another
- finding a job or functioning in a job
- making ends meet financially

Understand that even the most basic ADLs can be challenges for a client with a disability. You can help by assisting a client with a disability to meet these challenges successfully each day.

3. Define terms related to disabilities and explain why they are important

The terms used to describe people with disabilities have changed. For example, it used to be common to call a person in a wheelchair a "cripple." Now most people find that term offensive. Some find even the term "disabled" offensive, implying that they are less competent than others. You must be sensitive to the terms used to describe your clients.

Many people with disabilities want to be viewed and described as people first, rather than identified by their disability. Thus, someone may prefer to be called "a person who is deaf" rather than "a deaf person." Someone else may prefer the term "hearing-challenged," while others may prefer "hearing-impaired."

Avoid using terms that may be offensive. Find out how your clients refer to their disability, and use those terms. Be sensitive in discussing any

Clients with Disabilities

disability. Remember, you should only discuss your clients with the care team and, if appropriate, the family.

4. Identify social and emotional needs of persons with disabilities

People with disabilities have the same social and emotional needs we all have. However, some disabilities make it more difficult to meet those needs. Understand and help meet these needs when appropriate. As discussed in chapter 8, basic social and emotional needs include:

- independence

- dignity

- social interaction

- a sense of worth

Help your clients with disabilities do all they can for themselves. Give them opportunities to show what they can do. Do not take over a task just because you can do it faster or better. The sense of independence, dignity, social interaction, and self-worth are all boosted when the client is able to perform a task for himself. On the other hand, do not push a client beyond his or her abilities. Humiliation and failure do not help fulfill social or emotional needs. Treat all clients with respect.

5. Explain how a disability may affect sexuality and intimacy

Disability can affect sexual desires, needs, and abilities. Clients may be sensitive about how an illness or injury has affected their sexuality. Remember that sexual desire may not have been lessened by a disability, although ability to meet sexual needs may have been limited. Many people confined to wheelchairs can have sexual and intimate relationships, though adjustments may have to be made. Do not assume you know what impact a physical disability has had on sexuality. Be sensitive to privacy needs. Do not judge any sexual behavior you see (Fig. 17-3).

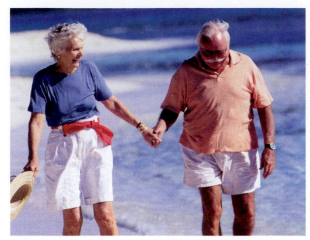

Fig. 17-3. Human beings continue to have sexual needs throughout their lives.

6. Identify skills you have already learned that can be applied to clients with disabilities

Many of the basic skills you have learned or will learn in other sections of this book apply to working with clients with disabilities:

- communication (chapter 4)

- safety and body mechanics (chapter 6)

- safe and comfortable transfers, ambulation, and body positioning (chapter 12)

- assisting with ADLs (chapter 13)

- taking vital signs and specimens (chapter 14)

- housekeeping and meal preparation (chapter 21 and chapter 23)

- skin care (chapter 15)

There are some adjustments you will make for each client. Generally, you should find that working with a client who is disabled is no different than working with any of your clients. Treat each person as an individual and with respect. You will be on your way to providing excellent care for all clients.

7. List five goals to work toward when assisting clients who have disabilities

1. **Promote self-care and independence.** Ask your client how much assistance he or she

needs to perform certain tasks. Tell your client about the goals of the care plan. Involve him or her in how assigned tasks should be performed. Ask your client about personal preferences (Fig. 17-4). Self-care and independence cannot be accomplished without the client.

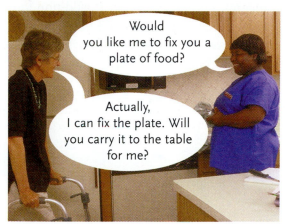

Fig. 17-4. By asking your client about personal preferences, you will find ways to promote dignity, independence, and self-care.

2. **Assure the client's safety**. Be aware of accidents that commonly occur in the home. Most can be avoided if you think ahead. Remember that each client is an individual with special needs. Think critically about each client's abilities and disabilities. Safety concerns vary depending on the disability. For example, clutter on the floor could cause falls for clients with impaired vision. Look over the home each day for things that might be unsafe. Being able to foresee problems is very important. Use good body mechanics when you are working. Encourage your clients to do the same to avoid injury (see chapter 6).

3. **Promote the client's health and comfort**. Help your clients by maintaining nutrition and hydration and by assisting with personal care. The care plan and your assignment sheet will include instructions for this type of care. To provide further comfort, watch and listen to the client. Think about how you might feel in similar situations to better anticipate your client's needs. You may see, for example, that an extra pillow under the client's arm would help keep his

shoulder from drooping. Some clients with disabilities may be unable to communicate their wishes to you.

4. **Maintain the client's dignity and self-worth**. Never discuss a client with anyone other than a member of the healthcare team or, if appropriate, the client's immediate family (see chapter 3 for more on client confidentiality). Treat a client who is disabled with the same respect you would give any client. Recognize that a person with a disability may have many feelings about his or her situation. Be sensitive to these feelings. Find ways to make your clients feel good about themselves. Remember to allow and encourage the client to direct how and when care is provided.

5. **Maintain the stability of the client's household**. Disability can disrupt the stability of a home, causing insecurity, anxiety, and disorder. You are in the home longer than any member of the healthcare team. Help maintain the stability of the household by being punctual and dependable. Respect the schedules of the family. Work cheerfully, calmly and efficiently. In addition, act as a role model by showing acceptance of and encouragement for the client.

8. Identify five qualities of excellent service needed by clients with disabilities

When asked what qualities they need and value most in home health workers, people with disabilities list the following:

1. **Punctuality**: Being on time for all scheduled visits makes a big difference to a client who needs your assistance.

2. **Reliability**: Clients with disabilities may depend on your help to meet basic needs, so being reliable is essential.

3. **Responsiveness to needs**: A client's needs may change, and you should be willing (with the approval of your supervisor) to adapt your service to be most helpful.

4. **Continuity**: Constantly changing caregivers may be disruptive or inconvenient for people with disabilities.

5. **Positive attitude**: Your cheerful and encouraging attitude is important to clients with disabilities (Fig. 17-5).

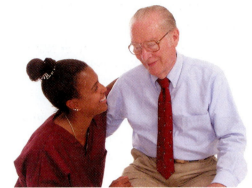

Fig. 17-5. Being cheerful and encouraging is something that will be expected of you.

9. Explain how to adapt personal care procedures to meet the needs of clients with disabilities

The guidelines below will help you understand the special needs clients with various disabilities may have. Always adapt your care to the individual client's needs. The care team works together to discover and address the needs a client may have. You will be with the client more than anyone else. It is very important to report your observations to your supervisor.

Developmental Disabilities

Developmental disabilities refer to disabilities that are present at birth or emerge during childhood. A developmental disability is a chronic condition that restricts physical or mental ability. These disabilities prevent a child from developing mentally or physically at a "normal" rate. Often, your role is to help these clients by giving family caregivers a break. Home health aides help teach clients self-care and assist with ADLs. They also provide a role model for families in dealing with the disability.

Mental Retardation. Mental retardation is the most common developmental disorder.

Approximately 1% of the general population has mental retardation. There are different degrees of mental retardation. It is neither a disease nor a psychiatric illness. People with mental retardation develop at a below-average rate. They have below-average mental functioning. They experience difficulty in learning and may have problems adjusting socially. In addition to their special needs, clients who are mentally retarded have the same emotional and physical needs that others have (Fig. 17-6).

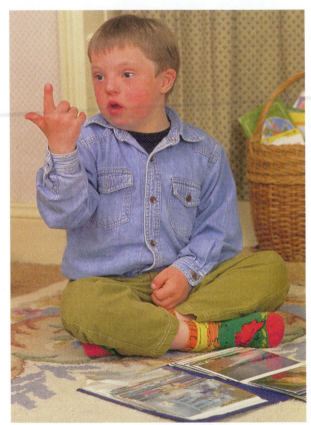

Fig. 17-6. People who are mentally retarded have the same emotional and physical needs as others do.

For clients who are mentally retarded, the main goal of care is to help the person have as normal a life as possible. For a person with mental retardation, this means recognizing her individuality, basic human rights, and physical and emotional needs, as well as special needs.

GUIDELINES
Mental Retardation

𝟡 Treat adult clients as adults, regardless of the behavior they exhibit.

- 🅖 Praise and encourage often, especially positive behavior.

- 🅖 Help teach the client to perform ADLs by dividing a task into smaller units.

- 🅖 Promote independence, but also assist clients with activities and motor functions that are difficult.

- 🅖 Encourage social interaction.

- 🅖 Repeat words you use to make sure they understand.

- 🅖 Be patient.

Down Syndrome. People who are born with Down syndrome experience different degrees of mental retardation, along with physical symptoms. A person with Down syndrome typically has a small skull, a flattened nose, short fingers, and a wider space between the first two fingers of each hand and the first two toes of each foot. As with other types of mental retardation, a person with Down syndrome can become fairly independent.

GUIDELINES
Down Syndrome

- 🅖 Provide the same type of care and instruction for a Down syndrome client as for any other person with mental retardation.

- 🅖 Praise and encourage often, especially positive behavior.

- 🅖 Help train the client to perform ADLs by dividing a task into smaller units.

Cerebral Palsy. People with cerebral palsy have suffered brain damage either while in the uterus or during birth. They may have both physical and mental disabilities. Damage to the brain stops the development of the child or causes disorganized or abnormal development. Muscle coordination and nerves are affected. People with cerebral palsy may lack control of the head, have difficulty using the arms and hands, have poor balance or posture, be either stiff and spastic or limp and flaccid, and may have speech impairment. Intelligence may also be affected.

GUIDELINES
Cerebral Palsy

- 🅖 Allow the client to move slowly. People with cerebral palsy take longer to adjust their body position and may repeat movements several times.

- 🅖 Maintain the client's body in as normal an alignment as possible.

- 🅖 Talk to the client, even if he or she cannot speak. Be patient and listen.

- 🅖 Use touch as a form of communication.

- 🅖 Avoid activities that are tiring or frustrating.

- 🅖 Be gentle when handling parts of the body that may be painful (Fig. 17-7).

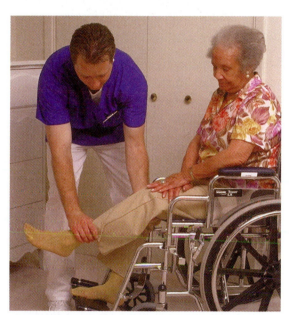

Fig. 17-7. Be gentle when moving body parts of a client who has cerebral palsy.

- 🅖 Promote independence and encourage socialization.

Spina Bifida (*spy-na BIF-e-da*). Spina bifida literally means "split spine." When part of the backbone is not well enough developed at birth, the spinal cord may bulge out of the person's back. Spina bifida can cause a range of disabilities. Some babies born with spina bifida will be able to walk and will experience no lasting disabilities. Others may be in a wheelchair and/or may have little or no bladder or bowel control. In some cases, complications of spina bifida may cause brain damage.

Clients with Disabilities

GUIDELINES
Spina Bifida

- If the client is an adult, provide assistance with range of motion exercises and ADLs. Help perform light housecleaning duties.
- If an infant or child has spina bifida, perform tasks that help the parents manage and stabilize the home.
- Be a positive role model for the family and the client in learning to deal with the client's disabilities.

Physical Disabilities

Physical disabilities that are not developmentally related are the result of disease or accident. These clients must adjust physically, as well as mentally, to a gradual or sudden loss of ability.

Muscular Dystrophy (MD) and Amyotrophic (a-me-o-TRO-fic) Lateral Sclerosis (ALS). MD refers to a number of progressive diseases that cause a variety of physical disabilities due to muscle weakness. Most forms of MD are present at birth or become apparent during childhood. Many forms of MD are very slow to progress. Often people with MD can live to middle or even late adulthood.

ALS, often called Lou Gehrig's disease, is a progressive disease that causes muscle atrophy (weakening or wasting) and eventually leads to death. A person may be diagnosed with ALS at any age. The average time a person lives with ALS is between three and five years, though some people can live longer. Physical disabilities may begin with muscle weakness in the limbs or throat. Because ALS is progressive, disabilities get worse. Eventually, people with ALS may have to breathe and be fed with the assistance of ventilators and tubes.

GUIDELINES
MD or ALS

- In the early stages of these diseases, assist with ADLs or range of motion exercises.
- In the more advanced stages, assist with skin care and positioning and perform ADLs for the client.

Multiple Sclerosis (MS). MS is a progressive disease that affects the central nervous system. Clients with MS may have widely varying abilities. Multiple sclerosis is usually diagnosed when a person is in his or her early twenties to thirties. It progresses slowly and unpredictably. Symptoms include blurred vision, tremors, poor balance, and difficulty walking. Weakness, numbness, tingling, incontinence, and behavior changes are also symptoms. MS can eventually cause blindness, contractures, and loss of function in the arms and legs.

GUIDELINES
Multiple Sclerosis

- Assist with housekeeping duties and with ADLs.
- Be patient with self-care and movement. Allow the client enough time to perform tasks.
- Prevent falls, which may be due to a lack of coordination, fatigue, and vision problems.

Parkinson's Disease. Parkinson's disease is a progressive disease. It causes a section of the brain to degenerate. It affects the muscles, causing them to become stiff. In addition, it causes stooped posture and a shuffling gait, or walk. Tremors or shaking make it very difficult for a person to perform ADLs such as eating and bathing. A person with Parkinson's may have a mask-like facial expression.

GUIDELINES
Parkinson's Disease

- Clients are at a high risk for falls. Protect clients from any unsafe areas and conditions.
- Assist with ADLs as needed.
- Encourage self-care.

Spinal Cord and Head Injuries. Diving, sports injuries, falls, car and motorcycle accidents, industrial accidents, war, and criminal violence are common causes of these injuries. Problems from these injuries range from mild confusion or temporary memory loss to coma, paralysis, and death.

Head injuries can cause permanent brain damage. Clients who have had a head injury may

have the following problems: mental retardation, personality changes, breathing problems, seizures, coma, memory loss, loss of consciousness, **paresis** (*pa-REE-sis*), and **paralysis** (*pa-RAL-a-sis*). Paresis is paralysis, or loss of ability, that affects only part of the body. Often, paresis is used to mean a weakness or loss of ability on one side of the body.

The effects of spinal cord injuries depend on the force of impact and where the spine is injured. The higher the injury on the spinal cord, the greater the loss of function. People with head and spinal cord injuries may have **paraplegia**, or loss of function of lower body and legs. These injuries may also cause **quadriplegia**, in which the person is unable to use his legs, trunk, and arms (Fig. 17-8).

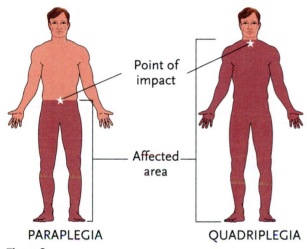

Point of impact

Affected area

PARAPLEGIA   QUADRIPLEGIA

Fig. 17-8.

Rehabilitation is necessary for clients with spinal cord injuries. It will help them to maintain muscle function that remains and to live as independently as possible. Clients will need emotional support as they adjust to their disability. Their specific needs will vary.

GUIDELINES
Head or Spinal Cord Injury

g Give emotional support, as well as physical assistance. Frustration and anger may surface as they attempt to deal with the reality of their lives. Do not take it personally.

g Safety is very important. Be very careful that clients do not fall or burn themselves.

Because clients who are paralyzed have no sensation, they are unable to feel a burn.

g Perform good skin care. It is essential to prevent pressure sores when mobility is limited.

g Assist clients to change positions every two hours to prevent pressure sores.

g Assist with range of motion exercises and bowel and bladder training if necessary.

Hearing Impairment or Deafness. Persons who have impaired hearing or are deaf may have lost their hearing gradually, or they may have been born deaf. If they have a gradual hearing loss, they may not be conscious of it. Signs of hearing loss include the following:

- speaking loudly
- leaning forward when someone is speaking
- cupping the ear to hear better
- responding inappropriately
- asking the speaker to repeat what has been said
- speaking in a monotone
- avoiding social gatherings or acting irritable in the presence of people who are having a conversation
- suspecting others of talking about them or of deliberately speaking softly

People who have hearing impairment may use a **hearing aid**, they may read lips, or use sign language. A hearing aid is a battery-operated device that amplifies sound. People with impaired hearing also closely observe the facial expressions and body language of others to add to their knowledge of what is being said.

GUIDELINES
Hearing Impairment

g If the person has a hearing aid, make sure he or she is wearing it and that it is working properly (Fig. 17-9). Wash the external ear piece daily with soap and water, and dry it thoroughly. Make sure hearing aid is positioned correctly and placed in the correct ear.

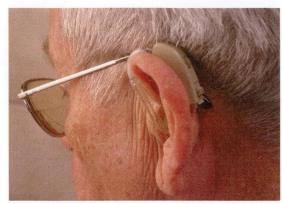

Fig. 17-9. Make sure hearing aids are turned on.

ⓖ Reduce or eliminate any background noise, such as televisions, radios, and loud speech. Close doors if you have to.

ⓖ Be sure to get the client's attention before speaking. Do not startle clients by approaching from behind. Walk in front of them or touch them lightly on the arm to let them know you are near.

ⓖ Speak clearly, slowly, and while directly facing the person (Fig. 17-10). Do not shout.

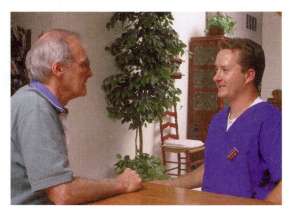

Fig. 17-10. Speak face-to-face in good light.

ⓖ Lower the pitch of your voice.

ⓖ If your client hears better out of one ear, communicate from that side.

ⓖ Use short sentences and simple words.

ⓖ Repeat words or rephrase sentences and ideas.

ⓖ Avoid long, tiring conversations.

ⓖ Be supportive.

In addition, some hearing-impaired clients have speech problems and may be difficult to understand. Do not pretend you understand if you do

not. Ask your client to repeat what was said. Observe the lips, facial expressions, and body language. Then tell your client what you think you heard. You can also request that the client write down important words.

Vision Impairment. Like hearing impairment, vision impairment can affect people of all ages. It can exist at birth or develop gradually. It can occur in one eye or in both. It can also be the result of injury, illness, or aging.

Some vision impairment causes people to wear corrective lenses. These can be contact lenses or eyeglasses. **Farsightedness** is the ability to see objects in the distance better than objects nearby. It develops in most people as they age. **Nearsightedness** is the ability to see things near but not far. It may occur in younger persons. Some people need to wear eyeglasses all the time. Others only need them to read or for activities, such as driving, that require seeing distant objects.

People over the age of 40 are at risk for developing certain serious vision problems. These include cataracts, glaucoma, and blindness. When a **cataract** develops, the lens of the eye becomes cloudy, preventing light from entering the eye (Fig. 17-11). Vision blurs and dims initially. Vision is eventually lost entirely. This disease process can occur in one or both eyes. It is corrected with surgery, in which a permanent lens implant is usually performed.

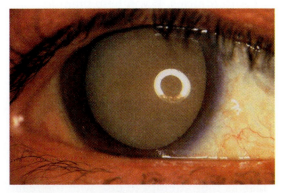

Fig. 17-11. When a cataract develops, the lens of the eye becomes cloudy. This prevents light from entering the eye.

Glaucoma is a disease that causes the pressure in the eye to increase. This eventually damages

the retina and the optic nerve. It causes blindness. Glaucoma can occur suddenly, causing severe pain, nausea, and vomiting. It can also occur gradually, with symptoms that include blurred vision, tunnel vision, and blue-green halos around lights. Glaucoma is treated with medication and sometimes surgery.

GUIDELINES
Vision Impairment

- Identify yourself immediately when you enter the room. Do not touch the client until you have said your name.
- Do not leave a room without telling your client that you are going.
- Do not change the position of furniture and other objects.
- Provide adequate lighting at all times.
- When you enter a new room with the client, orient him or her to where things are.
- Keep doors entirely open or entirely shut, never partly open.
- Use the face of an imaginary clock as a guide to explain the position of objects that are in front of the client (Fig. 17-12).

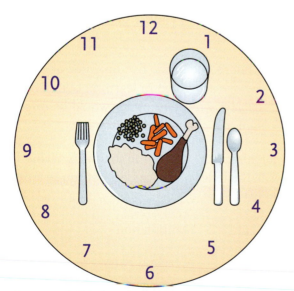

Fig. 17-12. Use the face of an imaginary clock to explain the position of objects.

- If your client needs guidance in getting around, walk slightly ahead. Let the client touch or grasp your arm lightly.

- Some clients may need assistance with cutting food and opening containers.
- Talking books (books on tape), large-print books, and Braille books are available. Learning to read Braille, however, takes a long time and requires special training.

If the client has glasses, make sure they are clean and that he or she wears them. Clean glass lenses with water and soft tissue. Clean plastic lenses with a special cleaning fluid and lens cloth. Also, make sure that glasses are in good condition and fit correctly.

If the client is able, it is best to leave contact lens care to him or her.

Amputation. Amputation is the removal of some or all of a body part, usually a foot, hand, arm or leg. Amputation may be the result of an injury or disease.

After amputation, some people feel that the limb is still there, or they feel pain in the part that has been amputated. This is called "**phantom sensation.**" It may persist for a short time or for several years. The pain or sensation, which is caused by remaining nerve endings, is real. It should not be ignored or ridiculed.

GUIDELINES
Amputation

- Clients who have had a body part amputated must make many physical, psychological, social, and occupational adjustments to their disability. Be supportive.
- Assist clients in performing their ADLs.
- You may also be trained by your supervisor to help clients use a **prosthesis**, or artificial limb (Fig. 17-13).
- Observe the skin on stump for signs of skin breakdown caused by pressure and abrasion. Report any redness or open areas.
- Keep a prosthesis and the skin under it dry and clean.
- Never try to repair a prosthesis. Report any problems with it to your supervisor.

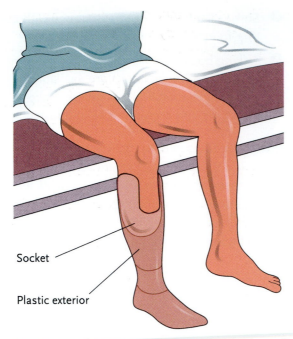

Socket

Plastic exterior

Fig. 17-13. Prostheses are specially fitted, expensive pieces of equipment.

- 🄶 Never display negative feelings regarding the stump during care.
- 🄶 Take care when handling a prosthesis. They are very expensive.

10. List important changes to report and document about for a client with disabilities

Again, each client is an individual and will have different abilities. As with any client, report changes to your supervisor and document it in your notes. For example, if a client with some vision impairment is suddenly unable to see anything, report this immediately.

Be very careful to observe and report changes in the skin. This is particularly true for clients with disabilities that affect mobility. Pressure sore prevention is an important role of the home health aide.

Emotional changes should also be observed and reported. Clients may be at risk for depression. Report any signs of depression, including moodiness, weight loss or gain, fatigue, or withdrawal.

Chapter Review

1. Name three reasons a person may be born with a disability.

2. Do you know anyone with a disability? What are his or her daily challenges?

3. Why is it important to be aware of and sensitive to your clients' preferred terms for referring to their disabilities?

4. Why should you not take over a task for a disabled client when you know you could do it better and faster?

True or False. Mark each statement with either a "T" for true or "F" for false.

5. ___ Clients may be sensitive about how an injury has affected their sexuality.

6. ___ People confined to wheelchairs cannot have sexual relationships.

7. Is working with a disabled client dramatically different from working with other clients?

8. Describe one thing you can do to promote each of the five goals outlined in learning objective 7.

9. Choose one of the five qualities of excellent service described in learning objective 8 and explain why you think it would be important to a client with a disability.

Matching. For each of the following terms, write the letter of the correct definition from the list below.

10. _____ Amputation

11. _____ Cerebral Palsy

12. _____ Down Syndrome

13. _____ Farsightedness

14. _____ Glaucoma

15. _____   Hearing Impairment

16. _____   Mental Retardation

17. _____   Multiple Sclerosis

18. _____   Muscular Dystrophy

19. ____   Nearsightedness

20. ____   Parkinson's disease

21. ____   Spina Bifida

22. ____   Spinal Cord Injury

a.   This disability comes from suffering brain damage in the uterus or during birth. Development is abnormal, and muscle coordination and nerves are affected.

b.   This disability occurs when the backbone is not well enough developed at birth, and the spinal cord may bulge out of the person's back. In some cases, it may cause brain damage.

c.   This condition causes below-average intellectual abilities, though there are different degrees of it. Children may be slow to develop.

d.   People with this disability experience different degrees of mental retardation. They typically have a small skull, flattened nose, and short fingers.

e.   This disability depends on the severity of trauma suffered by the client. Quadriplegia and paraplegia are examples.

f.   This is the ability to see objects nearby better than objects in the distance.

g.   People with this disability may use a hearing aid, read lips, or use sign language.

h.   This is a progressive disease affecting the central nervous system. It is usually diagnosed in a person's early 20s or 30s.

i.   This disease causes pressure in the eye to increase, thereby damaging the retina and optic nerve. It eventually causes blindness.

j.   This refers to a number of progressive diseases that cause a variety of physical disabilities. Most forms are present at birth.

k.   This is the ability to see objects in the distance better than objects nearby.

l.   This is the removal of some or all of a body part, resulting from an accident or because the body part is badly diseased.

m.   This is a progressive disease of the nervous system. It causes a shuffling gait and tremors.

23. Why is it important to observe a client's skin changes?

24. Why should any emotional changes in a client be reported?

18

Mental Health and Mental Illness

1. Identify five characteristics of mental health

Mental health is the normal functioning of emotional and intellectual abilities. Characteristics of a person who is mentally healthy include the abilities to

- get along with others (Fig. 18-1)
- adapt to change, care for self and others, and give and accept love
- deal with situations that cause anxiety, disappointment, and frustration
- take responsibility for decisions, feelings, and actions
- control and fulfill desires and impulses appropriately

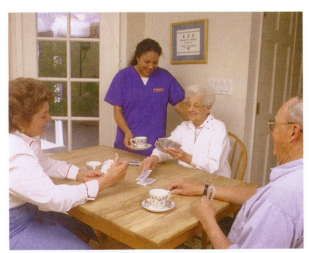

Fig. 18-1. The ability to interact well with other people is a characteristic of mental health.

2. Identify four causes of mental illness

Although it involves the emotions and mental functions, **mental illness** is a disease. It is similar to any physical disease. It produces signs and symptoms and affects the body's ability to function. It responds to appropriate treatment and care. Mental illness disrupts a person's ability to function at a normal level in the family, home, or community. It often produces inappropriate behavior. Some signs and symptoms of mental illness include confusion, disorientation, agitation, and anxiety.

However, signs and symptoms like those of mental illness can occur when mental illness is not present. A personal crisis, temporary physical changes in the brain, side effects from medications, interactions among medications, and severe change in the environment may cause a **situation response**. In a situation response, the signs and symptoms are temporary.

Mental illness can be caused or made worse by chronic stress from any of the following conditions:

1. **Physical factors.** Physical illness, disability, or aging can cause stress that may lead to mental illness. Substance abuse or a chemical imbalance can also lead to mental illness. Self-respect and self-worth are the building blocks of mental health. They are

challenged when ill or disabled people have difficulty with their activities of daily living (ADLs). They may become fearful of the future. They may be concerned about their dependency on others.

2. **Environmental factors**. Weak interpersonal or family relationships, or traumatic early life experiences (such as suffering abuse as a child) can lead to mental illness.

3. **Heredity**. Mental illness can occur repeatedly in some families. This may be due to inherited traits or family influence.

4. **Stress**. Different people can tolerate different levels of stress. People have different ways of coping with stress. When the amount of stress becomes too great and a person cannot cope with it, mental illness may arise.

3. Distinguish between fact and fallacy concerning mental illness

A **fallacy** (*FAL-a-see*) is a false belief. The greatest fallacy about mental illness is that people who are mentally ill can control it. Mentally ill people cannot simply choose to be well. Mental illness is a disease like any other physical illness. Mentally healthy people are able to control their emotions and responses. Mentally ill people usually do not have this control. Knowing mental illness is a disease helps you work with mentally ill clients.

> **Fact**: Mental illness is a disease like any physical illness. People with mental illness cannot control their illness.
>
> **Fallacy**: People with mental illness can control their illness or choose to be well.

4. Explain the connection between mental and physical wellness

Mental health is important to physical health. The ability of mentally healthy people to reduce

stress can help prevent some physical illnesses (Fig. 18-2). It can help them cope if illness or disability occur. Mental health can help protect and improve physical health. The reverse is also true. Physical illness or disability can cause or worsen mental illness. The stress these conditions create takes a toll on mental health.

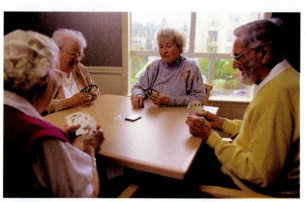

Fig. 18-2. Social interaction can promote mental and physical health.

5. List guidelines for communicating with mentally ill clients

Different types of mental illness will determine how well clients are able to communicate. Treat each client as an individual. Tailor your style of communication to the situation. Use the following guidelines to communicate with clients who are mentally ill (Fig. 18-3).

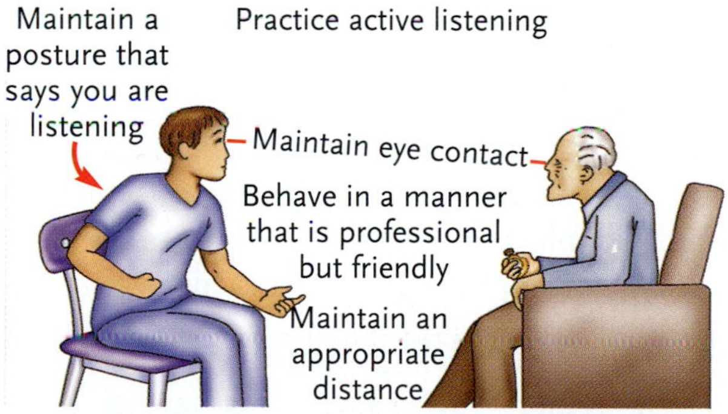

Maintain a posture that says you are listening

Practice active listening

Maintain eye contact

Behave in a manner that is professional but friendly

Maintain an appropriate distance

Fig. 18-3. Practice good communication skills with mentally ill clients.

GUIDELINES
Mental Illness

🅖 Do not talk to adults as if they were children.

🅖 Use simple, clear statements and a normal tone of voice.

Mental Health and Mental Illness

18

ⓖ Be sure that what you say and how you say it show respect and concern.

ⓖ Sit or stand at a normal distance from the client. Be aware of your body language.

ⓖ Be honest and straightforward, as you would with any client.

ⓖ Avoid arguments.

ⓖ Maintain eye contact.

ⓖ Listen carefully.

6. Identify and define common defense mechanisms

Defense mechanisms are unconscious behaviors used to release tension or cope with stress. They help to block uncomfortable or threatening feelings. All people use defense mechanisms at times. However, people who are mentally ill use them to a greater degree. An overuse of these mechanisms prevents a person from understanding their emotional problems and behaviors. If a person is unable to recognize problems, he or she will not address them. The problems may get worse.

Common defense mechanisms are listed below:

Denial: Completely rejecting the thought or feeling—"I'm not upset with you!"

Projection: Seeing feelings in others that are really one's own—"My teacher hates me."

Displacement: Transferring a strong negative feeling to a safer situation. For example, an unhappy employee cannot yell at his boss for fear of losing his job. He later yells at his wife.

Rationalization: Making excuses to justify a situation—After stealing something, saying "Everybody does it."

Repression: Blocking unacceptable thoughts or painful feelings from the mind—For example, not remembering sexual abuse.

Regression: Going back to an old, usually immature behavior—For example, throwing a temper tantrum as an adult.

7. Describe the symptoms of anxiety, depression, and schizophrenia

There are many degrees of mental illness, from mild to severe. A person with severe mental illness may lose touch with reality and become unable to communicate or make everyday decisions. Some people with mild mental illness, however, seem to function normally. They may sometimes become overwhelmed by stress or unreasonably emotional. Many symptoms of mental illness are simply extreme behaviors most people occasionally experience. Being able to recognize such behavior may make it easier to understand clients who are mentally ill.

Anxiety-related Disorders. Anxiety (*ang-ZYE-i-tee*) is uneasiness or fear, often about a situation or condition. When a mentally healthy person feels anxiety, he or she can usually identify the cause. The anxiety fades once the cause is removed. A mentally ill person may feel anxiety all the time. He or she may not know the reason for feeling anxious. Physical symptoms of anxiety-related disorders include shakiness, muscle aches, sweating, cold and clammy hands, dizziness, fatigue, racing heart, cold or hot flashes, a choking or smothering sensation, or a dry mouth (Fig. 18-4).

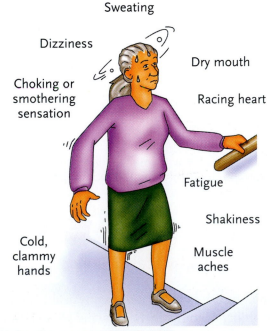

Sweating

Dizziness

Dry mouth

Choking or smothering sensation

Racing heart

Fatigue

Shakiness

Cold, clammy hands

Muscle aches

Fig. 18-4. **Common symptoms of anxiety.**

Phobias (*FOH-bee-uhs*) are an intense form of anxiety. Many people are very afraid of certain things or situations. Examples include being afraid of dogs or being afraid of flying. For a mentally ill person, a phobia is a disabling terror. It prevents the person from participating in normal activities. For example, the fear of being in a confined space, **claustrophobia** (*claws-tro-FOH-bee-a*), may make using an elevator a terrifying experience.

Other types of anxiety-related disorders include **panic disorder**, in which a person is terrified for no apparent reason. **Obsessive compulsive disorder** is the name for obsessive behavior a person uses to cope with anxiety. For example, a person may wash his hands over and over again as a way of dealing with guilt. Anxiety-related disorders may also be brought on by a traumatic experience. This type of anxiety is known as **post traumatic stress disorder**.

Depression. Clinical depression is a serious mental illness. It may cause intense mental, emotional, and physical pain and disability. Depression also makes other illnesses worse. If left untreated, it may result in suicide. The National Institute of Mental Health lists depression as one of the most common conditions associated with suicide in older adults.

Clinical depression is not a normal reaction to stress. Sadness is only one sign of this illness. Not all people who have depression complain of sadness or appear sad. Other common symptoms of clinical depression include (Fig. 18-5)

- pain, including headaches, abdominal pain, and other body aches
- low energy or fatigue
- **apathy** (*A-pah-thee*), or lack of interest in activities
- irritability
- anxiety
- loss of appetite
- problems with sexual functioning and desire
- sleeplessness, difficulty sleeping, or excessive sleeping

- guilt
- difficulty concentrating
- repeated thoughts of suicide and death

Depression can occur in conjunction with other illnesses. Common examples are cancer, HIV or AIDS, Alzheimer's disease, and diabetes. Depression is very common in the elderly population.

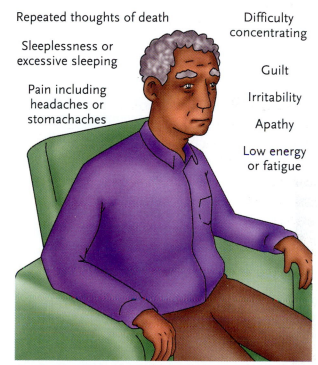

Fig. 18-5. Common symptoms of clinical depression.

There are different types and degrees of depression. **Major depression** may cause a person to lose interest in everything he once cared about. **Manic depression** causes a person to swing from periods of deep depression to periods of extreme activity. Characteristics of these episodes include high energy, little sleep, big speeches, rapidly changing thoughts and moods, inflated self-esteem, overspending, and poor judgment.

People cannot overcome depression through sheer will. Depression is an illness like any other illness. It can be treated very successfully. People who suffer from depression need compassion and support. Know the symptoms so that you can recognize the beginning or worsening of depression. Any suicide threat should

18

Mental Health and Mental Illness

be taken seriously and reported immediately. It should not be regarded as an attempt to get attention.

Schizophrenia (*skit-zo-FRAY-nee-a*). Contrary to popular belief, schizophrenia does not mean "split personality." Schizophrenia is a brain disorder that affects a person's ability to think and communicate clearly. It also affects the ability to manage emotions, make decisions, and understand reality. Treatment makes it possible for many people to lead relatively normal lives.

Some of the symptoms of schizophrenia are easy to observe (Fig. 18-6). **Hallucinations** (*ha-loo-sin-AY-shuns*) are illusions a person sees or hears. A person may see someone or something that is not really there, or hear a conversation that is not real. **Delusions** (*de-LOO-zhuns*) are persistent false beliefs. For example, a person may believe that other people are reading his thoughts. **Paranoid** (*PAIR-a-noyd*) **schizophrenia** is a form of the disease that centers mainly on hallucinations and delusions. Not all cases of hallucinations or delusions are related to schizophrenia.

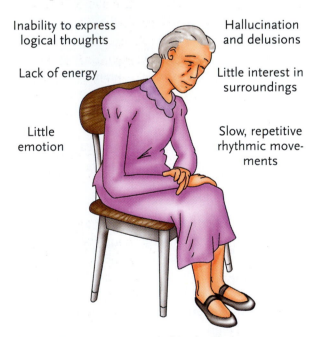

Inability to express logical thoughts

Lack of energy

Little emotion

Hallucination and delusions

Little interest in surroundings

Slow, repetitive rhythmic movements

Fig. 18-6. Common symptoms of schizophrenia.

Other symptoms of schizophrenia include disorganized thinking and speech. This makes a person unable to express logical thoughts.

Disorganized behavior means a person moves slowly, repeating gestures or movements. People with schizophrenia may also show less emotion. They may seem to have less interest in the things around them, and have a lack of energy.

8. Explain how medications can help a client who is mentally ill

It is extremely important to remember that mental illness can be treated. Medication and psychotherapy are common treatment methods. Medication can have a very positive effect. It may allow mentally ill people to function more completely.

Drugs used to treat mental illness must be taken properly to promote benefits and reduce side effects. HHAs may be assigned to observe clients taking their medications.

9. Explain your role in caring for clients who are mentally ill

Personal care of clients who are mentally ill is similar to care for any client. The care plan will tell you what care to perform. You will also have some special responsibilities, including the following guidelines:

GUIDELINES
Caring for Mentally Ill Clients

- Observe clients carefully for changes in condition or abilities. Document and report your observations.

- Support the client and the family. Coping with mental illness can be very frustrating. Your positive, professional attitude encourages the client and the family. If you need help coping with the stress of caring for someone who is mentally ill, speak to your supervisor.

- Encourage clients to do as much as possible for themselves. Progress toward independence may be very slow. Be patient, supportive, and positive.

g Help preserve the mentally ill client's role and authority in the family. Remember that you are not replacing the client. You are only filling in until the client is well enough to resume his or her role in the family.

Abilities vary among people who are mentally ill. Clients should do as much as possible for themselves. However, a stable home environment is important in managing many forms of mental illness. By assisting the family with meeting their basic needs, you help the recovery process. This is true even if your care is not physically directed to the recovering person. For example, knowing that their children are being well cared for can greatly assist persons being treated for depression. You may be assigned to provide the following services:

- food shopping, meal planning, and preparation

- housecleaning and laundry

- assistance with ADLs and personal care such as bathing

- caring for children and other family members

10. Identify important observations that should be made and reported

Carefully observe your clients. Do not draw conclusions about the cause of the behavior. Report the facts of your observations, including what you saw or heard, how long the behavior lasted, and how frequently it occurred.

OBSERVING AND REPORTING
Mentally Ill Residents

- changes in ability

- positive or negative mood changes, especially withdrawal (Fig. 18-7)

- behavior changes, including changes in personality, extreme behavior, and behavior that does not seem appropriate to the situation

- comments, even jokes, about hurting self or others

- failure to take medicine or improper use of medicine

- real or imagined physical symptoms

- events, situations, or people that seem to upset or excite clients

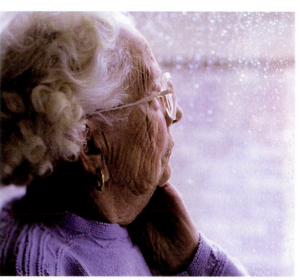

Fig. 18-7. Withdrawal is an important change to report.

11. List the signs of substance abuse

Substance abuse refers to the use of legal or illegal drugs, cigarettes, or alcohol in a way that is harmful to oneself or others. It is not necessary for a substance to be illegal for it to be abused (Fig. 18-8). Alcohol and cigarettes are legal for adults, but are often abused. Over-the-counter medications including diet aids and decongestants can be addictive and harmful. Even household substances such as paint or glue are abused, causing injury and death.

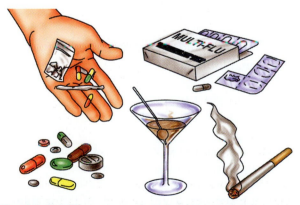

Fig. 18-8. Illegal drugs are not the only substances that are abused.

You may be in a position to observe the signs of substance abuse in your clients, their children, or other family members. Report these signs to your supervisor. You can report your observations without accusing anyone of abuse. Simply report what you see, not what you think the cause may be.

OBSERVING AND REPORTING
Substance Abuse

- O&R changes in personality, moodiness, strange behavior, disruption of routines
- O&R changes in physical appearance (red eyes, dilated pupils, weight loss)
- O&R odor of cigarettes, liquor, or other substances on breath or clothes
- O&R diminished sense of smell
- O&R loss of appetite
- O&R inability to function normally at school or work
- O&R need for money, or money missing from the home
- O&R alcohol or cigarettes missing from the home
- O&R new friends or companions, strange phone calls

Chapter Review

1. For each of the five characteristics of mental health, give one example of behavior that demonstrates the characteristic.

2. What are four possible causes of mental illness?

3. What is the most common fallacy about mental illness?

4. Why might a physical illness cause or make worse a mental illness?

5. List each of the defense mechanisms described in learning objective 6.

6. List three symptoms of each of the mental illnesses described in learning objective 7.

7. What are the most common treatments for mental illness?

8. List three care guidelines for mentally ill clients.

9. Why is assisting with home management helpful to a mentally ill client?

10. List five important observations to make about a mentally ill client.

True or False. Mark each statement with either a "T" for true or "F" for false.

11. ___ Because cigarettes and alcohol are legal, they cannot be abused.

12. ___ Some household substances are abused.

13. ___ If you suspect substance abuse, you have no choice but to directly accuse the abuser.

14. ___ If your client's teenage daughter often smells of alcohol and has a new set of friends, the best thing you can do is to stay out of it and say nothing.

19

New Mothers, Infants and Children

1. Explain the growth of home care for new mothers and infants

New mothers and their babies used to stay in the hospital for several days after delivery. Today, new restrictions by insurers and the popularity of natural childbirth techniques have changed that. Many new mothers and their babies are sent home as early as 24 hours after an uncomplicated delivery. Thus, new mothers today return home more tired and uncomfortable. They are less confident feeding and handling their babies when than women were in the past. Home care helps ease the transition from hospital to home. It allows the mother to rest and recover.

Home health aides also assist with household management when an expectant mother is put on **bed rest** by her doctor. Bed rest is ordered if a woman shows signs of early labor, has a history of miscarriage or premature deliveries, or is extremely ill. Stopping all activity and staying in bed helps prevent labor from starting before the baby is ready to be born. An expectant mother may have to stay mostly in bed for a period of a few weeks up to a few months.

2. Identify common neonatal disorders

Neonatal (*nee-oh-NAY-tal*) is the medical term

for newborn. Doctors who specialize in caring for newborn babies are called **neonatologists** (*nee-o-nay-TAH-loh-jists*). A newborn baby is sometimes called a **neonate** (*NEE-oh-nayt*).

While most babies are born healthy, some babies are born with diseases or disorders that require special care. Babies born prematurely or at low birth weight, or who are injured during birth, will also need special care.

The most common neonatal disorders include the following:

- prematurity (birth more than three weeks before due date)
- low birth weight
- cerebral palsy
- cystic fibrosis
- Down syndrome
- viral or bacterial infections
- susceptibility to sudden infant death syndrome (SIDS)

3. Identify ways of assisting a new mother with her transition to the home

Care for a new mother will be spelled out in the care plan. Each situation will be different. The care needed will depend on the mother's condi-

tion, the baby's condition, and the situation in the home. Care will depend on how much support the mother has from her husband, family, or others.

A new mother may need the following types of assistance:

- basic care for the baby: feeding, diapering, bathing

- basic care for herself: rest, meal preparation, and comfort measures such as heat, ice, or sitz baths

- light housekeeping and laundry

- care of older children

- meal planning and shopping for the family

In some cases, special care for the mother or baby may be needed. You may be asked to assist the mother in caring for a **cesarean section** (*se-SAYR-ee-an*) incision or an **episiotomy** (*e-pee-zee-AHT-o-mee*). A cesarean section is a birthing procedure in which the baby is delivered through an incision in the mother's abdomen. An episiotomy is an incision sometimes made in the perineal area during vaginal delivery.

If the baby is on a monitor (for pulse and respiration) or receiving oxygen, you may be asked to monitor the equipment. Sometimes, a new mother needs help in establishing or continuing breastfeeding.

4. List important observations to report and document

Your supervisor should instruct you about observations to make. You may be documenting the baby's or the mother's vital signs regularly. You may also be documenting how much and how often the baby eats, how long the baby nurses, the baby's sleeping patterns, and how many diapers are changed.

Document and/or report any observations that seem important to you. In addition, pay attention to the following:

The home: Is it clean, healthy, and safe?

The family: Are older children maintaining their regular routines? Do the husband and other family members know how they can help?

The mother: Is she able to rest? Does she seem to be handling everything? Is she depressed, crying, or moody? Watch for signs of **postpartum** (after birth) **depression**, similar to signs of depression described in chapter 18.

The baby: Is the baby eating regularly, wetting and soiling the diapers, and sleeping well? Does the baby have good color?

The baby's room or space: Is there a safe place for the baby to sleep? Is the crib, bassinet, or bed free of pillows or excess bedding that could cause suffocation? Is the room temperature comfortably warm?

5. Explain guidelines for safely handling a baby

Wash your hands thoroughly before touching a baby or any baby supplies. Preventing the spread of germs is extremely important around a newborn baby. See that all visitors and family members wash their hands frequently, especially before touching or holding the baby. People with colds or signs of illness should stay away from a newborn, or wear a mask to prevent transmission of disease.

Always lift and hold a baby safely, according to the procedure below. Newborn babies cannot hold their heads up without assistance. Leaving the head unsupported can cause injury. Be sure all visitors and family members hold the baby safely.

Never leave a baby in an unsafe location or position. **The only safe place to leave a baby is in a crib with the side rails up or in an adult's arms.** Do not leave babies in swings, carriers, seats or on blankets on the floor unless you can see them at all times. Never put seats, swings or carriers on tables, chairs, or countertops. Even

when changing a baby's diaper, never leave the baby on a table or countertop without keeping at least one hand on the baby at all times. Letting go, even for one second, can be dangerous. Never leave a baby or any child alone in a bath.

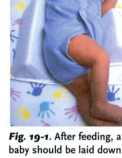

Never put a baby down on his or her abdomen if the baby is too young to lift its head to breathe. Babies should be placed on their backs or propped on their sides with a rolled blanket or towel (Fig. 19-1). The side position is best after a feeding in case the baby vomits.

Fig. 19-1. After feeding, a baby should be laid down on its side. A rolled towel or blanket should be placed behind the baby's back for support.

Crib mattresses should be firm. Infants should not be placed on a blanket, comforter, pillow, or sheepskin. These items can cause suffocation and may contribute to SIDS, which occurs when a baby stops breathing and dies.

Supervise older children and pets around babies. Jealousy can cause even well-behaved children and pets to harm babies. Older children may not mean to hurt a baby, but may not know how to touch or handle a baby.

Picking up and holding a baby

1. Wash your hands.

2. Reach one hand under the baby and behind his head and neck. Cradle the head and neck in your hand. Support the head at all times when lifting or holding a newborn.

3. With the other hand, support the baby's back and bottom (Fig. 19-2).

4. There are several ways to hold a baby safely: the **cradle hold**, the **football hold**, and **upright** against your chest (Figs. 19-2 through 19-4). Always be sure the baby's head and neck are supported.

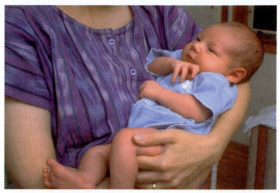

Fig. 19-2. The cradle hold is with the baby's head and neck resting in the crook of one elbow and the legs in the other arm. You must support the baby's back with one or both hands.

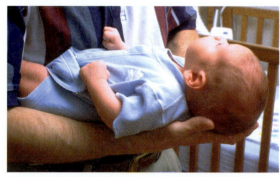

Fig. 19-3. The football hold is accomplished by holding the baby's head in one hand and supporting the baby's back with the arm on the same side of your body. The baby's body will lie along the side of your body.

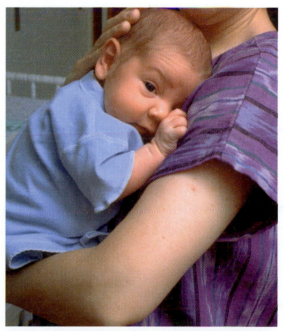

Fig. 19-4. When holding a baby upright against your chest, you must support the baby's head, neck, and back with one hand while keeping the other arm under the baby's bottom to support its weight.

19

New Mothers, Infants, and Children

6. Describe guidelines for assisting with feeding a baby

Assisting with Breastfeeding

Many pediatricians encourage mothers to breastfeed, or nurse, their babies. Breastfeeding provides the perfect nutrition for infants. The decision to breast- or bottle feed is a personal one that each mother must make for herself. If a mother chooses to try breastfeeding, she may need support while learning how to breastfeed. Many professionals recommend that women try breastfeeding for two weeks before deciding whether to continue or stop. The first two weeks may be challenging for the mother. Your support can help her get off to a good start.

Discuss with the mother how much help she wants or needs. Ask her questions to determine her experience with and knowledge of breastfeeding: Did you breastfeed your other children? If yes, for how long? If no, what made you decide to do so now? Did the nurses in the hospital teach you about breastfeeding? Did you take any newborn classes before delivery? The mother may only want you to help her get into position. Or, she may need your coaching throughout the process. Make sure she knows that breastfeeding consultants can help solve breastfeeding problems. Report any problems you observe or the client shares with you.

Women have different breastfeeding styles. Some are very comfortable and will nurse anytime, in the presence of others. Others may want more privacy while nursing. Be sensitive to individual preferences. A calm setting where the mother can relax will help her body provide the most milk for the baby.

GUIDELINES
Helping a Mother with Breastfeeding

ⓖ Remind the mother to wash her hands. Help her get in position for breastfeeding, usually sitting upright in a comfortable chair or in bed supported by pillows. Provide a low footrest if possible, and a pillow for the

mother's lap (Fig. 19-5). Some mothers are able to breastfeed while lying down. Others, however, find this more difficult, especially with a newborn baby.

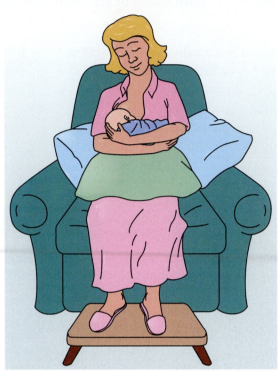

Fig. 19-5. A new mother usually prefers to nurse in an upright, sitting position. Provide support with pillows and a footrest.

ⓖ Provide for privacy. Close the door and occupy older children if necessary.

ⓖ Change the baby's diaper if necessary before bringing him to the mother. If desired, use a towel or blanket to cover the mother's breast and baby's head after baby has latched on.

ⓖ If necessary, remind the mother how to hold the nipple and areola between thumb and forefinger to allow baby to latch on. If baby does not latch on right away, have the mother stroke his cheek with her nipple.

ⓖ Good nutrition and plenty of fluids are important for nursing mothers. Offer frequent drinks of water, juice, or milk, and snacks as needed. Instruct the mother not to eat spicy foods, chocolate, or caffeinated beverages. They may affect the breast milk.

ⓖ Observe the baby nursing to be sure he stays latched on properly (Fig. 19-6). If necessary, have the mother use one hand to

hold the breast tissue away from the baby's nose.

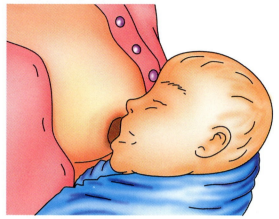

Fig. 19-6. When the baby is properly latched on to the mother's nipple, his mouth covers much of the areola. The nipple is sucked straight out rather than at an angle. This ensures the best milk flow and prevents the nipples from becoming sore.

- When it is time to switch from one breast to the other, the mother can break the suction by pressing down on the breast above the nipple or by gently putting her finger in the baby's mouth.

- Help the mother burp the baby when switching breasts and when finishing the feeding.

- Change the baby's diaper after the feeding. Help the mother lay the baby down safely.

- Many women find it helpful to tie a ribbon or place a pin on the side the baby last fed on. This helps them remember to start the baby's feeding on that side next time, so the breasts will be emptied more evenly.

Assisting with Bottle Feeding

Many women choose to bottle-feed their babies some or all of the time. Infant formula is commercially prepared and provides the nutrition babies need. There are many brands and types of formula. If you are doing the shopping, know exactly which type you need to buy. The three most common types are ready-to-feed formula, concentrated liquid formula, and powdered formula (Fig. 19-7).

Ready-to-feed or **prepared** formula is sold in bottles or cans. This formula is ready to use. Do

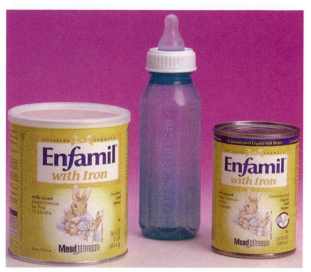

Fig. 19-7. Baby formula is available ready-to-feed in cans or bottles, concentrated in cans, or powdered in cans.

not dilute it or mix it with water. If the formula comes in a bottle, simply shake, unscrew the cap, and screw on a standard nipple and ring. Discard any formula remaining in the bottle after feeding. If the ready-to-feed formula comes in a can, shake the can before opening it with a sterilized can opener. Pour into sterile bottles. Store remaining formula in the can, covered and refrigerated, for no more than two days. Ready-to-feed formula is the most convenient to use. It is also the most expensive.

Concentrated formula is sold in small cans. It must be mixed with sterile water before using. Shake the can and open it with a sterile can opener. Measure an amount into a marked bottle and add an equal amount of sterile water. Screw on the nipple and ring, and shake to mix. Sterile water can be purchased in small bottles or in gallon jugs. You can also make sterile water by bringing water to a boil and then cooling. Store unused concentrate in the can, covered and refrigerated, for no more than two days.

Powdered formula is sold in one- or two-pound cans. It is carefully measured and mixed with sterile water. A scoop is included in the can for measuring. Mix the powder and sterile water in sterile bottles or a sterilized pitcher or covered container. Follow the directions on the package carefully. Once mixed, the formula can

be stored for two days in the refrigerator. Shake before feeding. Powdered formula is the most difficult to use, but is usually the cheapest to buy.

Before feeding, bottles should be warmed. To heat, immerse the bottle in warm tap water for several minutes. Bottles or formula just out of the refrigerator will take longer to warm. Never use the microwave to warm bottles. This can create hot spots in the liquid that can burn the baby (Fig. 19-8). Always shake the bottle after warming and shake a few drops of formula onto the inside of your wrist. It should feel warm, not hot or cold.

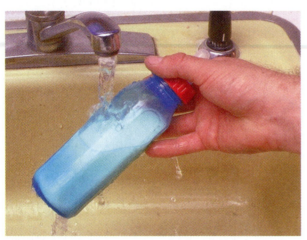

Fig. 19-8. Warm bottles in warm tap water—not in the microwave!

Sterilizing bottles

Equipment: clean bottles, nipples, and rings to be sterilized (these should be washed in hot, soapy water using a bottle brush, and allowed to drain), large kettle filled halfway with water, tongs, clean dish or paper towels to set sterile bottles on

1. Wash your hands.

2. Bring water to a boil and put bottles, nipples, and rings in. Use tongs to push bottles under water.

3. Bring water to boil again and boil for five minutes.

4. Using tongs, remove bottles, nipples, and rings, draining the water into the pot. Set everything on the clean towels. When dry, store in a clean, dry cabinet.

5. Discard water.

Assisting with bottle feeding

1. Wash your hands.

2. Prepare bottle and formula as directed.

3. Sit in a comfortable chair and hold the baby safely in either the cradle hold or football hold.

4. Stroke the baby's lips with the bottle nipple until he opens his mouth. Put the bottle nipple in the baby's mouth.

5. Be sure the baby's head is higher than his body during feeding. Also make sure the nipple stays full of milk so the baby does not swallow air (Fig. 19-9).

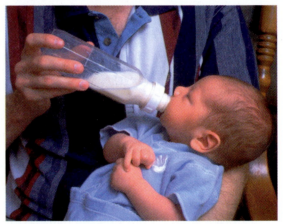

Fig. 19-9.

6. Talk or sing to the baby while feeding. Feedings are the high points of his days and should be special times.

7. When baby is through or has stopped sucking, burp him (see procedure below). Resume feeding or, if finished, change the diaper (see procedure later in chapter). Put the baby down safely.

8. Wash your hands and document the feeding, how much was consumed, and any other observations.

9. Throw out unused formula left in bottle. Wash the bottle, nipple, and ring in hot soapy water with a bottle brush, and allow to dry. Sterilize before using again.

Babies must be burped after each feeding to release air swallowed during feeding. Burping prevents babies from developing gas. Gas can be very uncomfortable for them. Burping in the middle of a feeding may allow a baby to eat more.

Burping a baby

1. Wash your hands.

2. Assemble equipment: a clean towel, cloth diaper, or burp pad.

3. Pick up the baby safely. There are two different positions to use for burping. Most people like to hold the baby against the shoulder to burp (Fig. 19-10). However, babies who are very small, who have breathing problems, or who tend to choke or vomit should be held on the lap with the head supported by holding the baby's chin with the thumb and forefinger (Fig. 19-11). This position allows you to watch the baby for signs of respiratory distress, especially color changes, or spit-up. Whichever position you use, put the burp pad under the baby's chin to catch any spit-up.

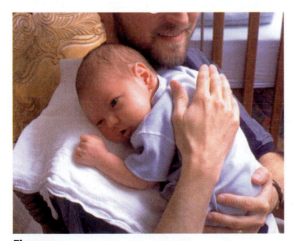

Fig. 19-10.

4. With the baby in a safe and comfortable position, pat the baby's back gently with your flat hand. Concentrate on the area between the shoulder blades. Some people like to pat up and down the baby's back. Others like to massage the back using an upward motion with the flat hand. Use any technique that

works for you. The more relaxed and comfortable the baby is, the sooner the burp will come.

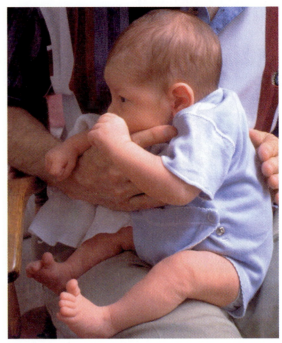

Fig. 19-11.

5. After the baby has burped, return him or her to a safe position or resume feeding.

7. Explain guidelines for bathing and changing a baby

Keeping a baby clean is important to his health. Follow the guidelines for safely handling a baby. In addition, remember the following:

- Because you could come into contact with body fluids, wear disposable gloves when bathing or changing a baby. Remember, however, that gloves can make a wet baby slippery! Be very careful when handling a baby during a bath.

- Whether bathing or changing a baby, keep one hand on the infant at all times. Have all supplies ready so you **never** have to take both hands off the baby.

- Give baths in a warm place.

- Close doors and windows to prevent drafts. Dry the baby's head immediately after washing hair.

- Be very careful about bath temperature. Always test the temperature of the water (either on the inside of your wrist or with a bath thermometer).

- Keep the baby's bottom dry. Be sure the area is thoroughly dried after a bath. Moisture contributes to diaper rash. Dry the bottom after changing a diaper. Leaving the diaper off for a few moments when changing the baby allows air to circulate and helps prevent diaper rash.

- Do not use powder unless directed to do so. Babies who are very small, premature, or who have breathing problems, can be harmed by inhaling baby powder.

Giving an infant sponge bath

Equipment: disposable gloves, clean basin, blanket or towel to pad surface, washcloth and towel, baby cleanser or mild soap, baby shampoo or mild shampoo, cotton hat, lotion or oil, cotton ball or cotton-tipped swabs and alcohol, diaper ointment if used, clean diaper, clean clothes or sleeper, clean receiving blanket

1. Wash your hands.

2. Put on gloves. Be careful—gloves make the baby slippery!

3. Give the bath in a warm place. Use a blanket or towel to pad the surface the baby will lie on. Have all your supplies within reach. You will need to keep one hand on the baby during the entire bath. Remove caps from shampoo and cleanser to make it easier.

4. Fill the basin with warm water. Test the temperature on the inside of your wrist. Put the bottle of lotion or oil in the warm water to warm it.

5. With the baby still dressed, hold him or her in the football hold. Wet the washcloth and gently wipe the eyes, from the inner corner to the outer (Fig. 19-12). Then clean the rest of the face. Use only warm water—no soap.

6. To wash hair, hold the baby in the football hold with the head over the basin. Use the washcloth to wet the hair. Using a small

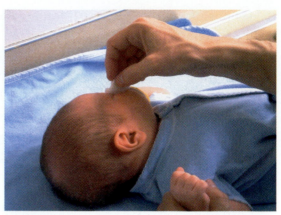

Fig. 19-12.

amount of shampoo, lather the baby's hair (Fig. 19-13). Rinse with the washcloth. Pat the head dry immediately with the towel. Put a cotton hat over the baby's head. Much heat is lost through the head. Be careful to keep the head warm.

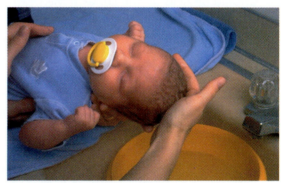

Fig. 19-13.

7. Lay the baby down on the padded surface. Always keep at least one hand on the baby.

8. Undress the upper body. Wash the neck, chest, back, arms and hands using the washcloth and small amounts of soap. Rinse using the washcloth and water from the basin (Fig. 19-14). Pat dry. Cover the upper body with a towel.

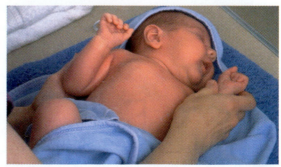

Fig. 19-14.

9. Undress the lower body, removing the diaper. Wash the baby's abdomen and legs. Rinse. Pat dry.

10. Wash the perineal area last. For a girl, wipe the perineal area from front to back. For a boy who has recently been circumcised, do not wash the area of the circumcision. Follow special instructions to care for the circumcision.

11. Wash the baby's bottom thoroughly and dry the entire area completely with the towel. Moisture can contribute to diaper rash.

12. As gently and quickly as possible, rub lotion over the baby's body. Avoid the cord if it has not yet healed. Use lotion on the face only if skin is very dry. Be extremely careful not to get any lotion near the eyes. Keep the baby covered except for the part you are rubbing.

13. Diaper and dress the baby. Wrap baby in blanket and put him or her down safely.

14. Put used towels and washcloth in the laundry. Discard water. Clean basin and store. Store other supplies. Discard gloves.

15. Wash your hands.

16. Document the bath, including any observations.

Giving an infant tub bath

In addition to the supplies listed in the procedure above for a sponge bath, you will need a large basin or baby bath tub. You may also bathe a baby in a clean sink. Follow the first six steps in the procedure for a sponge bath for preparing the bath and washing the baby's face and hair.

1. Lay the baby down on the padded surface and undress him or her completely. Immerse baby in the tub or basin. Support the head and neck above water with one hand at all times (Fig. 19-15).

2. Using the washcloth and small amounts of soap, wash the baby from the neck down.

3. Remove the baby from the bath and lay him or her down on the padded surface. Keep

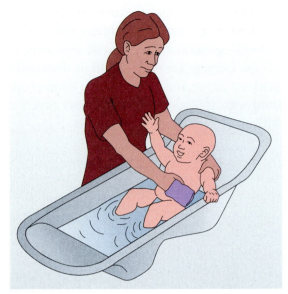

Fig. 19-15.

one hand on the baby at all times. Cover baby immediately with a towel and pat dry (Fig. 19-16).

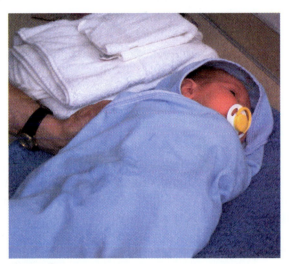

Fig. 19-16.

4. Apply lotion, keeping the baby covered as much as possible.

5. Diaper, dress, and wrap the baby in a receiving blanket. Put him or her down safely.

6. Put used linens in the laundry. Discard bath water. Clean and store basin. Store all supplies. Discard gloves.

7. Wash your hands.

8. Document the bath, including any observations.

Diapers catch the baby's urine and feces. Children wear diapers until they are toilet trained—generally between two and three years of age. Diapers are either cloth or disposable, made of paper and plastic. Cloth diapers are used with special waterproof diaper covers or with diaper pins and plastic pants.

A newborn will need between six and ten diaper changes in 24 hours. As babies get older, they use fewer diapers each day. The appearance, consistency, and smell of a baby's feces will depend on what he or she is fed. Some newborn babies have loose bowel movements with every feeding, as many as eight a day. Others have different schedules. Babies must be changed frequently to avoid diaper rash or irritation.

Changing cloth or disposable diapers

Equipment: clean disposable diaper or clean cloth diaper, diaper cover or pins, and plastic pants, wipes or a washcloth wet with warm water, diaper ointment or oil if used, clean clothes if clothes are soiled or wet

1. Wash your hands.

2. Put on gloves.

3. Change the diaper in a warm place. You need a padded surface, which may be a special changing table or a countertop. Never turn your back on the baby. Always keep one hand on baby at all times. Have supplies within reach.

4. Undress the baby as necessary and remove wet or soiled diaper. Set it aside for handling later.

5. Clean the perineal area with wipes or washcloth. Remove all traces of feces. Spread the legs to clean thoroughly. For girls, wipe from front to back and spread the labia to clean as needed.

6. Let air circulate on the bottom for a moment. Exposure to air prevents diaper rash. Apply ointment or oil as directed.

7. For disposable diapers: Unfold the diaper and expose tapes. Place the diaper flat under the baby's bottom with the tapes in back. Bring the front of the diaper up between the baby's legs and bring the back sides around and over the front (Fig. 19-17). Peel tapes open and tape the side of the diaper securely to the front.

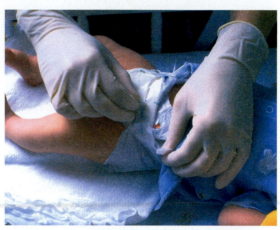

Fig. 19-17. A disposable diaper is fastened with adhesive or Velcro tape attached to the back sides of the diaper.

8. For cloth diapers with diaper cover: Fold the diaper in thirds lengthwise. Then open out the back corners about three inches (Fig. 19-18). Lay the back of the diaper inside the back of the diaper cover (the back of the diaper cover has the tabs extending from it). Place the diaper and cover underneath the baby's bottom. Bring the front of the diaper and cover up through the baby's legs. Bring the tabs around from the sides to the front of the diaper cover and use them to close the cover securely over the diaper. Check that all the edges of the diaper are tucked under the cover.

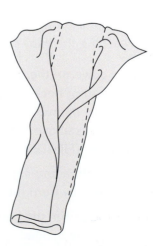

Fig. 19-18.

19

New Mothers, Infants, and Children

9. For cloth diapers with pins and plastic pants: Fold the diaper lengthwise in thirds, then open out the back corners about three inches. Place the diaper under the baby's bottom and bring the front of the diaper up between the baby's legs. Fold down the front of the diaper to the inside (next to baby's skin) so that the diaper covers the genitals and lower abdomen. Bring the corners of the diaper around the baby's sides and pin them to the front of the diaper. Hold your fingers inside the diaper next to baby's skin when pinning to avoid sticking the baby (Fig. 19-19). You do not need to pin through all layers. Just pin enough to fasten the back of the diaper to the front. When diaper is securely pinned, put plastic pants over the diaper to keep urine from leaking.

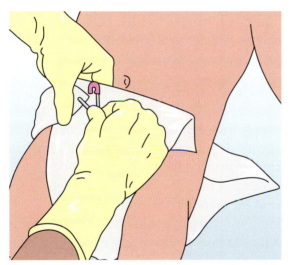

Fig. 19-19.

10. Dress the baby in clean clothes and put him down safely.

11. Dispose of diaper properly. Disposable diapers can be rolled into a ball (dirty side in), sealed with tapes, and disposed of in a special trash bag in a sealed container to prevent odors. Cloth diapers may need to be soaked before washing or removal by a diaper service. Check with the baby's mother or your supervisor for instructions.

12. Remove gloves.

13. Wash your hands.

14. Clean changing area and store supplies.

15. Wash hands again as needed.

16. Document any observations, including unusual color, consistency, or odor.

8. Explain guidelines for special care

At birth, the **umbilical** (*um-BIL-i-kul*) **cord** that connected the baby to the placenta (*pla-SEN-ta*) inside the mother's uterus (*YOU-ter-us*) is cut. The stump of the cord remains attached to a newborn's navel for up to three weeks. Proper care of the cord stump is necessary to prevent infection and allow healing.

- With every diaper change, moisten the cord with rubbing alcohol. Use a cotton ball or cotton-tipped swabs soaked in rubbing alcohol to swab the area around the navel and cord. This helps the stump dry up and fall off.

- Never pull on or handle the cord. It will fall off by itself. The baby will feel no pain when the cord falls off.

- Keep diapers folded down away from the cord to allow air to circulate and prevent irritation (Fig. 19-20).

- Do not give an infant a tub bath until the cord has fallen off.

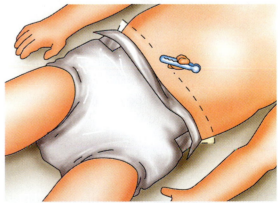

Fig. 19-20. Keep diapers folded down away from the cord to allow air to circulate and to prevent irritation.

Taking an infant's axillary or tympanic temperature

An infant's temperature is typically taken by the axillary or tympanic methods. Rectal tempera-

tures are no longer recommended due to the chance of damaging rectal tissue. Oral temperatures are never taken for infants because the method is too difficult and dangerous.

Equipment: mercury-free or glass thermometer, disposable probe cover, if needed

1. Wash your hands.

2. Be sure thermometer is clean. Put on disposable probe cover, if used. Shake thermometer down to below the lowest number.

3. For axillary temperature: Undress the upper body on one side. Lay the baby on a padded surface. Place the tip of the thermometer under the arm and hold the baby's arm close to his body, so the thermometer tip touches skin on all sides (Fig. 19-21). Keep thermometer in place for 3 to 5 minutes for a glass thermometer, or until the signal sounds for a digital thermometer.

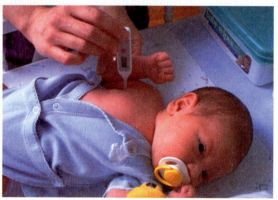

Fig. 19-21.

4. For tympanic temperature: Lay the baby on his side. Pull the outside of the ear gently toward the back of the head. Insert the thermometer tip into the ear, pointing toward the opposite eye (Fig. 19-22). Be sure the ear is sealed by the thermometer. Press the button and hold for one second.

5. For all methods, remove the thermometer and read the temperature. Keep one hand on the baby at all times.

6. Dress the baby and put him down safely.

7. Clean and store thermometer and supplies.

8. Wash your hands.

9. Document temperature.

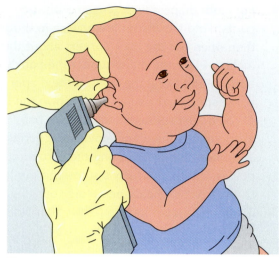

Fig. 19-22.

Circumcision (*SIR-kum-si-zjun*) is the removal of part of the foreskin of the penis. It is commonly performed on male babies. Some religions require circumcision. Other parents choose to have their baby circumcised for hygienic or social reasons.

The circumcision is usually performed in the hospital or at the doctor's office when the baby is only days old. Afterwards, the circumcision site needs special care to heal. This usually includes covering the tip of the penis with a gauze pad rubbed with petroleum jelly to prevent the diaper from irritating the site. However, some types of circumcision require different care. Follow your supervisor's instructions carefully.

Some babies who need special care will have medical equipment in the home. You will probably not be responsible for operating or handling the equipment. However, it is helpful to be familiar with various items. Always follow your supervisor's instructions before touching any medical equipment.

Apnea monitor. Apnea (*AP-nee-a*) is the state of not breathing. Some babies may stop breathing for periods of time due to immaturity of the lungs or other reasons. The apnea monitor alerts parents or caregivers if breathing has stopped. Many apnea monitors also monitor heart rate.

Ventilator or oxygen equipment. Some babies with breathing problems need to be given oxygen. Oxygen is considered a medication. In most states it cannot be given by a home health aide. In addition, home health aides are not allowed to change the amount of oxygen being given. As always, be careful when working around oxygen, as it is flammable. Follow your supervisor's instructions carefully when working in a home where oxygen is in use.

You may have contact with children in several ways. You may be assigned to care for a client's children when the client is unable to care for them. In this case you are a substitute for the parent. In other cases, the child may be the client and is suffering from a disease or disability that requires home care. In either case, it is important to understand some basic principles of caring for and working with children.

9. Identify special physical, mental, and emotional needs of children

Children have the same basic physical and emotional needs as adults (see chapter 8). They also have some special physical, mental, and emotional needs. Children's growing bodies need adequate and nutritious food and fluids, exercise, fresh air, and plenty of sleep. Their developing minds need to be stimulated by age-appropriate activities, opportunities for learning, and chances for increasing independence. Emotionally, children need love and affection, reassurance, encouragement, security and guidance. They also need consistent and constructive discipline. In addition, children need protection from injury and illness. Chapter 10 describes child development in more detail.

Children with disabilities have the same physical and emotional needs as other children (Fig. 19-23). Remember to treat these children as children first. Disabilities may make normal social contact with other children difficult. However, it is important for children with disabilities to interact with others their own age. Chapter 17 has information on special needs.

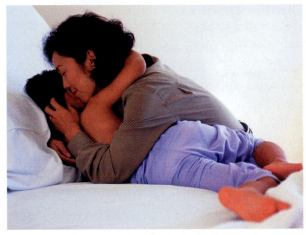

Fig. 19-23. Children with disabilities have the same emotional needs as other children. They need love and acceptance, reassurance, encouragement, security and guidance, and consistent and constructive discipline.

10. List symptoms of common childhood illnesses and the required care

Most childhood illnesses are caused by bacterial or viral infections. These include colds, flu, and various infections causing fever, diarrhea, vomiting, or coughs. You can help prevent illness by preventing the spread of infection in the home. Handwashing, cleaning, and disinfection are the best ways to control infection (see chapter 5). Treatment for some of the most common symptoms of childhood illnesses is described below.

Fever. Fever may indicate serious illness. It should always be reported to your supervisor. Rest and fluids are recommended for fevers. Treatment for a fever may also include acetaminophen, or a lukewarm bath or sponging. Home health aides never give any medication, including over-the-counter medications. You can assist by making sure the family caregiver follows a doctor's dosage instructions for all medications. The strength of over-the-counter drugs varies in infant, children, and adult formulas. It is especially important to follow dosage instructions. For example, infant acetaminophen is stronger than children's acetaminophen, so the dosage is smaller. Too much can cause liver damage or failure. In general, children should not be given aspirin, as it has been associated with some serious disorders.

19

New Mothers, Infants, and Children

19

New Mothers, Infants, and Children

Diarrhea. Diarrhea, or frequent loose or watery bowel movements, can have many causes. In children, it is often caused by a virus. Cramps and abdominal pain may accompany diarrhea. Children with diarrhea should rest and drink plenty of clear liquids, including water, broth, and diluted juices. Doctors may recommend electrolyte-replacement drinks to prevent dehydration. Usually, children with diarrhea should avoid solid foods until the problem subsides. Then they may follow the BRAT diet: bananas, rice, applesauce, and toast. Other starchy foods, such as pasta or crackers, are also allowed. Milk products, fruits, vegetables, and fatty foods should be avoided until the bowels return to normal.

Vomiting. The treatment for vomiting is similar to the treatment for diarrhea, including rest and clear liquids, and later the BRAT diet.

Always call your supervisor if symptoms continue. Follow instructions in the care plan or your assignment sheet carefully.

11. Identify guidelines for working with children

The following suggestions may help you establish a trusting and honest relationship with the children in your care.

Introduce yourself. Treat children as important members of the family, and worthy of your notice. Be friendly, tell the children your name, and explain why you are there.

Maintain routine. As much as possible, stick with the family's regular schedule. The comfort of a routine can help ease the stress children may feel if someone in their household needs home care.

Give comfort. Children who are hurt, angry, or sad may need a hug, a pat, or soothing words to make them feel more secure (Fig. 19-24).

Offer encouragement and praise. Praise and encouragement contribute to the child's sense of

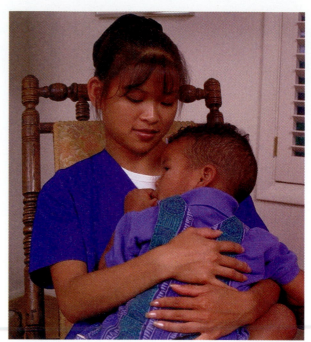

Fig. 19-24.

self-worth and self-confidence. Word your praise so that it does not belittle other children.

Do not make comparisons. Children should not be compared to each other.

Use positive phrases. Children often respond better to guidance such as, "Let's try it this way…" rather than "no" or "don't."

Listen. Pay attention when children attempt to communicate. Do not interrupt them or deny their feelings. Help them to express what they are feeling by using your communication skills.

Answer. Respond to children's questions immediately, willingly, and clearly. If you do not know the answer or are not sure you are the right person to answer it, tell the child. Bring the child's question to the appropriate person.

Do not force children to eat. Like adults, children do not always feel like eating. Do not allow a meal to become a power struggle. Children are usually motivated to eat when meals are simple but attractive and contain their favorite foods.

Involve children in household activities. Children feel capable and responsible when they are given household tasks to perform

(Fig. 19-25). Like all people, they like to feel they are making a contribution to the family.

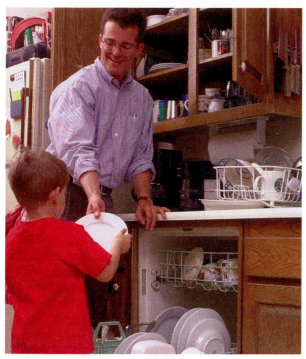

Fig. 19-25. Help children contribute.

Encourage children to play. Children need to exercise and socialize with other children. Playing helps children express themselves and be creative. Exercise is important for their growth and health. Socialization is especially important for children who are learning social skills.

Recognize individual needs. Not all children are the same. They have different needs for sleep, food, and exercise. They grow and develop at different paces.

Be nonjudgmental. As with any client, you must accept a child regardless of disabilities or problems.

12. List the signs of child abuse and neglect and know how to report them

Child abuse is the physical, sexual, or psychological mistreatment of a child. Children who are abused can range in age from infant to adolescent. **Sexual abuse** of children includes inappropriate touching of a child's body, sexual contact, or penetration. **Psychological abuse** includes verbal abuse, such as name-calling, social isolation, and seclusion. **Child neglect** is the conscious or unconscious failure to provide for the needs of a child. Children who are neglected may not receive adequate food, water, medications, supervision, or shelter.

Children should never be harmed, threatened, or teased. They must be treated with respect and concern. Adults must talk to children calmly and quietly and give them positive comments, praise, and encouragement.

Child abuse or neglect can come from anyone who is responsible for a child's care. This includes parents, guardians, paid caregivers, teachers, friends, or relatives. The law requires that health professionals must report suspected child abuse. **If you observe or suspect abuse or neglect, or if a child reports that someone has abused or neglected him or her, you must immediately report this to your supervisor.** You and your agency can get into trouble for not reporting suspected abuse or neglect. Follow your employer's procedures for reporting suspected abuse.

OBSERVING AND REPORTING
Child Abuse

If you observe any of these signs of child abuse or neglect, or if you suspect abuse or neglect, speak to your supervisor immediately.

- Child has burns, cuts, bruises, abrasions, or fractured bones.
- Child stares vacantly or watches intensely.
- Child is extremely quiet.
- Child avoids eye contact. In some cultures, however, it is the norm to avoid eye contact.
- Child is afraid of adults.
- Child behaves aggressively.
- Child exhibits excessive activity or hyperactivity. Some hyperactive children, however, have a chemical imbalance that produces this behavior.
- Child tells you that someone is abusing him or her.

Chapter Review

1. Why are new mothers often more tired and uncomfortable when they get home than women were in the past?

2. What kind of doctor specializes in working with newborns?

3. List five things you may do to assist a new mother.

4. What might you be asked to routinely document in caring for a newborn and mother?

5. What should you always do before picking up a baby?

6. Where are the only safe places to leave a baby?

7. Why must you support a baby's head when you hold him/her?

8. Why should a baby NOT be put to sleep on its stomach or on a blanket or comforter?

9. Why are women encouraged to try breast-feeding?

10. How should you warm a bottle?

11. How do you mix concentrated formula?

12. For what length of time can you refrigerate ready-to-feed formula?

13. How does burping help a baby?

14. Why should you have all supplies ready before bathing or changing a baby?

15. How can you test the temperature of a baby's bath water?

16. How many diaper changes will a newborn typically need in 24 hours?

17. What should you do to care for the umbilical cord stump every time you change a baby's diaper?

18. What does circumcision care generally require?

19. Why is it important to treat children with disabilities as children first?

20. Name each of the three symptoms outlined in learning objective 10 and describe at least one common treatment for each.

21. If a child asks you a question and you do not know the answer, what should you do?

22. Why is maintaining routine important for children?

23. How does playing help children?

24. List six common signs of child abuse.

19

New Mothers, Infants, and Children

20

Common Chronic and Acute Conditions

1. Define arthritis and identify treatments and care guidelines

Arthritis (*ar-THRYE-tis*) is a general term that refers to **inflammation**, or swelling, of the joints. It causes stiffness, pain, and decreased mobility. Arthritis may be the result of aging, injury, or an **autoimmune illness**. During an autoimmune illness, the body's immune system attacks normal tissue in the body. There are several types of arthritis.

Osteoarthritis (*AH-stee-oh-ar-thrye-tis*). Osteoarthritis is a common type of arthritis that affects the elderly. It may occur with aging or as a result of joint injury. Hips and knees, which are weight-bearing joints, are usually affected. However, joints of the fingers, thumbs, and spine can also be affected. Pain and stiffness seem to increase in cold or damp weather.

Rheumatoid Arthritis (*ROOM-a-toyd ar-THRYE-tis*). Rheumatoid arthritis can affect people of all ages. Joints become inflamed, red, swollen, and very painful (Fig. 20-1). Movement is eventually restricted. Fever, fatigue, and weight loss are also symptoms. Rheumatoid arthritis usually affects the smaller joints first, then progresses to larger ones. Other parts of the body that may be affected are the heart, lungs, eyes, kidneys, and skin.

Arthritis is generally treated with some or all of the following:

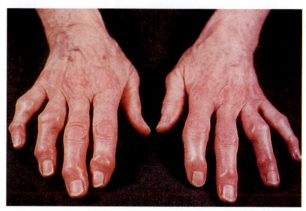

Fig. 20-1. Rheumatoid arthritis. (Photo courtesy of Frederick Miller, MD)

- anti-inflammatory medications such as aspirin or ibuprofen

- local applications of heat to reduce swelling and pain

- range of motion exercises

- a regular exercise and/or activity routine

- diet to reduce weight or maintain strength

GUIDELINES
Caring for Clients with Arthritis

- Watch for stomach irritation or heartburn caused by aspirin or ibuprofen. Some clients cannot take these medications. Report signs of stomach irritation immediately.

- Encourage activity. Gentle activity can help reduce the effects of arthritis. Follow the care plan instructions carefully. Use canes or other walking aids as needed.

ⓖ Adapt activities of daily living (ADLs) to allow independence. Many devices are available to allow clients to bathe, dress, and feed themselves even when they have arthritis. Choose clothing that is easy to put on and fasten. Suggest handrails and safety bars for the bathroom. Special utensils are available to make it easier for clients to feed themselves (Fig. 20-2).

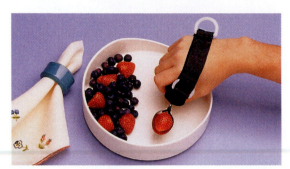

Fig. 20-2. Special equipment can help a person with arthritis remain independent. (Photo courtesy of North Coast Medical, Inc., www.ncmedical.com, 800-821-9319)

ⓖ Treat each client as an individual. Arthritis is very common among elderly clients. Do not assume that each client has the same symptoms and needs the same care.

ⓖ Help maintain client's self-esteem by encouraging self-care. Maintain a positive attitude. Listen to the client's feelings. You can help him or her remain independent for as long as possible.

2. Define cancer and list eight risk factors for cancer

Cancer is a general term used to describe many types of malignant tumors. A **tumor** (*TOO-mer*) is a cluster of abnormally growing cells. **Benign** (*bee-NINE*) **tumors** grow slowly in local areas. They are considered non-cancerous. **Malignant** (*ma-LIG-nant*) **tumors** grow rapidly and invade surrounding tissues.

Cancer invades local tissue, and it can spread to other parts of the body. When cancer spreads from the site where it first appeared, it can affect one or more other body systems. In general, treatment is more difficult and cancer is more deadly after this has occurred. Cancer

often appears first in the breast, colon, rectum, uterus, prostate, lungs, or skin.

There is no known cure for cancer. However, some treatments are effective. They are discussed later in the chapter.

Risk factors for cancer include the following:

- tobacco use (Fig. 20-3)

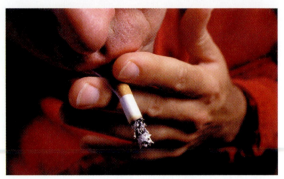

Fig. 20-3. Tobacco use is considered a risk factor for cancer.

- exposure to sunlight
- excessive alcohol use
- exposure to some chemicals and industrial agents
- some food additives
- radiation
- poor nutrition
- lack of physical activity

When Smokers Quit

Within 20 minutes of smoking that last cigarette, the body begins a series of changes that continues for years.

20 minutes
- Blood pressure drops to normal.
- Pulse rate drops to normal.
- Body temperature of hands and feet increases to normal.

8 hours
- Carbon monoxide level in blood drops to normal.
- Oxygen level in blood increases to normal.

24 hours
- Chance of heart attack decreases.

48 hours
- Nerve endings start re-growing.
- Ability to smell and taste is enhanced.

2 weeks to 3 months
- Circulation improves.
- Walking becomes easier.
- Lung function increases up to 30 percent.

1 to 9 months
- Coughing, sinus congestion, fatigue, shortness of breath decrease.
- Cilia re-grow in lungs, increasing ability to handle mucus, clean the lungs, reduce infection.
- Body's overall energy increases.

1 year
- Excess risk of coronary heart disease is half that of a smoker.

5 years
- Lung cancer death rate for average former smoker (one pack a day) decreases by almost half.
- Stroke risk is reduced to that of a nonsmoker 5-15 years after quitting.
- Risk of cancer of the mouth, throat and esophagus is half that of a smoker's.

10 years
- Lung cancer death rate is similar to that of nonsmokers.
- Precancerous cells are replaced.
- Risk of cancer of the mouth, throat, esophagus, bladder, kidney and pancreas decreases.

15 years
- Risk of coronary heart disease is the same as that of a nonsmoker.

Source: American Cancer Society, Centers for Disease Control and Prevention

3. List seven warning signs of cancer

When diagnosed early, cancer can often be treated and controlled. The American Cancer Society has identified seven warning signs of cancer:

1. Change in bowel or bladder habits
2. A sore that does not heal
3. Unusual bleeding or discharge from a body opening
4. Thickening or lump in the breast or else-where
5. Indigestion or difficulty swallowing
6. Obvious change in a wart or mole
7. Nagging cough or persistent hoarseness

4. Identify common treatments for cancer

People with cancer can often live longer and sometimes recover when treated using the following methods. These treatments are most effective when tumors are discovered early. Often these treatments are combined.

Surgery. Surgery is the front line of defense for most forms of cancer. It is the key treatment for malignant tumors of the skin, breast, bladder, colon, rectum, stomach, and muscle. Surgeons attempt to remove as much of the tumor as possible to prevent cancer from spreading.

Chemotherapy. Chemotherapy refers to medications given to fight cancer. Certain drugs destroy cancer cells and limit the rate of cell growth. However, many of these drugs are toxic to the body. They destroy healthy cells as well as cancer cells. Chemotherapy can have severe side effects, including nausea, vomiting, diarrhea, hair loss, and decreased resistance to infection.

Radiation. Radiation therapy directs radiation to a limited area to kill cancer cells. However, other normal or healthy cells in its path are also destroyed (Fig. 20-4). By controlling cell growth, radiation can reduce pain. Radiation can cause the same side effects as chemotherapy. The skin of the area exposed to radiation may become sore, irritated, and sometimes burned.

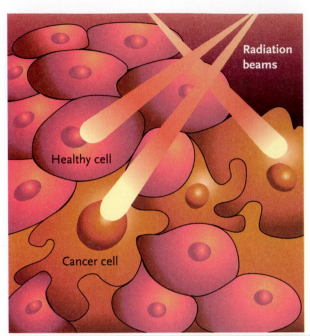

Fig. 20-4. Radiation is targeted at cancer cells, but it also destroys some healthy cells in its path.

5. Describe care guidelines for the client who has cancer

Coping with cancer can be a tremendous challenge. Keep the following guidelines in mind when working with clients who have cancer.

GUIDELINES
Caring for Clients with Cancer

- **Each case is different**. Cancer is a general term and refers to many separate situations. Clients may expect to live many years or only several months. Treatment affects each person differently. Do not make assumptions about a client's condition.

- **Communication**. Clients may want to talk or may avoid talking. Respect each client's needs. Listen if a client wants to share feelings or experiences with you. However, never push a client to talk. Be honest. Never tell a client "everything will be okay." Be sensitive. Remember that cancer is a disease, and we do not know its cause. Maintain a positive attitude and focus on concrete details. For example, comment if a client seems stronger, or notice that the sun is shining outside.

- **Nutrition**. Good nutrition is extremely important for clients with cancer. Follow the care plan instructions and your assignments carefully. Clients frequently have poor appetites. Encourage a variety of food. In general, clients should be served four to six meals a day. Serve favorite foods that are high in nutrition. Liquid nutrition supplements may be used in addition to, not in place of, meals. If nausea or swallowing is a problem, foods such as soups, gelatin, or starches may appeal to the client. Use plastic utensils for a client receiving chemotherapy. It makes food taste better. Metal utensils cause a bitter taste.

- **Pain control**. Cancer can cause terrible pain, especially in the late stages. Watch your client for signs of pain. Observe the client's use of pain medication. Assist with comfort measures, including repositioning and providing distractions such as conversation, music, or reading materials (Fig. 20-5). Report to your supervisor if pain seems to be uncontrolled.

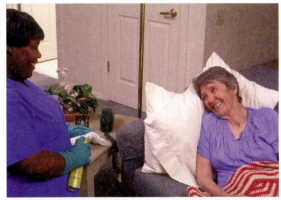

Fig. 20-5. Distractions such as conversation can help a client with cancer deal with pain.

- **Skin care**. Use lotion regularly on dry or delicate skin. Do not apply lotion to areas receiving radiation therapy. Offer back rubs to provide comfort and increase circulation. For clients who spend many hours in bed, egg crate mattress covers or sheepskins may be more comfortable. Moving to a chair for some period of time may improve comfort as well. Clients who are very weak or immobile need to be repositioned every two hours.

20

Common Chronic and Acute Conditions

⑧ **Oral care**. Help clients brush and floss teeth regularly. Medications, nausea, vomiting, or mouth infections may cause a bad taste in the mouth. You can help ease discomfort by using a soft-bristled toothbrush, rinsing with baking soda and water, or using a prescribed rinse. Do not use a commercial mouthwash. The alcohol in it can further irritate a client's mouth.

⑧ **Self-image**. People with cancer may suffer from low self-image because they are weaker and their appearance has changed. For example, hair loss is a common side effect of chemotherapy. Assist with grooming if desired. Your concern and interest can help improve self-image.

⑧ **Psychosocial needs**. If visitors help cheer your client, encourage them and do not intrude. If some times of day are better than others, suggest this to the client's friends or family. Support groups exist for people with cancer and their families. Check with your supervisor for referrals in your area. It may help a person with cancer to think of something besides cancer and treatment for a while. Pursue other topics and get to know what interests your clients have. As always, report any signs of depression immediately (see chapter 18).

⑧ **Family assistance**. Caring for a person with cancer at home can be very difficult for family members. Be alert to needs that are not being met or stresses created by the illness. Report your observations. Know the resources available in your area.

OBSERVING AND REPORTING
Cancer

Report any of the following to your supervisor:

- increased weakness or fatigue
- weight loss
- nausea, vomiting, diarrhea
- changes in appetite
- fainting
- signs of depression (see chapter 18 for a discussion of these signs)
- confusion
- blood in stool or urine
- change in mental status
- changes in skin integrity
- new lumps, sores, or rashes
- increase in pain, or pain unrelieved by current measures

6. Identify community resources available to people with cancer and their families

Numerous services and support groups are available for people with cancer and their families or caregivers. Hospitals, hospice programs, churches, and synagogues offer many resources, including meal services, transportation to doctors' offices or hospitals, counseling, and support groups. Check the local yellow pages under "cancer," or call the local or state chapter of the American Cancer Society. Also contact your local Area Agency on Aging.

7. Describe diabetes and identify its signs and complications

In **diabetes mellitus** (*dye-a-BEE-tees mel-EYE-tus*), commonly called diabetes, the pancreas (*PAN-kree-as*) does not produce enough insulin (*IN-su-lin*). **Insulin** is the substance the body needs to convert **glucose** (*GLOO-kohs*), or natural sugar, into energy for the body. Without insulin to process glucose, these sugars collect in the blood. This causes problems with circulation and can damage vital organs.

Diabetes commonly occurs in people with a family history of the illness, in the elderly, and in people who are obese. Two types of diabetes have been identified:

1. **Type I**, or insulin-dependent diabetes mellitus (IDDM), is often called juvenile diabetes because it most often appears before age 20. It will continue throughout a person's life. However, a person can develop Type I dia-

20

Common Chronic and Acute Conditions

betes up to age 40. Type I diabetes is treated with insulin and a special diet.

2. **Type II**, or noninsulin-dependent diabetes mellitus (NIDDM) appears in adults. It can usually be controlled with diet and/or oral medications. This type is also called adult-onset diabetes. Type II diabetes usually develops slowly. It is the milder form of diabetes mellitus. It typically develops around age 35. It often occurs in obese individuals or those with a family history of Type II diabetes.

People with diabetes mellitus may have the following signs and symptoms (Fig. 20-6):

- increased thirst
- increased hunger
- weight loss
- elevated levels of blood sugar
- presence of sugar in the urine
- increased frequency of urination

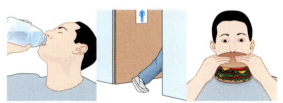

Fig. 20-6. Increased thirst, hunger, and urination are all symptoms of diabetes.

Diabetes can lead to the following complications:

- Changes in the circulatory system can cause heart attack and stroke, reduced circulation to the extremities, poor wound healing, and kidney and nerve damage.

- Damage to the eyes can cause impaired vision and blindness.

- Good foot care is vitally important for people with diabetes. Poor circulation and impaired wound healing may result in leg and foot ulcers, infected wounds, and gangrene. Gangrene can lead to amputation.

- Insulin shock and diabetic coma can be life-threatening. Learn to recognize signs of each.

Diabetes

Report any of the following to your supervisor:

- skin breakdown
- change in appetite (client overeating or not eating enough)
- weight changes
- changes in mental status
- increase or decrease in urine output
- visual changes
- change in mobility
- change in sensation

8. Describe the differences between insulin shock and diabetic coma, and list care for each

Insulin shock and diabetic coma are complications of diabetes that can be life-threatening. Discuss each individual client's status with your supervisor. **Insulin shock**, or **hypoglycemia** (*hye-poh-glye-SEE-mee-a*), can result from either too much insulin or too little food. It occurs when a dose of insulin is administered and the person skips a meal or does not eat all the food required. Even when a regular amount of food is eaten, physical activity may rapidly metabolize the food so that too much insulin is in the body. Vomiting and diarrhea may also lead to insulin shock in people with diabetes.

The first signs of insulin shock include feeling weak or different, nervousness, dizziness, and perspiration. These signal that the client needs food in a form that can be rapidly absorbed. A lump of sugar, a hard candy, or a glass of orange juice should be consumed right away. The client who is diabetic should always have a quick source of sugar handy. Contact your supervisor if the client has shown early signs of insulin shock.

The following are signs and symptoms of insulin shock:

- hunger

- weakness
- rapid pulse
- headache
- low blood pressure
- perspiration
- cold, clammy skin
- confusion
- trembling
- nervousness
- blurred vision
- numbness of the lips and tongue
- unconsciousness

Diabetic coma, also known as **acidosis** (*a-sid-OH-sis*) or **hyperglycemia** (*high-per-glye-SEE-mee-a*), is caused by having too little insulin. It can result from undiagnosed diabetes, going without insulin or not taking enough, eating too much food, not getting enough exercise, or physical or emotional stress.

The signs of diabetic coma include increased thirst or urination, abdominal pain, deep or labored breathing, and breath that smells sweet or fruity. Call your supervisor immediately if you suspect your client is experiencing diabetic coma or insulin shock. Know and follow your agency's policies and procedures for when to call emergency services.

Other signs and symptoms of diabetic coma include the following:

- hunger
- weakness
- rapid, weak pulse
- headache
- low blood pressure
- dry skin
- flushed cheeks
- drowsiness
- slow, deep, and labored breathing
- nausea and vomiting
- abdominal pain

- sweet, fruity breath odor
- air hunger, or client gasping for air and being unable to catch his breath
- unconsciousness

9. List care guidelines for the client with diabetes

Diabetes must be carefully controlled to prevent complications and severe illness. When working with clients with diabetes, follow care plan instructions carefully.

GUIDELINES
Caring for Clients with Diabetes

Follow diet instructions exactly. The intake of carbohydrates, including breads, potatoes, grains, pasta, and sugars, must be regulated. Meals must be eaten at the same time each day. The client must eat everything that is served. If a client refuses to eat what is directed, or if you suspect that he or she is not following the diet when you leave, report this to your supervisor. More information on diet for a person with diabetes is provided later in this chapter.

Encourage your client to follow his or her exercise program. A regular exercise program is important. It affects how quickly our bodies use the food we eat. Exercise also helps improve circulation. Exercises may include walking or other active exercise (Fig. 20-7). It may also include passive range of motion exercises. Assist with exercises as necessary. Try to make it fun. A walk can be a chore or it can be the highlight of the day.

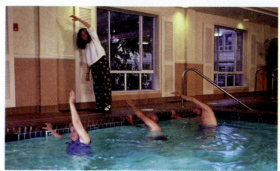

Fig. 20-7. Following an exercise program is very important for diabetic clients.

g Observe the client's management of insulin doses. Doses are calculated exactly. They should be administered at the same time each day. Home health aides are not permitted to inject insulin. However, you may be asked to bring the insulin and supplies to the client, to check the expiration date, to store the insulin (usually in the refrigerator), and/or to keep a record of where on the body the insulin was injected.

g Perform urine and blood tests as directed (Fig. 20-8). Sometimes the care plan will specify a daily blood or urine test to determine sugar or insulin levels. Not all states allow home health aides to do this. Know your state's rules. Your agency will train you. Perform tests only as directed.

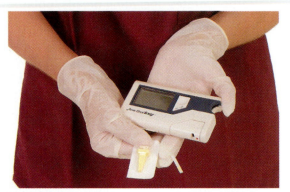

Fig. 20-8. This equipment measures glucose levels in the blood.

g Perform foot care only as directed. Because poor circulation occurs in diabetics, even a small sore on the leg or foot can grow into a large wound. It can result in amputation. Careful foot care, including regular inspection, is very important. The goals of diabetic foot care are to check for signs of irritation or sores, to promote blood circulation, and to prevent infection.

In addition to daily foot care, encourage diabetic clients to wear comfortable, well-fitting shoes that do not hurt their feet. To avoid cuts or injuries to the feet, diabetics should never go barefoot. Cotton socks are best because they absorb sweat. Home health aides should **never trim or clip any client's toenails, but especially not a diabetic client's toenails. Only a nurse or doctor should trim a diabetic client's toenails.**

Providing foot care for the diabetic client

Equipment: basin of warm water, mild soap, washcloth, soft towel, lotion, cotton balls, cotton socks, shoes or slipper, gloves if client has broken skin

1. Wash your hands.

2. Explain the procedure to the client, speaking clearly, slowly, and directly, maintaining face-to-face contact whenever possible.

3. Provide privacy for the client.

4. Put on gloves if the client has broken skin.

5. Using the washcloth and soap, wash the feet gently. Rinse with the warm water.

6. Pat the feet dry gently, wiping between the toes.

7. Starting at the toes and working up to the ankles, gently rub lotion into the feet with circular strokes. Your goal is to increase circulation, so take several minutes on each foot.

8. Observe the feet, ankles, and legs for dry skin, irritation, blisters, redness, sores, corns, discoloration, or swelling.

9. Help client put on socks and shoes or slippers.

10. Put used linens in the laundry. Pour water into the toilet. Clean and store basin and supplies.

11. Remove gloves if worn.

12. Wash your hands.

13. Document the procedure, including any abnormalities you observed on the feet or legs.

10. Describe a meal plan for the client with diabetes

People with diabetes must be very careful about what they eat. To keep their blood glucose levels near normal, they must eat the right amount of the right type of food at the right time. To make it easier to keep track of what they should eat, diabetics often follow meal plans and use exchange lists.

A dietitian, working with the client, creates a **meal plan** that includes all the right types and amounts of food for each day. The client uses **exchange lists**, or lists of similar foods that can substitute for one another, to make up a menu. For example, the meal plan might call for one starch and one fruit to be eaten as a snack. Looking at the exchange list, the client may choose which starch and fruit he wants to eat. The list has many choices, from bagels to biscuits to pretzels. The equivalent serving size for each food is also given, so the person will get the right amount of carbohydrates, protein, and fat to meet their requirements. Using meal plans and exchange lists, a person with diabetes can control his diet while still making his own food choices.

You will not be responsible for making up meal plans. A dietitian will create meal plans, provide exchange lists, and train the client to use them. If you are assigned to prepare food for the client, however, you should follow the diet exactly. If you observe the client not following his or her diet, report it to your supervisor.

Sample Meal Plan and Exchange List

The following is a sample meal plan and a partial exchange list a person with diabetes might use. Keep in mind that this is only an example. A client's diet may also be under other restrictions. The diet will vary according to the client's daily caloric needs. Actual exchange lists contain many more choices than the sample below.

Sample Meal Plan

- Breakfast (to be eaten between 7:30 and 8:30 a.m.): two starches, one milk, one fruit, one fat
- Snack (to be eaten between 10 and 11 a.m.): one milk
- Lunch (12:30 to 1:30 p.m.): one meat, one milk, two starches, one vegetable, one fruit
- Snack (3:00 to 4:00 p.m.): one vegetable, one milk

- Dinner (5:30 to 6:30 p.m.): three meats, one starch, two vegetables, one milk, two fats
- Snack (7:30 to 8:30 p.m.): one milk, one starch

Following the meal plan for what types of food and how many servings to eat, the person chooses specific foods and determines serving sizes using the exchange lists.

Exchange List Sample Items

- Starch list: 1 slice of bread, 1/2 bagel, 1/2 cup cereal, 1/2 cup pasta, 1/2 cup rice, 1 baked potato, 3 cups popcorn, 15-20 fat-free potato chips
- Milk list: 1 cup milk (skim, 1%, 2%, or whole, depending on other dietary guidelines), 3/4 cup yogurt
- Fruit list: 1/2 cup unsweetened applesauce, 1 small banana, 1/2 cup orange juice, 2 tablespoons raisins, 1 small orange, 1/2 cup canned pears
- Vegetable list: 1/2 cup cooked vegetables or vegetable juice, 1 cup raw vegetables (not included are corn, potatoes, and peas, which are on the starch exchange list instead)
- Meat list: 1 oz. meat, fish, poultry, or cheese, 1 egg, or 1/2 cup dried beans
- Fat list: 1 tsp margarine or butter, 2 tsps peanut butter, 2 tbsps sour cream, 1 tsp mayonnaise, 10 peanuts

11. Define cerebral vascular accident (CVA) and list common warning signs

The medical term for a stroke is a **cerebral vascular accident** (ser-EE-bral VAS-kyoo-lar AK-si-dent (CVA). CVA, or stroke, is caused when the blood supply to the brain is cut off suddenly by a clot or a ruptured blood vessel (Fig. 20-9). Without blood, part of the brain gets no oxygen. This causes brain cells to die. Brain tissue is further damaged by leaking blood, clots, and swelling that cause pressure on surrounding areas of healthy tissue.

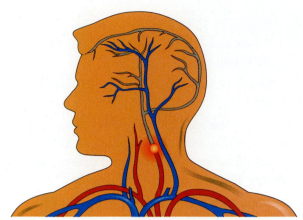

Fig. 20-9. A stroke is caused when the blood supply to the brain is cut off suddenly by a clot or ruptured blood vessel.

A **transient ischemic attack** (*TRAN-see-ent is-KEE-mik a-TAK*), or TIA, is a warning sign of a CVA. It is the result of a temporary lack of oxygen in the brain. Symptoms may last up to 24 hours. They include tingling, weakness, confusion, or some loss of movement in an extremity. These symptoms should not be ignored. Report any of these symptoms to your supervisor immediately.

A stroke may be preceded by symptoms. These symptoms include dizziness, ringing in the ears, headache, nausea, vomiting, slurring of words, and loss of memory. These symptoms should also be reported immediately.

Signs that a stroke is occurring include any of the following: loss of consciousness, redness in the face, noisy breathing, seizures, loss of bowel and bladder control, **hemiplegia** (*hem-i-PLEE-jee-a*), **hemiparesis** (*hem-i-pa-REE-sis*), **aphasia** (*a-FAY-see-a*), use of inappropriate words, elevated blood pressure, and slow pulse rate. Hemiplegia is paralysis on one side of the body. Hemiparesis is weakness on one side of the body. Aphasia is the inability to speak or to speak clearly.

The two sides of the brain control different functions. Symptoms depend on which side of the brain the stroke affected. Weaknesses on the right side of the body indicate that the left side of the brain was affected. Weaknesses on the left side of the body indicate that the right side of the brain was affected.

12. Describe six common physical changes in CVA clients

Strokes can be mild or severe. After a stroke, a client may experience any of the following:

- weakness or paralysis on one side of the body
- difficulty speaking or inability to speak
- difficulty understanding spoken or written words
- loss of sensations such as temperature or touch
- loss of bowel or bladder control
- confusion
- poor judgment
- memory loss
- loss of cognitive abilities
- tendency to ignore one side of the body
- difficulty swallowing

If the stroke was mild, the client may experience few, if any, of these effects. Physical therapy may help stroke victims regain physical abilities. Speech therapy and occupational therapy can also help a person learn to communicate and perform ADLs again.

13. Describe care guidelines and communication techniques for the CVA client

Clients who have had a stroke will need specific care for their disabilities. A client with hemiplegia will need different care than a client with speech loss. Follow the care plan and your assignments, but keep the following general guidelines in mind.

GUIDELINES
Caring for Clients Recovering from Stroke

- Clients with paralysis, weakness or loss of movement will usually receive physical therapy or occupational therapy. You may be asked to assist clients in performing exer-

cises. Range of motion exercises will help strengthen muscles and keep joints mobile. Clients may also need to perform leg exercises to improve circulation. Safety is important when post-CVA clients are exercising.

🅖 Adapt procedures when providing personal care for clients with one-sided paralysis or weakness. When helping with transfers or walking, stand on the weaker side. Always use a gait belt for safety.

🅖 Never refer to the weaker side as the "bad side," or talk about the "bad" leg or arm. Use the term "**weaker**" or "**involved**" to refer to the side with paralysis or paresis.

🅖 Clients with speech loss or communication problems may receive speech therapy. You may be asked to help. This includes helping clients to recognize written words or to speak words. Speech therapists will also evaluate a client's swallowing ability. They will decide if swallowing therapy or thickened liquids are needed.

🅖 Use verbal and nonverbal communication to express your positive attitude. Let the client know you have confidence in his or her abilities through smiles, touches, and gestures. Gestures and pointing can also help you convey information or allow the client to speak to you. More ideas for communicating with CVA clients are listed later in the chapter.

Experiencing confusion or memory loss is upsetting. People often cry for no apparent reason after suffering a stroke. Be patient and understanding. Your positive attitude will be important. Keeping a routine may help clients feel more secure.

Monitoring the home safety of clients who have had a stroke is essential. Clients who are unsteady, weak, or confused are at risk of falling. Clients with loss of sensation are at risk of burning themselves in the bathroom or at the stove. Some safety tips include:

- Remove any hazards from the home, including unnecessary clutter or throw rugs.

- Unplug appliances like toasters and coffee makers when not in use.

- Check the refrigerator and cabinets for spoiled food. A stroke may impair the senses of smell and taste.

- Report any suspected safety hazards to your supervisor.

- Follow instructions for safe client transfers using good body mechanics (see chapters 6 and 12).

- Always check on the client's body alignment. Sometimes an arm or leg can be caught and the client is unaware.

- Pay special attention to skin care and observe for changes in the skin if a client is unable to move.

Encourage independence and self-esteem. Let the client do things for him- or herself whenever possible, even if you could do a better or faster job. Make tasks less difficult for the client to do. Appreciate and acknowledge clients' efforts to do things for themselves even when they are unsuccessful. Praise even the smallest successes to build confidence.

GUIDELINES
Assisting Clients with One-sided Weakness with Transfers, Dressing, and Eating

When assisting with transfers, remember the following:

🅖 Support the involved side.

🅖 Lead with the uninvolved (stronger) side (Fig. 20-10).

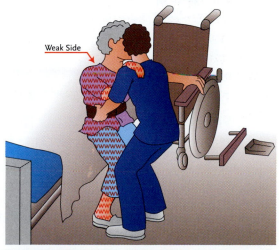

Weak Side

Fig. 20-10. When helping a client transfer, support the weak side while leading with the stronger side.

20

Common Chronic and Acute Conditions

- Follow the principles of good body mechanics (see chapter 6).

When assisting with dressing, remember the following:

- Dress weaker side first. Place the weaker arm or leg into the clothing first. This prevents unnecessary bending and stretching of the limb. Undress stronger side first. Lead with the stronger side. Then remove the weaker arm or leg from clothing to prevent the limb from being stretched and twisted.

- Use adaptive equipment to help client dress himself (see chapters 13 and 15).

- Encourage self-care.

When assisting with eating, remember the following:

- Place food in the client's field of vision (Fig. 20-11).

- Use assistive devices such as silverware with built-up handle grips, plate guards, and drinking cups (see chapter 15).

- Watch for signs of choking.

- Serve soft foods if swallowing is difficult.

- Always place food in the unaffected side of the mouth.

- Make sure food is swallowed before offering more bites.

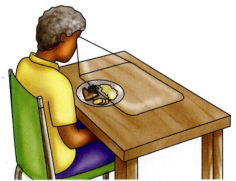

Fig. 20-11. A client who has had a stroke may have a limited field of vision. Make sure the client can see what you place in front of him.

GUIDELINES
Communicating with Clients Who Have Had a Stroke

- Keep your questions and directions simple.

- Phrase questions so they can be answered with a "yes" or "no".

- Agree on signals, such as shaking or nodding the head, or raising a hand or finger to indicate "yes" or "no".

- Use pictures, gestures, or pointing to communicate. Use communication boards or special cards to make communication easier (Fig. 20-12).

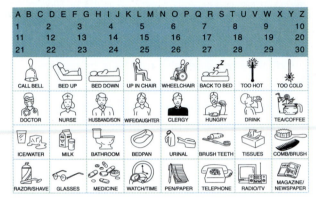

Fig. 20-12. A sample communication board.

- Use a pencil and paper if a client is able to write. A thick handle or tape wrapped around the pen may help the client hold it more easily.

- Keep a bell or other call signal within reach of clients. They can let you know when you are needed.

- Never talk about a client as if he or she were not there. Speak to all clients with respect.

Assisting with Rehabilitation

You will often help in the rehabilitation of a person who has suffered a stroke.

People who have had a stroke usually take a long time to recover. Therefore, it is important to work with them in stages or steps that allow them to master simple goals first. An example is strengthening a weak arm. By doing this you will help them gain confidence in their difficult fight to regain strength and ability.

Encourage the client to use and exercise the weaker side. Instruct him or her to use the strong arm or leg to assist the range of motion

exercises on the weak side. Rolling over onto the strong side first is recommended for changing positions. Remind recovering stroke clients to place the strong foot under the involved ankle when crossing the legs in preparation for rolling over or moving the leg (Fig. 20-13).

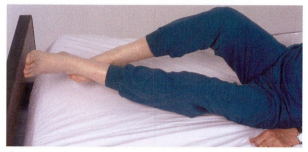

Fig. 20-13.

If the client is in a sitting position, place the elbow on an armrest to support the involved shoulder (Fig. 20-14).

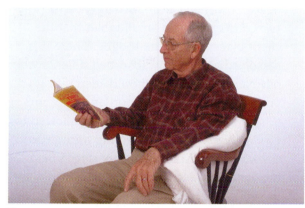

Fig. 20-14.

Ninety-degree flexion is a good position for the weak hip and knee. It is important to remember to position the involved side correctly. Often a person who has had a stroke cannot feel that one side of the body is weaker than the other (Fig. 20-15).

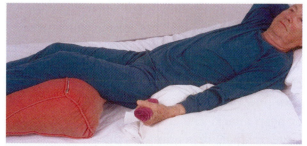

Fig. 20-15. In bed, the client's involved side should be properly supported.

14. Identify common circulatory disorders, their symptoms, and care guidelines

High Blood Pressure or Hypertension

When blood pressure consistently measures 140/90 or higher, a person is diagnosed as having **hypertension** (*high-per-TEN-shun*), or high blood pressure. If blood pressure is between 120/80 and 140/90 mmHg, then it called **pre-hypertension**. This means that the person does not have high blood pressure now but is likely to develop it in the future.

High blood pressure is caused by **atherosclerosis** (*ath-er-oh-skle-ROH-sis*), or a hardening and narrowing of the blood vessels (Fig. 20-16). It can also result from kidney disease, tumors of the adrenal gland, complications of pregnancy, and head injuries. High blood pressure can develop in persons of any age.

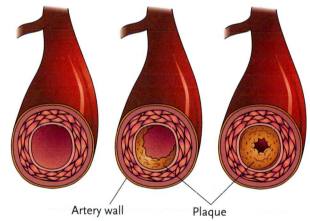

Artery wall   Plaque

Fig. 20-16. Arteries may become hardened, or narrower, because of a build-up of plaque. Hardened arteries cause high blood pressure.

Signs and symptoms of high blood pressure are not always obvious, especially in the early stages. Often it is only discovered when a blood pressure measurement is taken. Persons with the disease may complain of headache, blurred vision, and dizziness.

GUIDELINES
Caring for Clients with High Blood Pressure

- Because it can lead to serious conditions such as CVA, heart attack, kidney disease, or

20

Common Chronic and Acute Conditions

blindness, treatment to control high blood pressure is essential. Clients may take medication that lowers cholesterol or **diuretics** (*dye-you-RET-iks*). Diuretics are drugs that reduce fluid in the body.

g Clients may also have a prescribed exercise program or be on a special low-fat, low-sodium diet. You will probably be required to take frequent blood pressure measurements. You can also help by encouraging clients to follow their diet and exercise programs.

Coronary Artery Disease (CAD)

Coronary artery disease occurs when the blood vessels in the coronary arteries narrow. This reduces the supply of blood to the heart muscle and deprives it of oxygen and nutrients. Over time, as fatty deposits block the artery, the muscle that was supplied by the blood vessel dies. CAD can lead to heart attack or stroke.

The heart muscle that is not getting enough oxygen causes chest pain, or **angina pectoris** (*an-JYE-na PEK-tor-is*). The heart needs more oxygen during exercise or exertion, stress, excitement, or a heavy meal. In CAD, constricted blood vessels prevent the extra blood with oxygen from getting to the heart (Fig. 20-17).

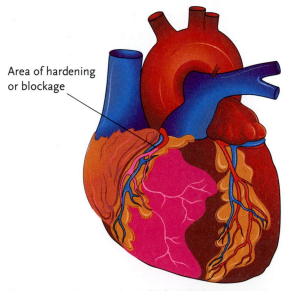

Area of hardening or blockage

Fig. 20-17. Angina pectoris results from the heart not getting enough oxygen.

The pain of angina pectoris is usually described as pressure or tightness in the left side of the chest or in the center of the chest behind the sternum or breastbone. Some people complain of pain radiating or extending down the inside of the left arm or to the neck and left side of the jaw. A person suffering from angina pectoris may perspire or appear pale. The person may feel dizzy and have difficulty breathing.

GUIDELINES
Caring for Clients with Angina Pectoris

g Rest is extremely important. Rest reduces the heart's need for extra oxygen. It helps the blood flow return to normal, often within three to fifteen minutes.

g Medication is also necessary to relax the walls of the coronary arteries. This allows them to open and get more blood to the heart. This medication, **nitroglycerin** (*nite-roh-GLIS-er-in*), is a small tablet that the client places under the tongue. There it is dissolved and rapidly absorbed. Clients who have angina pectoris should keep nitroglycerin on hand to use as soon as symptoms arise. Home health aides are not allowed to give any medication, including nitroglycerin. Call your supervisor if a client needs help taking the medication. Nitroglycerin is also available as a patch. Do not remove the patch. Inform your supervisor immediately if the patch comes off.

g Clients may also be required to avoid heavy meals, overeating, intense exercise, and exposure to cold or hot and humid weather.

Myocardial Infarction (MI) or Heart Attack

When blood flow to the heart muscle is completely blocked, oxygen and important nutrients fail to reach the cells in that region (Fig. 20-18). Waste products are not removed and the muscle cell dies. This is called a **myocardial infarction** (*mye-oh-KAR-dee-al in-FARK-shun*) or MI, or heart attack. The area of dead tissue may be large or small, depending on the artery involved.

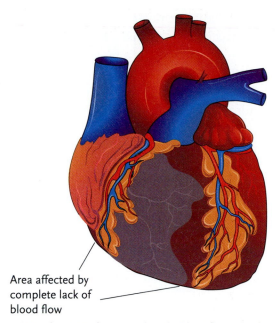

Area affected by complete lack of blood flow

Fig. 20-18. A heart attack occurs when the blood flow to the heart or a portion of the heart is cut off completely.

A myocardial infarction is an emergency that can result in serious heart damage or death. The following are signs and symptoms of MI:

- sudden, severe pain in the chest, usually on the left side or in the center behind the sternum

- a feeling of indigestion or heartburn

- nausea and vomiting

- **dyspnea** (*DISP-nee-a*) or difficulty breathing

- dizziness

- pale, gray, or **cyanotic** (*sye-a-NOT-ik*) skin; cyanotic skin is a bluish color, indicating lack of oxygen

- perspiration

- cold and clammy skin

- weak and irregular pulse rate

- low blood pressure

- anxiety and a sense of impending doom

The pain of a heart attack is commonly described as a crushing, pressing, squeezing, stabbing, piercing, vise-like pain, or "like someone is sitting on my chest." The pain may radiate down the inside of the left arm. A person may also feel it in the neck and/or in the jaw. The pain does not go away.

Caring for Clients Having or Recovering from a Heart Attack

g Someone having a heart attack must receive emergency treatment from medical personnel. This helps minimize damage and prevent further illness or death. Call 911 for emergency medical assistance immediately if a client is having a heart attack. If you are trained to perform cardiopulmonary resuscitation (CPR), do so if necessary when help is not available or until help arrives. Contact your supervisor after medical personnel arrive to take over care of the client.

g Generally, clients who have had a heart attack will be placed on a regular exercise program.

g Clients may be placed on a diet low in fat and cholesterol and/or a low-sodium diet.

g Medications may be prescribed to regulate heart rate and blood pressure.

g Clients recovering from a heart attack may be cautioned to avoid exposure to cold temperatures.

Congestive Heart Failure (CHF)

Coronary artery disease, heart attack, high blood pressure, or other disorders may all damage the heart. When the heart muscle has been severely damaged, the heart fails to pump effectively. Blood backs up into the heart instead of circulating. This is called **congestive heart failure**, or CHF. It can occur on one or both sides of the heart.

Signs and symptoms of congestive heart failure include the following:

- difficulty breathing; coughing or gurgling with breathing

- dizziness, confusion, and fainting

- pale or cyanotic skin

- low blood pressure

- swelling of the feet and ankles

- bulging veins in the neck

- weight gain

20

Common Chronic and Acute Conditions

20

Common Chronic and Acute Conditions

GUIDELINES
Caring for Clients with CHF

ⓖ Although congestive heart failure is a serious illness, it can be successfully treated and controlled. Medications can strengthen the heart muscle and improve its pumping.

ⓖ Medications help eliminate excess fluids. This means more frequent trips to the bathroom. Assist client as needed.

ⓖ A low-sodium diet may be recommended.

ⓖ A weakened heart pump may make it difficult for clients to walk, carry groceries, or climb stairs. Limited activity may be prescribed.

ⓖ Intake of fluids and output of urine may need to be measured (see chapter 14).

ⓖ Client may weigh daily at the same time to note weight gain from fluid retention.

ⓖ Elastic leg stockings may be applied to reduce swelling in feet and ankles.

ⓖ Range of motion exercises improve muscle tone when activity and exercise are limited (Fig. 20-19).

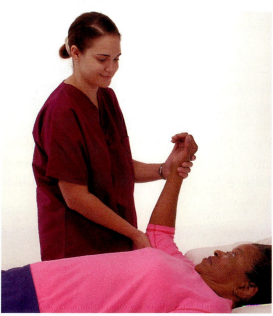

Fig. 20-19. Range of motion exercises improve muscle tone.

ⓖ Assistance with personal care and ADLs may need to be provided.

A common side effect of medications for CHF is dizziness, which may result from a lack of potassium. High-potassium foods and drinks such as bananas or raisins, orange juice, or other citrus juices can easily help this. These foods should be eaten as a preventive measure as well. The client care plan should mention the possible side effects of drugs and what signs or symptoms to report to your supervisor.

15. Define COPD and list care guidelines

Chronic obstructive pulmonary disease, or COPD, is a chronic disease. This means the client may live for years with it but never be cured. Clients with COPD have difficulty breathing, especially in getting air out of the lungs. There are four chronic lung diseases (see chapter 9) that are grouped under COPD. They include

- Chronic bronchitis
- Pulmonary emphysema
- Asthma
- Chronic bronchiectasis

Over time, a client with any of these lung disorders becomes chronically ill and weakened. There is a high risk for acute lung infections, such as pneumonia (see chapter 9). Sometimes medications for lung conditions are given directly into the lungs using sprays or inhalers (Fig. 20-20).

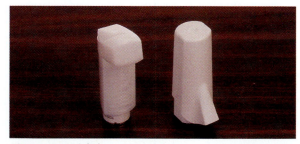

Fig. 20-20. An inhaler.

When the lungs and brain do not get enough oxygen, all body systems are affected. Clients may live with a constant fear of not being able to breathe. This can cause them to sit upright in an attempt to improve their ability to expand the lungs. These clients can have poor appetites. They usually do not get enough sleep.

All of this can add to their feelings of weakness and poor health. They may feel they have lost control of their bodies, and particularly their breathing. They may fear suffocation.

Clients with COPD may experience the following symptoms:

- chronic cough or wheeze
- difficulty breathing, especially when inhaling and exhaling deeply
- shortness of breath, especially during physical effort
- pale or cyanotic (blue) skin or reddish-purple skin
- mental confusion
- general state of weakness
- difficulty completing meals due to shortness of breath
- fear and anxiety

GUIDELINES
Caring for Clients with COPD

🅖 Colds or viruses can make clients very ill quickly. Always observe and report signs of symptoms getting worse.

🅖 Help clients sit upright or lean forward. Offer pillows to support them (Fig. 20-21).

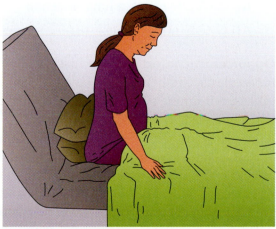

Fig. 20-21. It helps clients with COPD to sit upright and lean forward slightly.

🅖 Offer plenty of fluids and small frequent meals.

🅖 Encourage a well-balanced diet.

🅖 Keep oxygen supply available as ordered.

🅖 Being unable to breathe or fearing suffocation can be very frightening. Be calm and supportive.

🅖 Use good infection control, especially with handwashing by the client and the disposal of used tissues.

🅖 Encourage as much client independence with ADLs as possible.

🅖 Remind clients to avoid situations where they may be exposed to infections, especially colds and the flu.

🅖 Teach pursed-lip breathing. Pursed-lip breathing is placing the lips as if in a kiss and taking controlled breaths.

🅖 Encourage clients to save energy for important daily tasks. Encourage clients to rest during tasks.

OBSERVING AND REPORTING
COPD

Report any of the following to your supervisor:

- temperature over 101°F
- changes in breathing patterns, including shortness of breath
- changes in color or consistency of lung secretions
- changes in mental state or personality
- refusal to take medications as ordered
- excessive weight loss
- increasing dependence upon caregivers and family

16. Define HIV and AIDS and describe care guidelines

Acquired immunodeficiency (*im-YOU-noh-de-FISH-en-see*) **syndrome**, or **AIDS**, is an illness caused by the **human immunodeficiency virus**, or **HIV**. HIV attacks the immune system and gradually disables it. Eventually the HIV-infected person has weakened resistance to other

infections. Death is the result of these infections. However, medications help people live longer. HIV is a sexually transmitted disease. It can also be spread through the blood, from infected needles, or to a fetus from its mother. More information on high-risk behaviors for contracting HIV, avoiding HIV, and transmission of HIV is provided in chapter 9 and chapter 5 on infection control.

In general, HIV affects the body in stages. The first stage involves symptoms similar to flu, with fever, muscle aches, cough, and fatigue. These are symptoms of the body's immune system fighting the infection. As the infection worsens, the immune system overreacts and attacks not only the virus, but also normal tissue.

When the virus weakens the immune system in later stages, a cluster of problems may appear. These include opportunistic infections, tumors, and central nervous system symptoms that would not occur if the immune system were healthy. This stage of the disease is known as AIDS.

In the late stages of AIDS, damage to the central nervous system may cause memory loss, poor coordination, paralysis, and confusion. These symptoms together are known as **AIDS dementia complex**.

The following are the signs and symptoms of HIV infection and AIDS:

- appetite loss
- involuntary weight loss of 10 pounds or more
- vague, flu-like symptoms, including fever, cough, weakness, and severe or constant fatigue
- night sweats
- swollen lymph nodes in the neck, underarms, or groin
- excessive diarrhea
- dry cough
- skin rashes

- painful white spots in the mouth or on the tongue
- cold sores or fever blisters on the lips and flat, white ulcers on a reddened base in the mouth
- cauliflower-like warts (caused by the human papilloma virus) on the skin and in the mouth
- inflamed and bleeding gums
- bruising that does not go away
- susceptibility to infection, particularly pneumonia, but also tuberculosis, herpes, bacterial infections, and hepatitis
- **Kaposi's sarcoma**, a rare form of skin cancer that appears as purple or red skin lesions (Fig. 20-22)

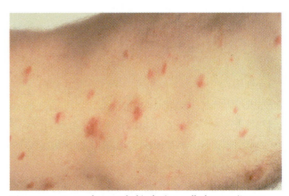

Fig. 20-22. A purple or red skin lesion called Kaposi's sarcoma can be a sign of AIDS.

- **pneumocystis pneumonia** (*new-moh-SIS-tis new-MOH-nee-a*), a lung infection
- AIDS dementia complex

Opportunistic infections, such as pneumonia, tuberculosis, and hepatitis, invade the body because the immune system is weak and unable to defend itself. These illnesses complicate AIDS. They further weaken the immune system. It is difficult to treat these infections because generally, over time, a person develops resistance to some antibiotics. These infections are frequently the cause of death in people with AIDS.

Persons who are infected with HIV are treated with drugs that slow the progress of the disease, but do not cure it. The medicines must be

taken at precise times. They have many unpleasant side effects. For some people, the medications work less well than for others. Other aspects of HIV treatment include relief of symptoms and prevention and treatment of infection.

You can help prevent the spread of HIV/AIDS by carefully following Standard Precautions (see chapter 5). Because the symptoms of HIV/AIDS may not appear for months or years, you and even the client him- or herself may not know the infection is present. You could be infected accidentally. But by following Standard Precautions and other infection control practices when working with all your clients, you will be safe from contracting HIV from clients.

GUIDELINES
Caring for Clients with HIV/AIDS

- Involuntary weight loss occurs in almost all people who develop AIDS. High-protein, high-calorie, and high-nutrient meals can help maintain a healthy weight.

- Some people with HIV/AIDS lose their appetites and have difficulty eating. These clients should be encouraged to relax before meals and to eat in a pleasant setting. Serve familiar and favorite foods. Report appetite loss or difficulty eating to your supervisor. If appetite loss continues to be a problem, the doctor may prescribe an appetite stimulant.

- It is extremely important to carefully follow guidelines for safe food preparation and storage when working with a client who has HIV/AIDS. Food-borne illnesses caused by improperly cooking or storing food can cause death for someone with HIV/AIDS (see chapter 23 for safe food handling practices). Wash your hands frequently, keep everything clean (especially countertops, cutting boards, and knives after they have been used to cut meat), thaw food in the refrigerator, and wash and cook foods thoroughly. When storing food, keep cold foods cold and hot foods hot, use small containers that seal tightly, check expiration dates, and remember "when in doubt, throw it out."

- Clients who have infections of the mouth and esophagus may require food that is low in acid and neither cold nor hot. Spicy seasonings should be removed. Soft or pureed foods may be easier to swallow. Drinking liquid meals and fortified drinks, such as milk shakes, may ease the pain of chewing. If loose stools result from this, liquid supplements that are high in fiber may be prescribed. Warm salt water or other rinses may help painful sores of the mouth. Good mouth care is essential.

- Someone who has nausea or vomiting should eat small, frequent meals, if possible. The person should eat slowly. The person should avoid high-fat and spicy foods, and eat a soft, bland diet. This includes mashed potatoes, noodles, rice, crackers, pretzels, toast, gelatin, and clear soups. Cold foods that have little odor are usually easier to eat than hot foods. When nausea and vomiting persist, liquids and salty foods should be encouraged, including clear soups, clear juices, ginger ale and colas, saltines, and pretzels. Clients should eat small, frequent meals and drink fluids in between meals. Care must be taken to maintain an adequate intake of fluids.

- Clients who have mild diarrhea may have frequent small meals that are low in fat, fiber, and milk products. If diarrhea is severe, the client's doctor may order a "BRAT" diet (a diet consisting of bananas, rice, apples, and toast). This diet is helpful for short-term use.

- Diarrhea rapidly depletes the body of fluids. Fluid replacement is necessary. Good rehydration fluids include water, juice, soda, and broth. Clients with diarrhea should avoid high-fiber foods, including seeds, nuts, wheat brans, whole wheat bread, and the skins of fruits and vegetables. They should also avoid fats, milk, cheese, ice cream, beans, cabbage, spicy foods, and caffeine.

- **Neuropathy** (*NOOR-oh-path-ee*), or numbness, tingling, and pain in the feet and legs is usually treated with pain medications.

Going without shoes or wearing loose, soft slippers may be helpful. If blankets and sheets cause pain, use a bed cradle to keep sheets and blankets from resting on the legs and feet (see chapter 12).

g Clients with HIV/AIDS may suffer from anxiety and depression. In addition, they often suffer the judgments of family, friends, and society. Some people blame them for their illness. People with HIV/AIDS may experience tremendous stress. They may feel uncertainty about their illness, health care, and finances. They may also have lost people in their social support network of friends and family (Fig. 20-23).

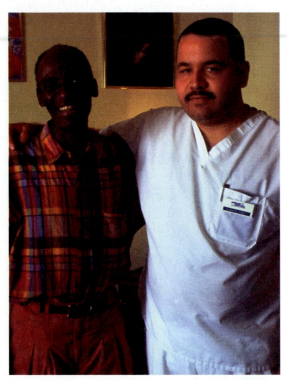

Fig. 20-23. Many people with AIDS have already lost family members or friends to the disease.

Clients with HIV/AIDS need support from others. This support may come from family, friends, religious and community groups, and support groups, as well as the healthcare team. Treat all your clients with respect. Help provide the emotional support they need.

g Withdrawal, apathy, avoidance of complex tasks, and mental slowness are symptoms that appear early in HIV infection. In addition, medications may cause side effects of

this type. Later, AIDS dementia complex may develop, causing further mental symptoms. There may also be muscle weakness and loss of muscle control, making falls a risk. Clients in this stage of the disease will need a safe environment and close supervision in their ADLs.

17. Describe normal changes of aging in the brain

As we age, we may lose some of our ability to think logically and quickly. This ability is called **cognition** (*kog-NI-shun*). When we lose some of this ability we are said to have **cognitive impairment** (*KOG-ni-tiv im-PAYR-ment*). Cognitive impairment affects concentration and memory. Elderly clients may lose their memories of recent events, which can be frustrating for them. You can help by encouraging them to make lists of things to remember and writing down names and phone numbers.

Other normal changes of aging in the brain include slower reaction time, difficulty finding or using the right words, and sleeping less.

18. Define dementia and recognize its causes

Dementia (*di-MEN-shee-a*) is a more serious loss of mental abilities such as thinking, remembering, reasoning, and communicating. As dementia advances, these losses make it difficult to perform ADLs such as eating, bathing, dressing, and toileting. **Dementia is not a normal part of aging.**

The following are a few of the common causes of dementia:

- Alzheimer's disease
- Multi-infarct or vascular dementia (a series of strokes causing damage to the brain)
- Lewy Body disease
- Parkinson's disease
- Huntington's disease

19. Describe Alzheimer's disease and identify its stages and related behaviors

Alzheimer's disease (AD) is a **progressive, degenerative**, and **irreversible disease**. It causes tangled nerve fibers and protein deposits to form in the brain, eventually causing dementia. Progressive and degenerative mean the disease gets worse, causing greater and greater loss of health and abilities. Irreversible means the disease cannot be cured. Thus, clients with Alzheimer's disease will never recover. They will need more care as the disease progresses.

Alzheimer's disease generally begins with forgetfulness and confusion. It progresses to complete loss of all ability to care for oneself. Each person with Alzheimer's will show different symptoms at different times. For example, one person with Alzheimer's may be able to read, but not be able to use the phone or remember her own address. Another person may have lost the ability to read, but still be able to do simple math. Skills a person has used constantly over a long lifetime are usually kept longer. Thus some people with Alzheimer's can cook or play a musical instrument with some help long after they have lost much of their memory. Look for these "preserved skills." Help your clients use and enjoy them as long as possible (Fig. 20-24).

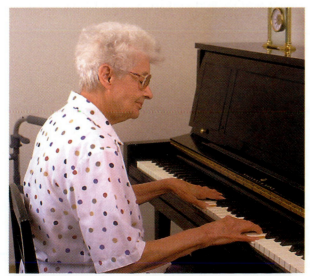

Fig. 20-24. Even when a person loses much of her memory, she may still keep skills she has used her whole life.

Encourage clients with AD to perform ADLs and keep their minds and bodies as active as possible. Working, socializing, reading, problem solving, and exercising should all be encouraged (Fig. 20-25). Having clients with AD do as much as possible for themselves may even help slow the progression of the disease. Look for tasks that are challenging but not frustrating. Help your clients succeed in performing them.

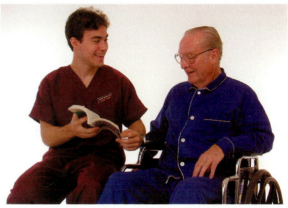

Fig. 20-25. Encourage reading and thinking activities for residents with AD.

General Progression of Alzheimer's Disease

Stage I

- recent (short-term) memory loss
- disorientation to time
- lack of interest in doing things, including work, dressing, recreation
- inability to concentrate
- mood swings
- irritability
- petulance: peevish, ill-humored, rude behavior
- tendency to blame others
- carelessness in personal habits
- poor judgment

Stage II

- increased memory loss, may forget family members and friends
- slurred speech
- difficulty finding right word, finishing thoughts, or following directions

- tendency to make statements that are illogical
- inability to read, write, or do math
- inability to care for self or perform ADLs without assistance
- incontinence
- dulled senses (for example, cannot distinguish between hot and cold)
- restlessness, wandering, and/or agitation (increase of these in the evening is called "sundowning")
- sleep problems
- lack of impulse control (for example: swears excessively or is sexually aggressive or rude)
- obsessive repetition of movements, behavior, or words
- temper tantrums
- hallucinations or delusions

Stage III

- total disorientation to time, place, and person
- apathy
- total dependence on others for care
- total incontinence
- inability to speak or communicate, except for grunting, groaning, or screaming
- total immobility/confined to bed
- inability to recognize family or self
- increased sleep disturbances
- difficulty swallowing, which produces risk of choking
- seizures
- coma
- death

20. Identify personal attitudes helpful in caring for people with AD or any dementia

The following attitudes will help you give the best possible care to your clients with AD:

Don't take it personally. Always remember that people with Alzheimer's do not have control over their words and actions. They may often be unaware of what they say or do. If a client with Alzheimer's doesn't recognize you, doesn't do what you say, ignores you, accuses you, or insults you, remember that it's the disease, not the person.

Put yourself in their shoes. Think about what it would be like to have Alzheimer's disease. Imagine being unable to perform ADLs. Treat clients with AD with dignity and respect, as you would want to be treated.

Work with the symptoms and behaviors you see. Each person with Alzheimer's disease is an individual. Clients with AD will not all show the same symptoms at the same times. Each client will do some things that others will never do. The best strategy is to work with the behaviors you see today. For example, an Alzheimer's client may want to go for a walk today, when yesterday she didn't seem able to get to the bathroom without help. If allowed by the care plan, try to go for a walk with her.

Work as a team. Always report and document your observations about your clients. Symptoms and behavior change from day to day. You are in a great position to give details about your clients' cases. Being with your clients frequently allows you to be the expert on each case. Make the most of this opportunity. You will be helping to give the best possible care.

Take care of yourself. Caring for someone with dementia can be exhausting—both emotionally and physically. Take care of yourself to continue giving the best possible care (Fig. 20-26).

Work with family members. Family members can be a wonderful resource. They can help you learn more about your client. They also provide familiarity and comfort to the person with Alzheimer's. Build relationships with family members and keep the lines of communication open. Home health aides are a big support to family members. Be a role model for appropri-

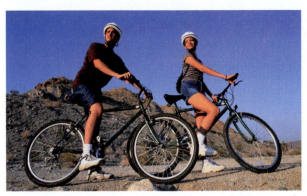

Fig. 20-26. Regular exercise is an important part of taking care of yourself.

ate behavior to assist the family in caring for the client.

Remember the goals of the client care plan. In addition to the practical tasks you will perform, the care plan will also call for maintaining clients' dignity and self-esteem. Help them to be as independent as possible.

21. List three strategies for better communication with Alzheimer's clients

1. **Speak in a low, calm voice, in a room with little background noise and distraction**. Many clients with AD become agitated easily; do everything you can to keep them calm. This means speaking in a quiet, slow manner. It may also mean eliminating noise and distractions, such as televisions or radios, and children or family members who are noisy.

2. **Repeat yourself, using the same words and phrases as often as needed**. When an Alzheimer's client does not understand what you are saying, repeat yourself using the same words. Remember that a person with Alzheimer's literally has tangles in the brain. It may take several repetitions for a message to get through. Keep messages simple. Break complex tasks into smaller, simpler ones.

    Repetition can also be reassuring for a person with Alzheimer's. In fact, many clients with AD will repeat words, phrases, ques-

tions, or actions frequently. This is called **perseveration**. If your client perseverates, do not try to stop him. Instead, answer his questions, using the same words each time, until he stops.

3. **Use pictures or gestures to communicate**. With some clients it may be more effective to use nonverbal communication. For example, use pictures, such as a drawing of a toilet on the bathroom door, and gestures, such as holding up a dress when you want to help your client dress. Usually it is most effective to combine verbal and nonverbal communication. For example, saying "Let's get dressed now," as you hold up clothes.

22. Describe a safe environment for a client with AD

Before you visit a client with Alzheimer's, a nurse should assess the home's safety. He will indicate changes to be made. Examples include using gates on stairways, putting locks on certain doors, and removing clutter. Report and document your observations.

When the client's condition changes, report this to your supervisor. Another visit will be made to reassess the home and make further changes. For example, if a client is no longer able to find the bathroom, signs can be posted on doors to indicate which room is which. If a client begins to wander, locks can be put on all doors and labels attached to clothing to identify the client who wanders away.

If you think additional changes need to be made, speak to your supervisor. When a client displays a new behavior, such as wandering, report it immediately.

Organizing the Home for the Client with AD

For disoriented clients:

*   Use signs to mark rooms, including stop signs on rooms that should not be entered.

- Use calendars and other reminders of day, date, and location.
- Put bells on the door to indicate when someone is coming or going.
- Keep pictures and familiar objects around.
- Put stickers or brightly colored tape on glass doors, large windows, or glass furniture (Fig. 20-27).

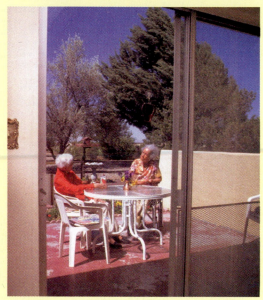

Fig. 20-27. Stickers or brightly colored tape on glass doors may help a disoriented client.

For the client who wanders:

- Use locks on doors. These can be installed low or high, so the client won't see them.
- Install alarms that go off when exit doors are opened.
- Have clients wear identification. Sew labels into clothes.
- Alert neighbors that client may wander. Show them a recent photo of the client.
- Keep a recent photo handy, as well as a piece of clothing the client has worn. These can help police and police dogs track a client who has wandered away.

For clients who pace:

- Remove clutter and throw rugs.
- Do not rearrange furniture.
- Do not wax floors.

- Be sure shoes and slippers fit and have nonslip soles.

For clients who have difficulty walking:

- Keep areas well lit, even at night.
- Block access to stairs with a gate placed at hip height (Fig. 20-28).

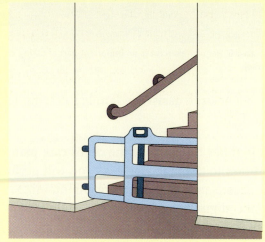

Fig. 20-28. A gate at the foot or head of the stairs will help prevent injuries. Place the gate at hip height to prevent the client from falling over it.

- Clear walkways of electrical cords.

General tips:

- Keep medications and other chemicals out of reach.
- Display emergency numbers, including poison control, and home address near the phone.
- Use red tape around radiators or heating vents to prevent burns.
- Check refrigerator and "hiding places" for spoiled food.
- Prevent kitchen accidents by removing knobs on stove, unplugging toasters and other small appliances, and supervising kitchen visits.

23. Explain how to assist with personal care and activities of daily living for the client with AD

Use the same procedures for personal care and ADLs for clients with Alzheimer's disease as you would with other clients. However, there

are some guidelines to keep in mind when assisting these clients. Three general principles will help you give your clients the best care:

1. Develop a routine and stick to it. Being consistent is very important when working with clients who are confused and easily upset.

2. Promote self-care. Help your clients to care for themselves as much as possible. This will help them cope with this difficult disease.

3. Take good care of yourself, both mentally and physically. This will help you give the best care.

GUIDELINES
Caring for Clients with AD

- Ensure safety by using nonslip mats, tub seats, and hand-holds.

- Schedule bathing when the client is least agitated. Be organized so the bath can be quick. Give sponge baths if the client resists a shower or tub bath.

- Always use the same steps, explaining in the same way every time.

- Assist with grooming. Help the people in your care feel attractive and dignified.

- Lay out clothes in the order in which they should be put on. Choose clothes that are simple to put on (Fig. 20-29).

- Set up a regular schedule for toileting and follow it. Never withhold or discourage fluids because a person is incontinent.

- Mark the restroom with a sign or a picture as a reminder to use it and where it is.

- Check skin regularly for signs of irritation.

- Document bowel movements.

- Prevent infections. Follow proper procedures for food preparation and storage, household management, and Standard Precautions.

- Observe the person's physical health. Report any potential problems. People with dementia may not recognize their own health problems.

- Maintain a daily exercise routine.

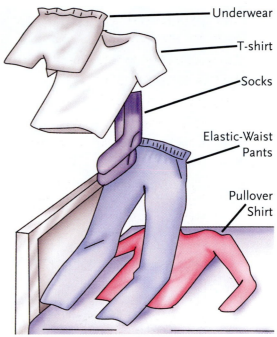

Fig. 20-29. Lay out clothes in the order in which they should be put on.

Underwear
T-shirt
Socks
Elastic-Waist Pants
Pullover Shirt

- Maintain the best nutrition.

- Schedule meals at the same time each day. Serve familiar foods. If restlessness prevents getting through an entire meal, try smaller, more frequent meals. Finger foods can allow eating while moving around.

- Offer one course at a time using one utensil at a time. If a client needs to be fed, do so slowly. Offer small pieces of food (Chapter 23 explains the procedure for feeding a client).

- Encourage fluids.

- Keep nutritious, bite-sized snacks nearby, especially favorites.

- Observe and report changes or problems in eating habits. Monitor weight accurately and frequently.

- Maintain self-esteem by encouraging independence in ADLs.

- Provide a daily calendar to encourage activities.

- Share in enjoyable activities, looking at pictures, talking, and reminiscing.

- Reward positive and independent behavior with smiles, hugs, warm touches, and thank yous (Fig. 20-30).

20

Common Chronic and Acute Conditions

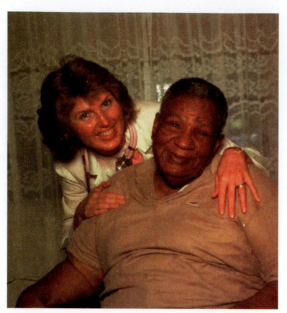

Fig. 20-30. Reward positive behavior with warm touches, smiles, and thank yous.

24. List eight difficult behaviors common in clients with AD and describe ways to manage each

Below are some common difficult behaviors that you may face when working with Alzheimer's clients. Remember that each client is different. Work with each client as an individual. Report behavior in detail to your supervisor.

1. **Agitation**. A client who is excited, restless, or troubled is said to be **agitated**. Situations that lead to agitation are **triggers**. Triggers may include change of routine or caregiver, new or frustrating experiences, or even violent television. Responses that may help calm a person who is agitated include the following:

   • Try to remove triggers. Keep routine constant. Avoid frustration.

   • Help client focus on a soothing, familiar activity, such as sorting things or looking at pictures.

   • Remain calm and use a low, soothing voice to speak to and reassure the client.

   • An arm around the shoulder, patting, or stroking may be soothing for some clients.

2. **Pacing and Wandering**. A client who walks back and forth in the same area is **pacing**. A client who walks aimlessly around the house or neighborhood is **wandering**. Pacing and wandering may have some of the following causes:

   • restlessness

   • hunger

   • disorientation

   • need for toileting

   • constipation

   • pain

   • forgetting how or where to sit down

   • too much daytime napping

   • need for exercise

Eliminate causes when you can. For example, provide nutritious snacks, encourage an exercise routine, and maintain a toileting schedule.

Responses to pacing and wandering include the following:

   • Let clients pace or wander in a safe and secure (locked) area where you can keep an eye on them, such as in a level, fenced yard (Fig. 20-31).

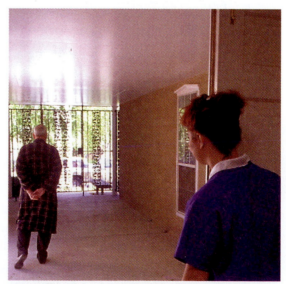

Fig. 20-31. Make sure a client is in a safe area if he paces or wanders.

   • Suggest another activity, such as going for a walk together.

3. **Hallucinations or Delusions**. A client who sees things that are not there is having **hallucinations**. A client who believes things that are not true is having **delusions**. You can respond to hallucinations and delusions in the following ways:

   - Ignore harmless hallucinations and delusions.

   - Reassure a client who seems agitated or worried.

   - Do not argue with a client who is imagining things. Remember that the feelings are real to him or her. Redirect client to other activities or thoughts.

   - Be calm. Reassure client that you are there to help.

4. **Sundowning**. When a person becomes restless and agitated in the late afternoon, evening, or night, it is called **sundowning**. Sundowning may be triggered by hunger or fatigue, a change in routine or caregiver, or any new or frustrating situation. Following are some effective responses to sundowning:

   - Remove triggers. Provide snacks or encourage rest.

   - Avoid stressful situations during this time. Limit activities, appointments, trips, and visits.

   - Play soft music.

   - Set a bedtime routine and keep it.

   - Recognize when sundowning occurs and plan a calming activity just before.

   - Eliminate caffeine from the diet.

   - Give a soothing back massage.

   - Distract the client with a simple, calm activity like looking at a magazine.

   - Maintain a daily exercise routine.

5. **Catastrophic Reactions**. When a person with AD overreacts to something in an unreasonable way it is called a **catastrophic** (kat-a-STRAH-fik) reaction. It may be triggered by any of the following:

   - fatigue

   - change of routine, environment, or caregiver

   - overstimulation (too much noise or activity)

   - difficult choices or tasks

   - physical pain

   - hunger

   - need for toileting

You can respond to catastrophic reactions as you would to agitation or sundowning. For example, remove triggers. Help the client focus on a soothing activity.

6. **Depression**. When clients become withdrawn, have no energy, do not want to eat or do things they used to enjoy, they may be **depressed**. Chapter 18 provides more information on depression and its symptoms. Depression may have many causes, including:

   - loss of independence

   - inability to cope

   - feelings of failure, fear

   - reality of facing a progressive, degenerative illness

   - chemical imbalance

You can respond to depression in a number of ways:

   - Report signs of depression to your supervisor immediately. It is an illness that can be treated with medication.

   - Encourage independence, self-care, and activity.

   - Talk about moods and feelings if your client is willing. Be a good listener.

   - Encourage social interaction.

7. **Perseveration or Repetitive Phrasing**. A client who repeats a word, phrase, question, or activity over and over is **perseverating** (per-SEV-er-ayt-ing). Repeating a word or phrase is also called **repetitive phrasing**. Such behavior may be caused by several factors, including disorientation or confusion. Respond to this with patience. Do not try to

silence or stop the client. Answer questions each time they are asked, using the same words each time.

8. **Violent Behavior**. A client who attacks, hits, or threatens someone is **violent**. Violence may be triggered by many situations, including frustration, overstimulation, or a change in routine, environment, or caregiver.

The following are appropriate responses to violent clients:

- Block blows but never hit back (Fig. 20-32).

- Step out of reach.

- Call for help if needed.

- Do not leave client in the home alone.

- Try to eliminate triggers.

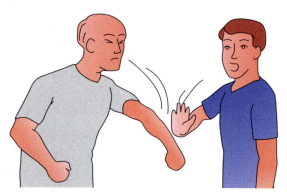

Fig. 20-32. Block blows but do not hit back.

- Use techniques to calm client as you would for agitation or sundowning.

25. Describe creative therapies for clients with AD

Although Alzheimer's cannot be cured, there are techniques to improve the quality of life for clients with AD. Follow the instructions in the client care plan and your assignments regarding creative therapies.

Reality Orientation

Reality orientation involves the use of calendars, clocks, signs, and lists to help clients remember who and where they are. It is useful in the early stages of AD when clients are confused but not totally disoriented. In later stages, reality orientation may only frustrate clients.

Example: Each day when you arrive at Mrs. Elkin's house, you show her the calendar and point out what day of the week it is. On the calendar or another piece of paper, you list all the things you will do today. For example, take a bath, go for a walk, eat lunch, and play cards. Whenever you speak to her, you call the client by her name, Mrs. Elkin. When assisting with tasks, you explain why you do things as you do. For example, "We use a tub seat in the shower so you don't have to stand up for so long, Mrs. Elkin."

Benefits: Using the calendar, making lists, and using names frequently all help your client stay in touch with the world around her. This will help her feel more in control of her life. It will also allow her to do as much as possible for herself. Explaining what you do and why you do it as you assist her will make her feel more like a participant in her care and less like an invalid.

Validation Therapy

Validation therapy means letting clients believe they live in the past or in imaginary circumstances. **Validating** means giving value to or approving. Make no attempt to reorient the client to actual circumstances. Explore the client's beliefs. Do not argue with him or her. Validating can provide comfort and reduce agitation. It is useful in cases of moderate to severe disorientation.

Example: Mr. Baldwin tells you he does not want to eat lunch today because he is going out to a restaurant with his wife. You know his wife has been dead for many years and that Mr. Baldwin can no longer eat out in restaurants. Instead of telling him that he is not going out to eat, you ask what restaurant he is going to and what he will have. You suggest that he eat a good lunch now because sometimes the service is slow in restaurants (Fig. 20-33).

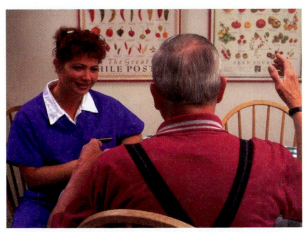
Fig. 20-33. Validation therapy accepts a client's fantasies without attempting to reorient him to reality.

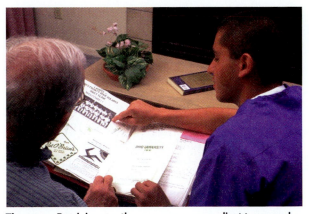
Fig. 20-34. Reminiscence therapy encourages a client to remember and talk about his past.

Benefits: By "playing along" with Mr. Baldwin's fantasy, you let him know that you take him seriously. You do not think of him as a crazy person or a child who does not know what is happening in his own life. You also learn more about your client. He used to enjoy eating out in restaurants. He liked to order certain dishes. Eating out is something he probably associates with being with his wife. These things can help you give Mr. Baldwin better care in the future.

Reminiscence Therapy

Reminiscence therapy involves encouraging your client to remember and talk about the past. Explore memories by asking about details. Focus on a time of life that was more pleasant. Work through feelings about a difficult time in the past. It is useful in many stages of Alzheimer's, but especially with moderate to severe confusion.

Example: Mr. Benavidez, an 82-year-old man with Alzheimer's, fought in World War II. In his home are many mementos of the war—pictures of his war buddies, a medal he was given, and more. You ask him to tell you where he was sent in the war. He tells you a little bit about being in the Pacific. You ask him more detailed questions about his experiences. Eventually he tells you a lot: the friends he made in the service, why he was given the medal, times when he was scared and how much he missed his wife and daughter (Fig. 20-34).

Benefits: By asking questions about Mr. Benavidez's experiences in the war, you show an interest in him as a person, not just as a client. You let him show you that he is a person who was competent, social, responsible, and brave. This boosts his self-esteem. You also learn that Mr. Benavidez cared very much for his wife and daughter. He probably would enjoy visits from his daughter now that he cannot get out as much.

Activity Therapy

Activity therapy uses activities the client enjoys to prevent boredom and frustration. These activities also promote self-esteem. Help the client take walks, listen to music, cook, read, or do other activities he or she enjoys (Fig. 20-35). It is useful throughout most stages of AD.

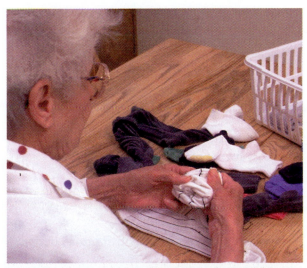
Fig. 20-35. Activities that are not frustrating can be helpful for clients with AD. They promote mental exercise.

Example: Mrs. Hoebel, a 70-year-old woman with AD, raised four children and ran a household for almost 50 years before being diagnosed with Alzheimer's. She loves cooking and baking. She misses being in the kitchen now that she cannot cook for herself. You learn that she always used to bake cookies at Christmas. You purchase some pre-made cookie dough and roll out the dough. Mrs. Hoebel uses her old cookie cutters to cut out the shapes. You bake the cookies for her, and another day she can decorate them.

Benefits: Mrs. Hoebel can enjoy an activity that always brought her pleasure. She feels competent, because you gave her small tasks, such as cutting out the cookies, that she could handle. You showed her that you care about her by taking the time to help her bake the cookies. She will associate positive feelings with you. That will make caring for her much easier.

Chapter Review

1. What are the causes of arthritis?

2. What type of medication might a client with arthritis take?

3. What health problems can anti-inflammatory medications cause?

4. Name one way you can help your client with arthritis as he or she performs ADLs.

5. What is a tumor?

6. What can a person do to greatly reduce his/her risk for lung cancer?

7. List the seven warning signs for cancer.

8. What is the first line of defense against most forms of cancer?

9. What are the side effects of chemotherapy and radiation?

10. How can you show sensitivity to a client who has cancer?

True or False. Mark each statement with either a "T" for true or "F" for false.

11. ___ Using a commercial mouthwash can help a client with cancer to maintain good oral care.

12. ___ It is appropriate for you to suggest to friends and family the best times of day to visit your client.

13. ___ Clients with cancer generally need three meals a day.

14. ___ It can help a client with pain if you provide distractions like conversation or music.

15. ___ You should not apply lotion to areas receiving radiation therapy.

16. Briefly describe the two types of diabetes.

17. Why is good foot care especially important for a client with diabetes?

18. List six signs or symptoms of diabetes that you need to report.

19. Explain what causes insulin shock.

20. Explain what causes diabetic coma.

21. Why is it important to follow diet instructions exactly for a diabetic client?

22. What things are you allowed to do with regards to insulin?

23. Why should a diabetic person not walk barefoot?

24. How does a client with diabetes make up a menu for each day?

25. What causes a CVA (stroke)?

26. What does TIA stand for?

27. What are some symptoms that may signal a coming stroke?

28. List five effects a client may experience after a stroke.

29. What terms should you use to refer to the weaker side of a person who has had a stroke?

30. What kinds of nonverbal communication can you use with a client who has had a stroke?

31. Why might some clients who have had strokes be at a greater risk of burning themselves?

32. In dressing a client with a one-sided weakness, which side should you dress first?

33. In which side of the mouth should food be placed if a client has a one-sided weakness?

34. What is hypertension? What does prehypertension mean?

35. List two care guidelines for a client who has high blood pressure.

36. List three care guidelines for a client with angina pectoris.

37. How is the pain of a heart attack usually described?

38. List four care guidelines for a client recovering from a heart attack.

39. List six care guidelines for a client who has CHF.

40. What are some effects of having COPD?

41. List four care guidelines for a client who has COPD.

42. How is HIV spread?

43. List seven care guidelines for a client who has AIDS.

44. What is dementia?

45. Alzheimer's disease is a progressive, degenerative, and irreversible disease. In your own words, what does this mean?

46. What type of skills does a person with Alzheimer's disease usually retain?

47. What can you encourage clients to do that may help slow the progression of AD?

48. For each of the personal attitudes described in learning objective 20, list one example of what you can do to demonstrate that attitude.

49. List each of the strategies for better communication with a client who has AD.

50. How would changes in an AD client's condition affect his or her safety in the house?

51. List 15 care guidelines for a client with AD.

52. A client with AD is having delusions that he is 19 years old again. What should his caregiver do?

53. A client with AD persists in asking her caregiver who she is. What should her caregiver do?

54. A client with AD suddenly becomes agitated and, without warning, tries to hit his caregiver. What should his caregiver do?

55. A client with AD becomes restless and agitated in the late afternoon. What should his caregiver do?

56. Describe each of the four creative therapies for AD.

20

Common Chronic and Acute Conditions

21

Clean, Safe and Healthy Environments

1. Describe how housekeeping affects physical and psychological well-being

Providing a safe, clean, and orderly environment has always been an essential part of home health care. Illness and disability cause great stress. Clients feel better physically and psychologically and recover more quickly when their homes and families receive care and support. Infection and accidents are prevented. In addition, families who lack some knowledge to manage their homes can be taught valuable household management skills. These skills include sanitation, safety, personal hygiene, nutrition, meal planning, shopping, child care, food preparation, communication skills, and specific healthcare techniques. You will be a role model for your clients and their families. Help them learn to accept greater responsibility.

2. List qualities needed to manage a home and describe general housekeeping guidelines

It takes efficiency, planning, knowledge, and skills to manage a household. You will need to know how to use your time and energy well. This is so that you do not neglect your primary responsibility—the personal care of the client.

Sensitivity is another important quality when caring for your clients' homes. You must re-

spect the customs, beliefs, and feelings of your clients and their families. How would you feel if a stranger were handling your personal items and possessions? How would you feel if you could no longer care for your home yourself?

Be sensitive when you ask members of the household for help with housekeeping as well. Know when it is appropriate to ask for assistance and how to ask for it in an appropriate way. Some family members may be experiencing such stress that they are unable to help at all.

Your assignments will vary. They may include simple cleaning and organizing of the client's room or general cleaning throughout the house. Some clients require management of all household functions, including finances. You may be required to dust, straighten, vacuum, sweep, wash dishes, clean the bathroom and kitchen, and do laundry. Your assignments will outline the specific duties to be performed (Fig. 21-1).

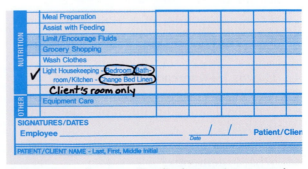

Fig. 21-1. Your assignments will outline home maintenance tasks you need to perform.

Your assignments may list specific days on which tasks should be performed or you may be allowed to make your own schedule. Flexibility is important and allows you to meet the client's and family's needs. If you receive requests for services not listed in your assignments or complaints about how tasks are done, contact your supervisor. Chapter 24 discusses in detail how to handle criticism and complaints.

Most agencies require that aides perform light housekeeping. This usually involves dusting, straightening, vacuuming or sweeping floors and floor coverings, cleaning bathrooms and the kitchen, and disposing of garbage and trash. Light housekeeping does not involve moving heavy furniture, washing windows, taking down drapes, cleaning the attic and basement, or mowing the lawn.

GUIDELINES
Housekeeping

- Invite family participation. Depending on their abilities and availability, clients and family members may be asked to participate in housekeeping tasks.

- Invite family and client input when you determine the tasks that need to be done and the methods used.

- Use cleaning materials and methods that are acceptable to and approved by clients and their families. Any efforts you make toward improving the home environment should coincide with the client's choices, lifestyle, and values.

- Be organized when performing tasks. Write out detailed daily and weekly schedules. Seek feedback from your supervisor and the client and family.

- Build some flexibility into the schedule to allow for changes in the client's condition, needs, appointments, or social activities.

- Organize cleaning materials and equipment by placing them in one closet. Place cleaning materials in a pail, a carrying bin that has a handle, a laundry basket, or a shopping bag

(Fig. 21-2). Do not leave cleaning equipment around the home.

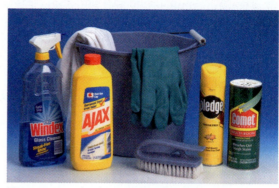

Fig. 21-2. Keep cleaning materials and equipment organized.

- Familiarize yourself with the cleaning materials and equipment. Read the labels and instruction booklets. Ask the client, family members, or your supervisor how the equipment works if you are unfamiliar with it.

- Maintain a safe environment as well as a clean and healthy one. Do not wax floors if your client is unsteady. Mop up spills immediately.

- Use housekeeping procedures and methods that promote good health. Many diseases may be transmitted through improper food handling, dishwashing, handwashing, and unclean bathrooms and kitchens.

- Observe the home environment for signs of infestation by roaches, rats, mice, lice, and fleas. These insects and animals are common carriers of disease. Controlling them is vital to family health and cleanliness.

- Use good body mechanics in performing home maintenance activities to prevent injury. Housecleaning can require a great deal of bending, standing, stooping, and lifting. Watch your posture. Kneel instead of stooping for long periods.

- Clean up and straighten up after every activity. Spills that have dried are difficult to remove later.

- Carry paper and a small pencil to make note of items that must be purchased or replaced. Maintain a shopping list on a bulletin board, refrigerator door, or other

convenient location, and encourage family members to use the list.

g Use your time wisely and efficiently. For example, prepare food while a load of wash is being done.

3. Describe cleaning products and equipment

Four basic types of home cleaning products are available in the market:

1. All-purpose cleaning agents can be used for many purposes and on several types of surfaces. These include countertops, walls, floors, and baseboards.

2. Soaps and detergents are used for bathing, laundering, and dishwashing.

3. Abrasive cleansers are used mostly to scour hard-to-clean surfaces.

4. Specialty cleaners are used to clean special surfaces, such as glass, metal, or ovens.

All cleaning products must be used properly. Cleaning products are chemicals, which can be irritating and can even cause burns. Some chemicals are poisonous when swallowed.

GUIDELINES
Using Household Cleaning Products

g Read and follow the directions on the label of every product you use. Cleaning products can harm the materials you are trying to clean.

g Do not mix cleaning products. This can cause a dangerous chemical reaction that may harm you or others. In particular, **never mix bleach or products containing bleach with ammonia. The fumes are toxic and can be fatal**.

g Open windows when cleaning to provide fresh air. Some cleaning products have fumes that are unpleasant or even harmful if you are exposed to them for a long time.

g Do not leave cleaning products on surfaces longer than the recommended time. Do not scrub too hard on some surfaces.

A basic set of cleaning tools generally includes two types:

1. Wet mops, pails, toilet brushes, and sponges are tools for softening and removing soil that has dried and hardened on washable surfaces.

2. A vacuum cleaner and attachments, carpet sweeper, dust mop, dust cloths, broom, and brush and dustpan are tools for removing dry dirt and dust.

Remember to be careful with equipment. Replacements can be expensive. Be familiar with the purpose and use of each piece of equipment. Keep it clean and in its proper place. Check the brushes and bags of vacuum cleaners frequently.

4. Describe proper cleaning methods for living areas, kitchens, bathrooms, and storage areas

Not all housekeeping tasks must be performed daily. Some tasks may be done weekly. Others only need to be done once a month or seasonally. Space out the special tasks. Do each cleaning job properly and efficiently. Do not take a lot of steps and do not reach, bend, and stoop unnecessarily. Experiment a little to find the most comfortable and effective way to do a job. Cleaning can be done when your client is resting, sleeping, or doing another activity. Care of the client is your primary responsibility. However, do not neglect housekeeping.

GUIDELINES
Straightening and Cleaning Living Areas

g Clear up clutter and put objects in their correct places.

g Pick up newspapers, magazines, and toys as needed.

g Empty wastebaskets and ashtrays daily.

g Make the beds each day.

g Keep essential and frequently used items, such as eyeglasses, tissues, a wastebasket, newspaper, magazines, and books, within

reach. Organize them on an accessible table, magazine rack, or hanging organizer (Fig. 21-3).

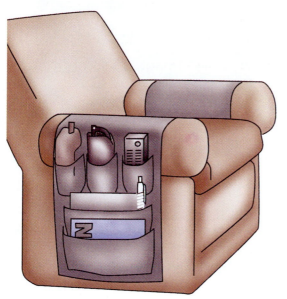

Fig. 21-3. A hanging organizer can help reduce clutter while keeping important items handy.

ⓖ Dust once a week or when necessary. If your client has allergies, you may need to dust daily.

ⓖ Vacuum floors and rugs once a week or more often if indicated. When vacuuming rugs, use long strokes and go over each area repeatedly. If the home does not have a vacuum, use a broom to sweep the floors and rugs. Take care not to raise much dust.

ⓖ Floors covered with vinyl, ceramic tile, and linoleum may be washed. Wood floors may not. Some floor coverings should be cleaned with water only. Check with the client or family before you begin. After removing loose dirt or crumbs with a vacuum or broom, wash floors with a cloth or mop dipped in warm, sudsy water. Dry the floor after you have washed it or close off the area for the time it takes for the floor to dry (Fig. 21-4). Wet or waxed floors are slippery and are frequent causes of falls in the home.

Handling food on contaminated surfaces, improper dishwashing, and contaminated food storage areas may transmit many diseases. Roaches, rats, and mice may cause disease and

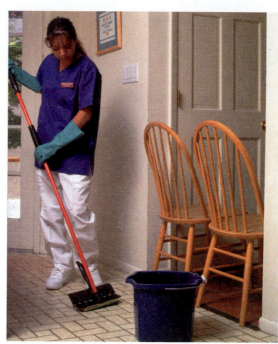

Fig. 21-4. Close off the area for the time it takes for the floor to dry.

allergy by contaminating food with their saliva or through their droppings. Pest control is vital to health and cleanliness. Always report pest control problems to your supervisor.

GUIDELINES
Cleaning the Kitchen

ⓖ Clean the kitchen after every use. Ask family members to do the same. Do not wait until the end of the day to clean up. Daily kitchen cleaning tasks include washing dishes, wiping surfaces, taking out garbage, and storing leftover food. Weekly tasks include cleaning the refrigerator and washing the floor. Cleaning cabinets, drawers, and other storage areas is usually done a few times a year.

ⓖ Wash dishes in hot, soapy water using liquid dish detergent. Rinse them in hot water. When working with clients who have an infectious disease or a cold, use boiling water for rinsing and add a tablespoon of chlorine bleach to the soapy water. The combination of heat and chlorine will kill **pathogens** (*PATH-o-jens*), or harmful microorganisms.

ⓖ Wash glasses and cups first, then silverware, plates, and bowls. Pots and pans are washed last. Rinse with hot water and dry on a rack.

4. Describe proper cleaning methods for areas in the home

Air drying dishes is more sanitary than drying with a dish towel.

ⓖ If the house has a dishwasher, learn how to correctly load and start it. Dishwashers save time. They can also sterilize dishes because of the high temperature used in washing and drying. Ask the client if you should scrape food from plates before placing in the dishwasher. Empty cups and glasses. Do not place dishes, cups, and flatware too close together. This keeps them from being washed thoroughly. Place dishes, cups, and glasses so that their eating or drinking surfaces are facing the water source.

ⓖ Do not wash the following items in the dishwasher: electrical appliances, certain plastic materials, wooden pieces or utensils, hand-painted or antique dishes, delicate china, crystal, cast iron, most pots and pans, and sharp or carbon steel knives. Use only a dishwasher detergent. Fill the well with only the amount recommended on the label.

ⓖ Clean the outside of the stove, the trays, and burners with hot, sudsy water or an all-purpose cleaner, and rinse. Ovens should be cleaned according to manufacturer's recommendations. Be sure to follow the directions. Do not spray the light bulb inside the oven with cleanser, or it may break. Soak the broiler pan immediately after use.

ⓖ The refrigerator should be totally cleaned once a week. However, you should wipe it out more frequently (Fig. 21-5). If the refrigerator is not a self-defrosting one, the freezer should be defrosted whenever necessary. One-half inch of frost usually means it should be defrosted. To defrost a freezer, turn the dial to the "off" position. Remove all food. Wrap frozen foods in newspapers to keep them from defrosting. Defrosting the freezer may take less time if you place pans of hot water in it. Do not use a knife to chip off the frost. This could damage the cooling unit.

ⓖ Mix two tablespoons of baking soda in one quart of warm water. Wipe the inside walls

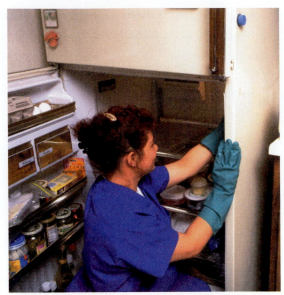

Fig. 21-5. The refrigerator should be totally cleaned once a week, but you should wipe it out more frequently.

of the refrigerator and freezer. Baking soda will remove odors. Wash the shelves and trays with warm, soapy water.

ⓖ Clean countertops, tables, and the stove each time they are used. Clean cabinet and drawer fronts and the refrigerator once a week. If a cutting board or other surface has been used to cut fresh meat, scrub the surface thoroughly with soap and bleach. Rinse well.

ⓖ An all-purpose cleaner may be needed to remove grease and cooked foods that have spilled or splashed on surfaces. Clean the sink with a cleanser such as scouring powder or cream.

ⓖ Never place food on soiled work or storage areas or in unclean containers. Keep food covered. Close lids of cartons and cover food storage containers to prevent contamination or infestation by insects and rodents. Place leftovers in covered containers and store them in the refrigerator immediately. Use them in two to three days.

ⓖ Vacuum, sweep, or dry mop the floor daily. Damp mop uncarpeted floors at least once a week, using hot water and a floor cleaner. Rinse the floor if the label recommends doing so. Dry the floor or close off the area until the floor dries to prevent accidents.

Ⓖ Dispose of garbage daily. To prevent odor and discourage insects and rodents, rinse out tin cans and bottles before placing them in the garbage pail or recycling bin. Follow the recycling procedures for your client's community. Periodically wash wastebaskets and trash cans with hot, soapy water.

Ⓖ Store all cleaning materials away from food, food preparation utensils, and food preparation areas. Keep them out of reach of children and confused clients.

A clean, organized, and odor-free bathroom is an important part of improving a family's hygiene and safety. Because it is moist and warm, the bathroom is a reservoir for the growth of microorganisms, mold, and mildew.

GUIDELINES
Cleaning the Bathroom

Ⓖ Involve the entire family in keeping the bathroom clean (Fig. 21-6). Always wash from clean areas to dirty areas, so you do not spread dirt into areas that have already been washed.

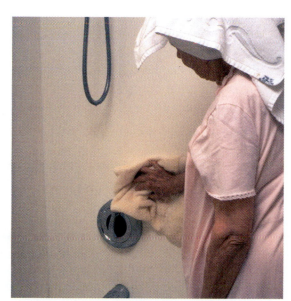

Fig. 21-6. Teach family members basic bathroom hygiene, such as wiping out the shower after each use.

Ⓖ Flush the toilet each time it is used.

Ⓖ Clean toothbrushes and toothbrush holders.

Ⓖ Scrub the tub and shower after use.

Ⓖ Remove hair from drain strainers.

Ⓖ Hang up all used towels to dry.

Ⓖ Put away toiletries.

Ⓖ Rinse the sink after brushing teeth, shaving, and washing.

Ⓖ Place soiled towels in the laundry hamper after they are dry.

The bathroom is the location of many home accidents. Make sure that all bathroom rugs are nonskid. Wipe up puddles of water immediately. If grab bars are not present and your client has difficulty moving about in the bathroom safely, report this to your supervisor.

Cleaning a bathroom

Equipment: disinfectant (a cleaning product that kills germs), scouring powder or scouring cream with bleach, sponge, toilet brush, glass cleaner, paper towels, disposable or rubber gloves

1. Put on gloves.

2. Using the disinfectant and sponge, wipe all surfaces and rinse as needed. Be sure to clean the sides, walls, and curtain or door of the shower or tub; the towel racks; holders for toilet paper, toothbrushes, and soap; and window sills.

3. Rinse sponge well or use a different sponge to wipe the outside of toilet bowl, seat, and lid. As a general cleaning rule, start with the cleanest surface first, then move to dirtier areas.

4. Use a different sponge to clean the bathtub, shower stall, and sink. Use scouring powder or cream for tile and porcelain, and disinfectant or all-purpose cleaner on other surfaces. Remember that scouring powder can scratch. Check with the client or a family member before using it. Be sure to scrub the sides, edges, and bottoms of all these areas. Clean faucets and scrub around their bases.

5. Scrub the inside of the toilet bowl with a brush and scouring powder containing bleach. Be sure to scrub under the rim. If you use a second, stronger toilet cleaner, flush the first cleaning product down the

4. Describe proper cleaning methods for areas in the home

drain first to avoid possible chemical reactions. Wash the toilet brush with a disinfectant solution. Store it in a plastic bag or holder after letting it air dry.

6. Vacuum or dry mop the floor first, then wash if the floor is tile or linoleum. Use an all-purpose floor cleaner in hot water. Wash the floor with a cloth or mop, taking special care to clean the areas at the base of the toilet and sink. Do not leave the floor wet. Dry it carefully to avoid accidents.

7. Clean the mirror and any glass or chrome surfaces using glass cleaner and paper towels or clean rags.

8. Place dry, soiled towels in the laundry hamper. Empty the waste can into a plastic or paper garbage bag and dispose of it. Replace toilet tissue and facial tissue when needed. Open the bathroom window for a short time, if possible, to air the room out. Once a week, wash out the waste can and laundry hamper, and launder the bath mats and rugs.

9. Store supplies.

10. Remove and dispose of gloves.

11. Wash hands.

12. Document the cleaning.

Cleaning and organizing storage areas will contribute to the order and organization of the home.

Cleaning and Organizing Storage Areas

- Every item in the home should have a storage place that is convenient for use. That means storage places should be as close as possible to where they are used (Fig. 21-7). For example, bath towels should be stored in or near the bathroom. Frequently used pots and pans and cooking utensils should be near the stove. Less frequently used items, such as popcorn poppers, should be stored in the less accessible storage places.

- Items that are frequently used should be easily seen and reached. When they are

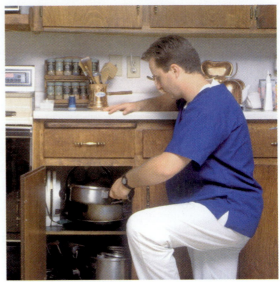

Fig. 21-7. Store items near where they will be used.

used, they should be immediately replaced. Items that are used together should be stored near each other. Arrange food on shelves according to category to save time in searching for items. Dangerous materials such as cleaning products should be stored out of reach of children and confused adults.

- Some storage areas only need to be cleaned occasionally. Remove the stored items and any shelf or drawer liners. Wipe the shelves and drawers with a damp cloth and all-purpose cleaner. Replace the liners or wipe them if they can be cleaned. Food storage areas and other storage areas that are used frequently should be cleaned more often.

- Do not change the client's or the family's storage arrangements without talking to them. If you think changes are needed, discuss your ideas with the family.

Cleaning Solution Ideas

Several types of cleaning solutions can be prepared from common household items when supplies are not available or when the family budget is restricted.

- Baking soda can be used instead of scouring powder. Baking soda can also be diluted with warm water to make a solution that will eliminate odors when used to clean surfaces.

- White vinegar can be used to remove lime or other mineral deposits on sinks, toilets, or chrome fixtures. White vinegar diluted with water can be used instead of glass cleaner. Mix solution using one part white vinegar to three parts water (1:3).

- Household bleach, diluted with four parts water, makes a strong disinfectant solution to clean bathroom surfaces. Diluted with nine parts water and stored in a spray bottle, bleach makes a milder disinfectant to use on kitchen counters. Do not spill or splash undiluted bleach or bleach solutions on carpets, clothing, or other surfaces that might be discolored.

5. Describe how to prepare a cleaning schedule

Most house-cleaning tasks should be done either immediately, daily, weekly, monthly, or less often. Take into account the care plan, your assignments, how much help is needed, and how much time you have in a particular home to prepare a cleaning schedule. You may not always stick to the schedule exactly. However, it will guide your work and help you get essential cleaning done. Establishing a schedule for cleaning can also help the family keep a housekeeping routine after your care has ended.

Creating a Cleaning Schedule

Below is a sample cleaning schedule. The client can do almost nothing around the house. Her daughter comes in several times a week, but no family members live with the client.

Cleaning Schedule for Mrs. Fontine

Immediately: Wipe counters, wash dishes, store food, clean spills, put away supplies.

Daily: Straighten up: make bed, sort mail, remove clutter, empty trash, etc. Clean bathroom. (One hour)

Weekly: Wash kitchen floors, wipe refrigerator, scrub sink, vacuum other floors, dust all surfaces, scrub bathtub. (Two to three hours)

Monthly: Clean out refrigerator, defrost freezer. (One hour)

Less often: Clean oven when needed. (One hour)

Cleaning schedules will be different for each client. Be flexible. You will need to adapt your schedule after you make it. Remember that client care is your first priority.

6. List special housekeeping procedures to use when infection is present

You must follow Standard Precautions with every client. This is true because you cannot know when infection is present (see chapter 5). However, when a client has a known infectious disease such as influenza, or one that weakens the immune system, such as AIDS or cancer, you need to take special precautions in housecleaning:

- Use disinfectant when cleaning countertops and surfaces in the kitchen and bathroom.

- Clean the client's bathroom daily. Have other family members use a different bathroom if possible.

- Use separate dishes and utensils for the infected client. In some cases, disposable dishes and utensils will be ordered.

- Wash dishes and utensils in the dishwasher or wash dishes in hot soapy water with bleach. Rinse in boiling water, and allow to air dry.

- Disinfect any surfaces that contact body fluids, such as bedpans, urinals and toilets.

- Frequently remove trash containing used tissues.

- Keep any specimens of urine, stool, or sputum in double bags and away from food or food preparation areas.

7. Explain how to do laundry and care for clothes

You may be expected to do hand or machine washing as part of an assignment. Clean clothes, bed linens, and towels are important for hygiene and comfort.

Laundry Products and Equipment. To do the laundry you will need laundry detergent, a washing machine or a basin for hand washing clothes, and a dryer or a clothesline and pins. The instructions for using washing machines are usually located on the inside of the machine lid.

In general, you will use all-purpose detergent. Some delicate fabrics, underwear, or stockings may require a special detergent. Some clients may prefer a non-detergent soap for use on baby clothes and diapers. Bleach, color brighteners, stain removers, and fabric softeners may also be used. Ask the client and family about their preferences for laundry products.

Pretreating. Pretreating means giving special treatment to items that have heavy soil, spots, and stains before washing them. Spots and stains should be treated immediately. The sooner they are treated, the easier they are to remove. Some oily stains harden with age and cannot be removed. Washing and ironing may set some stains, making them difficult or impossible to remove. If you can, identify the source of the stain and treat it according to a stain guide on the pretreating solution.

Bleach. Bleach is used with detergent. However, bleach cannot be used on all fabrics. Be familiar with the type of bleach and the fabric that is being washed. Three types of bleach are used in laundry: liquid chlorine, powdered chlorine, and oxygen or all-fabric bleach. Each type of bleach should be used with caution. Read the instructions on the container carefully.

Liquid chlorine bleaches are excellent stain removers. They whiten clothing. However, they can be very damaging. Bleach should always be diluted in water. Fill the washer, then add liquid bleach and stir the water before adding clothing. Never use liquid chlorine bleach on silk, spandex, wool, or any item that contains these fibers. Be careful not to spray or splash liquid chlorine bleach. It will remove color or damage fabric. Powdered chlorine bleach is more gentle than liquid, but it can also damage clothing. Either type of chlorine bleach is also an excellent disinfectant. Oxygen or all-fabric bleach is used on washable fabrics, but it is effective only in hot water.

Water Temperature. Read the washing instructions for all materials and garments (Fig. 21-8). Warm water is the safest temperature for most garments. However, some must be washed in cold to prevent shrinking or colors fading. Hot water is generally used for towels, bed linens, and white or colorfast cottons. Warm is usually used for permanent press, knit, synthetic, sheer, lace, acetate, fabric blends, washable rayons, and plastic. Cold water is used for brightly-colored fabrics or fabrics that are not colorfast.

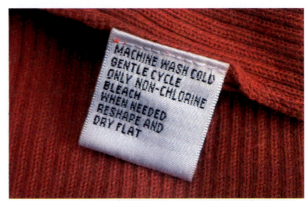

Fig. 21-8. A care tag gives washing and drying instructions. It can be found on most clothing.

Washing Action or Cycle. Use the normal setting on the washer for cottons, linens, rayons, sturdy permanent press, knits, synthetics, blends, and most other items. Set the washer on the slow or gentle setting for washable woolens, old quilts, curtains, and delicate or fragile items.

Drying Clothes. Settings on the dryer vary according to the model. Most dryers have a permanent press setting and a delicate setting. The more delicate a fabric, the lower the drying tem-

perature and the shorter the time in the dryer. Heavy items such as towels need higher temperature settings and a longer time in the dryer. Clean the lint filter each time you use the dryer. If your client does not have a clothes dryer, hang clothes on a clothesline using clothespins.

Folding. To reduce the amount of wrinkling, remove all clothes from the dryer immediately. Fold them neatly or place them on hangers. Set aside those that need to be ironed. Return other items to their drawers or closet.

Ironing. Before you begin to iron, check the label of the item for the recommended temperature. If the label does not recommend a particular setting or the fabric is a blend, use the lowest temperature on the iron. Take special care with pile fabrics, such as velvets and corduroy. They will keep their texture better if ironed on the wrong side over a towel. Dark fabrics, silks, acetates, rayons, linens, and some wools must be pressed on the wrong side to prevent them from becoming shiny. Use a pressing cloth to protect the fabric.

To prevent stretching, iron all fabrics lengthwise. Iron collars, cuffs, and garment facings first. Next, iron the sleeves, then the front and back. Hang or fold clothes immediately. Fasten all hooks and buttons and close zippers. Be sure clothes are completely dry before putting them away.

Maintaining Clothing. You may need to do basic mending or sewing occasionally. This is especially true if you are taking care of a family, an older person with impaired vision, or people who may not have the time or the ability to keep clothing and linens repaired. Some clients who can do their own mending may just need you to thread the needle.

Doing the laundry

1. Sort clothes carefully. Make separate piles of whites, colors, and bright colors. Check clothing labels for special washing instructions. Do not wash anything labeled "Dry Clean Only." If hand washing is recommended, do not wash in the machine.

2. As you sort laundry, check pockets and remove tissues, money, pens, and other items. Remove belts with buckles, trims, and nonwashable ornaments. Close zippers, buttons, and other fasteners. Check garments for stains and areas of heavy soil. If appropriate, mend or repair any holes, snags, rips, tears, pulled seams, and weak spots in garments and other items.

3. Pretreat spots and stains before washing. A small amount of liquid detergent or dry detergent dissolved in water can be worked in with an old toothbrush (Fig. 21-9). Pretreat or soak clothing as soon as possible for best results. If you know something is spotted, don't let it sit in the laundry hamper all week until you do the laundry.

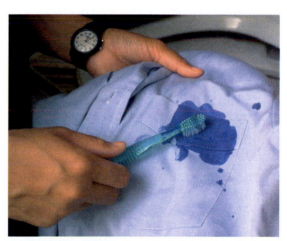

Fig. 21-9.

4. Use the correct water temperature: hot for whites, warm for colors, cold for bright colors.

5. Use the appropriate laundry product(s). Follow the washing instructions on the container.

6. Follow written instructions or client or family instructions for using the washer. Use the correct washing cycle for the load you are laundering.

7. Dry clothes completely either in a dryer or on a clothesline. If using an automatic dryer, follow the drying instructions on clothing la-

bels. Some fabrics require cooler temperatures.

8. Hand-wash items in warm or cool water, depending on the fabric and instructions. Use a mild detergent or special hand-washing liquid. Line dry or lay items flat on towels to preserve the shape of the garment.

9. Fold or hang clean laundry and sort into categories. Store in drawers or closets.

8. List special laundry precautions to use when infection is present

When a client has a known infectious disease, you must take special precautions when handling laundry:

*   Keep client's laundry separate from other family members'.

*   Handle dirty laundry as little as possible. Sort it and put it in plastic bags in the client's room or bathroom. Take it immediately to the laundry area.

*   Wear gloves and hold laundry away from your clothes and body when you are handling it (Fig. 21-10).

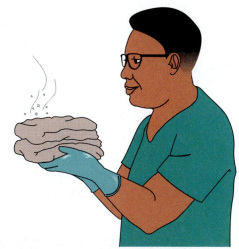

Fig. 21-10. Wear gloves and hold dirty laundry away from your clothes.

*   Use liquid bleach when fabrics allow.

*   Use agency-approved disinfectants in all loads.

*   Use hot water.

9. List guidelines for teaching housekeeping skills to clients' family members

In some assignments, you will be asked to teach housekeeping skills to family members. This prepares them to take over housekeeping and care when home care is discontinued. By teaching household management skills, you help families meet their daily needs and become more self-reliant.

GUIDELINES
Teaching Family Members

ⓖ   Get to know the family before starting to teach them. Understand their needs or problems before beginning.

ⓖ   Be patient. Give people time to learn new skills. Praise their efforts.

ⓖ   Keep teaching sessions brief.

ⓖ   Break down tasks into simple steps. Explain each step and demonstrate it.

ⓖ   Answer all questions.

ⓖ   Assist the person as necessary. Do not do the task for him or her.

ⓖ   Remember that each person is an individual and will learn in different ways. Customize your teaching to allow for these differences.

10. List three reasons careful bedmaking is important

When clients spend much or all of their time in bed, careful bedmaking is essential to their comfort, cleanliness, and health. Linens should always be changed after personal care procedures such as sponge baths, or any time bedding or sheets are damp, soiled, or in need of straightening. The following are three reasons why it is important that bed linens be changed frequently:

1. Sheets that are damp, wrinkled, or bunched up under a client are uncomfortable. They may prevent the client from resting or sleeping well.

2. Microorganisms thrive in moist, warm environments. Bedding that is damp or unclean encourages infection and disease.

3. Clients who spend long hours in bed are at risk for pressure sores. Sheets that do not lie flat under the client's body increase the risk of pressure sores because they cut off circulation.

Using Good Body Mechanics in the Home

Review the principles of body mechanics you learned in chapter 6. Remember the following additional tips when working in a home:

- Bend the knees, not the back, when lifting things from the floor or when kneeling to pick up objects.

- Carry heavy objects close to the body and distribute the weight evenly. For example, when carrying a basket of clothes, hold it directly in front of the body (Fig. 21-11).

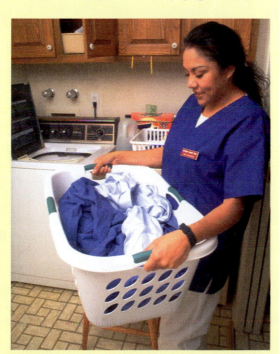

Fig. 21-11.

- Stand close to the work area. When possible, raise the work area to a comfortable level so you don't have to bend your back and neck to do the work.

- Try not to lift heavy objects. If you must move heavy objects such as furniture, try

pushing, pulling, or rolling, using the entire body.

- Avoid lifting heavy objects from the floor. For example, put the clothes basket on a chair before filling it (Fig. 21-12).

- Stand erect when doing tasks like washing dishes. Your knees may be slightly bent.

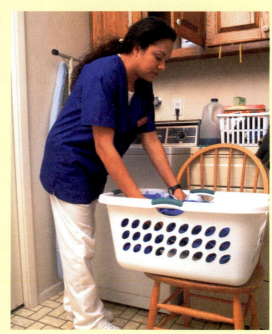

Fig. 21-12.

If a client cannot get out of bed, you must change the linens with the client in bed. When making the bed, be careful to use a wide stance with knees bent. Avoid bending from the waist, especially when tucking sheets or blankets under the mattress. Mattresses can be heavy, so remember to bend your knees to avoid injury. It is easier to make an unoccupied bed than one with a client in it. If the client can be moved temporarily to a chair or other comfortable spot, your job will be easier.

Making an occupied bed

Equipment: clean linen: mattress pad, fitted or flat bottom sheet, waterproof bed protector if needed, cotton draw sheet, flat top sheet, blanket(s), pillowcase(s), gloves, laundry hamper or basket

1. Wash your hands.

2. Explain the procedure to the client, speaking clearly, slowly, and directly, maintaining face-to-face contact whenever possible.

3. Provide privacy if the client desires it.

4. Place clean linen on clean surface within reach (e.g., bedside stand or chair).

5. If the bed is adjustable, adjust bed to a safe working level, usually waist high. If the bed is movable, lock bed wheels.

6. Put on gloves.

7. Loosen top linen from the end of the bed or working side. Cover the client with a cotton bath blanket or the loosened top sheet on the bed.

8. You will make the bed one side at a time. Raise side rail on far side of bed. This protects the client from falling out of the bed while you are making it. After the raising side rail, ask the client to roll towards the raised side rail. If the client cannot roll to the side without assistance, assist him or her to turn onto his or her side, moving away from you toward raised side rail (Fig. 21-13).

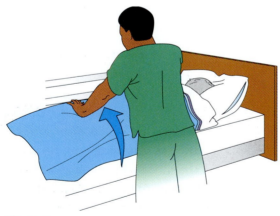

Fig. 21-13.

9. On the opposite side of the bed, with the client's back to you, loosen the bottom soiled linen, mattress pad, and protector if present.

10. Roll bottom soiled linen toward client, tucking it snugly against the client's back.

11. Place and tuck in clean bottom linen, finishing with bottom sheet free of wrinkles. If you are using a flat bottom sheet, leave enough overlap on each end to tuck under the mattress. If the sheet is only long enough to tuck in at one end, tuck it in securely at the top of the bed. Make hospital corners to keep bottom sheet wrinkle-free (Fig. 21-14).

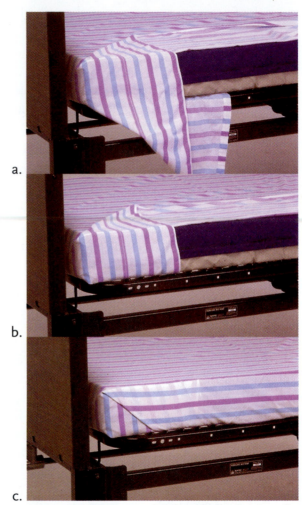

a.

b.

c.

Fig. 21-14. Hospital corners help keep the flat sheet smooth under the client.

12. Smooth the bottom sheet out toward the client. Be sure there are no wrinkles in the mattress pad. Roll the extra material toward the client and tuck it under the client's body.

13. If using a waterproof pad, unfold it and center it on the bed. Tuck the side near you under the mattress. Smooth it out toward the client, and tuck as you did with the sheet.

14. If using a draw sheet, place it on the bed. Tuck in on your side, smooth, and tuck as you did with the other bedding.

10. List three reasons careful bedmaking is important

15. Assist client to turn onto clean bottom sheet toward you. Protect the client from any soiled matter on the old linens. Raise side rail nearest you.

16. Move to other side of the bed and lower the side rail.

17. Loosen the soiled linen. Roll linen from head to the foot of bed. Avoid contact with your skin or clothes. Place it in a hamper or basket. Never put it on the floor or furniture. Never shake it. Soiled bed linens are full of microorganisms that should not be spread to other parts of the room.

18. Pull and tuck in clean bottom linen just like the other side, finishing with bottom sheet free of wrinkles (Fig. 21-15).

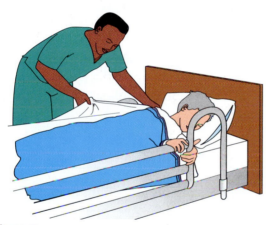

Fig. 21-15.

19. Ask client to turn onto his or her back. Keep client covered and comfortable, with a pillow under the head.

20. Unfold the top sheet and place it over the client. Ask the client to hold the top sheet. Slip the blanket or old sheet out from underneath. Put it in the laundry hamper.

21. Place a blanket over the top sheet, matching the top edges. Tuck the bottom edges of top sheet and blanket under the bottom of the mattress, making square corners on each side. Loosen the top linens over the client's feet. This prevents pressure on the feet. At the top of the bed, fold the top sheet over the blanket about six inches.

22. Remove the pillow. Do not hold it near your face. Remove the soiled pillowcase by turn

ing it inside out. Place it in the laundry hamper. Remove your gloves.

23. With one hand, grasp the clean pillowcase at the closed end and turn it inside out over your arm. Next, using the same hand that has the pillowcase over it, grasp one narrow edge of the pillow. Pull the pillowcase over it with your free hand (Fig. 21-16). Do the same for any other pillows. Place them under your client's head or as client desires.

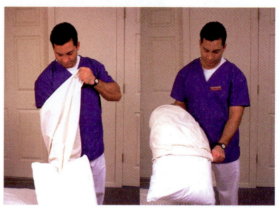

Fig. 21-16.

24. If you raised an adjustable bed, be sure to return it to its lowest position. Put any signaling device within the client's reach. Carry laundry hamper to laundry area.

25. Wash your hands.

26. Document the procedure and any observations.

Making an unoccupied bed

Equipment: clean linen: mattress pad, fitted or flat bottom sheet, waterproof bed protector if needed, cotton draw sheet, flat top sheet, blanket(s), pillowcase(s), gloves, laundry hamper or basket

1. Wash your hands.

2. If the bed is adjustable, adjust bed to a safe working level, usually waist high. If the bed is movable, lock bed wheels.

3. Put on gloves.

4. Loosen soiled linen. Roll soiled linen (soiled side inside) from head to foot of bed. Avoid contact with your skin or clothes. Place it in a hamper or basket. Remove your gloves.

Clean, Safe and Healthy Environments

5. Remake the bed, spreading mattress pad and bottom sheet, tucking under. Make hospital corners to keep bottom sheet wrinkle-free. Put on mattress protector and draw sheet, smooth, and tuck under sides of bed.

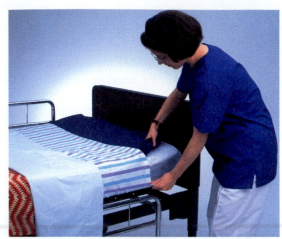

Fig. 21-17. Multiple layers of bedding, including a draw sheet, are used for clients who spend a lot of time in bed.

6. Place top sheet and blanket over bed. Center these, tuck under end of bed and make hospital corners. Fold down the top sheet over the blanket about six inches. Fold both top sheet and blanket down so client can easily get into bed. If client will not be returning to bed immediately, leave bedding up.

7. Remove pillows and pillowcases. Remove gloves. Put on clean pillowcases (as described in procedure above). Replace pillows.

8. If you raised an adjustable bed, be sure to return it to its lowest position. Put any signaling device within the client's reach. Carry laundry hamper to laundry area.

9. Wash your hands.

10. Document the procedure and any observations.

A **closed bed** is a bed completely made with the bedspread and blankets in place. A closed bed is turned into an **open bed** by folding the linen down to the foot of the bed. Most clients are out of bed most of the day. A closed bed is made until it is time for the client to go to sleep. Then an open bed is made.

11. Identify hazardous household materials

Any of the following household materials can have harmful effects:

- household bleach
- cleaning products
- aerosol or spray cans
- paint
- chemicals such as turpentine or paint thinner
- medicines, both prescription and over-the-counter
- hair spray
- nail polish remover

These products should be kept in separate cabinets with childproof latches or locks, or up out of the reach of children. If a client is confused, mark these cabinets with signs that indicate danger.

Chapter Review

1. What skills are important in household management?

2. What home maintenance assignments might you receive?

3. What are some housekeeping tasks you should NOT be asked to perform?

4. Why is it important to read the instructions for cleaning products?

5. Why should you not mix cleaning products?

6. What two parts of a vacuum cleaner should you check often?

7. How often should wastebaskets and ashtrays be emptied?

8. How should you clean the floors if the home does not have a vacuum?

9. What should you do when washing dishes for clients who have an infectious disease or cold?

10. How frequently should the refrigerator be cleaned?

11. Leftover food should be eaten in what time frame?

12. What items should you not wash in the dishwasher?

13. Ideally, where should storage places be located?

14. Describe why it is important to make a cleaning schedule even if you may not always be able to stick to it exactly.

15. How frequently should you clean the bathroom of a client with an infectious disease?

16. List two guidelines for dealing with the dishes and utensils of a client with an infectious disease.

True or False. Mark each statement with a "T" for true or an "F" for false.

17. ___ Bleach cannot be used on all fabrics.

18. ___ A stain should be pretreated as quickly as possible.

19. ___ Hot water is usually used for permanent press items.

20. ___ Before ironing, you should check the label of the item for the recommended temperature.

21. ___ Clothes will look best if you fold them right after they're done in the dryer.

22. ___ Items like towels should be dried on high heat.

23. For a client with an infectious disease, what cleaners might you use when washing clothes and linens?

24. List four guidelines to follow when teaching family members housekeeping skills.

25. When should bed linens be changed?

26. Where should hazardous household materials be kept?

22

Clients' Nutritional Needs

1. Describe the importance of good nutrition and list the six basic nutrients

Good nutrition is very important. **Nutrition** is how the body uses food to maintain health. Our bodies need a well-balanced diet containing essential nutrients and plenty of fluids. This helps us grow new cells, maintain normal body function, and have energy for activities.

Good nutrition in childhood and early adulthood helps ensure good health later in life. For those who are ill or elderly, a well-balanced diet helps maintain muscle and skin tissues and prevent pressure sores. A good diet promotes the healing of wounds. It also helps us cope with physical and emotional stress.

The Six Basic Nutrients

The body needs the following nutrients for growth and development:

1. **Protein**. Proteins are part of every body cell. They are essential for tissue growth and repair. Proteins are also an alternate supply of energy for the body. Excess proteins are excreted by the kidneys or stored as body fat.

Sources of protein include fish, seafood, poultry, meat, eggs, milk, cheese, nuts, peas, and dried beans or legumes (Fig. 22-1). Whole grain cereals, pastas, rice, and breads contain some proteins of lower quality. They must be complemented by a small quantity of the more complete proteins. Beans and rice or cereal and milk are examples of complementary proteins.

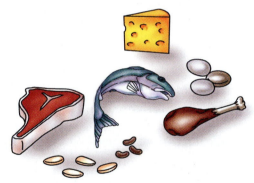

Fig. 22-1. Sources of protein.

2. **Carbohydrates**. Carbohydrates (*kar-boh-HIGH-drayts*) supply the fuel for the body's energy needs. They supply extra protein and help the body use fat efficiently. Carbohydrates also provide **fiber**, which is necessary for bowel elimination.

Carbohydrates can be divided into two basic types: complex and simple carbohydrates. **Complex carbohydrates** are found in foods such as bread, cereal, potatoes, rice, pasta, vegetables, and fruits. **Simple carbohydrates** are found in foods such as sugars, sweets, syrups, and jellies. Simple carbohydrates do not have the same nutritional value as complex carbohydrates do (Fig. 22-2).

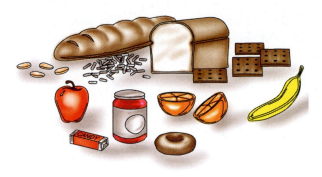

Fig. 22-2. Sources of carbohydrates.

3. Fats. Fat helps the body store energy. Body fat also provides the body with insulation. It protects body organs. In addition, fats add flavor to food and are important for the absorption of certain vitamins. Excess fat in the diet is stored as fat in the body.

Examples of fats are butter, margarine, salad dressings, oils, and animal fats found in meats, fowl, and fish (Fig. 22-3). Monounsaturated vegetable fats (including olive oil and canola oil) and polyunsaturated vegetable fats (including corn and safflower oils) are healthier kinds of fats. Saturated fats, including animal fats like butter, lard, bacon and other fatty meats, are not as healthy. They should be limited in most diets.

4. Vitamins. Vitamins are substances the body needs to function. The body cannot produce most vitamins. They can only be obtained from food. Vitamins A, D, E, and K are fat-soluble vitamins. This means they are carried and stored in body fat. Vitamins B and C are water-soluble vitamins that are broken down by water in our bodies. They cannot be stored in the body. They are eliminated in urine and feces.

5. Minerals. Minerals form and maintain body functions. They provide energy and regulate

VITAMIN	SOURCE	FUNCTION
Vitamin A	dark green and yellow vegetables, such as broccoli and turnips	assists with skin and eye development, keeps the skin healthy, helps the eyes adjust to dim light, helps the linings of the respiratory and digestive tracts resist infection
Vitamin C	fruits such as oranges, strawberries, grapefruit, cantaloupe; and vegetables such as broccoli, cabbage, brussels sprouts, and green peppers	assists with healing wounds and building bones and teeth, holds cells together, strengthens the walls of blood vessels, and helps the body absorb iron
Vitamin B2 or riboflavin	milk, milk products, lean meat, green leafy vegetables, eggs, breads, and cereals	helps cells use oxygen, which allows them to release energy from food; important for protein and carbohydrate metabolism; needed for growth, healthy eyes, skin, and mucous membranes
Vitamin B3 or niacin	lean meat, poultry, fish, peanuts and peanut butter, whole grain breads and cereals, peas, beans, and eggs	important for protein, carbohydrate and fat metabolism, appetite, and the functioning of the skin, tongue, nervous system, and digestive system; helps cells use oxygen for energy
Vitamin D	milk, butter, liver, and fish liver oils; also obtained by exposing the body to direct sunlight, which interacts with the cholesterol in the skin	responsible for the body's absorption of the minerals calcium and phosphorus and contributes to the formation of healthy bones; especially important to growing children and women who are pregnant or breastfeeding
Thiamin	lean pork, dried beans, peas, whole grain and enriched breads and cereals, and certain types of nuts	helps the body obtain energy from foods

Table 22-1. Source and function of essential vitamins.

22

Clients' Nutritional Needs

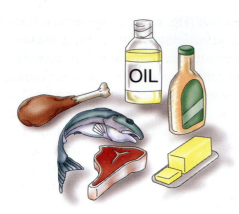

Fig. 22-3. Sources of fat.

processes. Zinc, iron, calcium, and magnesium are examples of minerals. Minerals are found in many foods.

6. **Water**. Because one-half to two-thirds of our body weight is water, we need 6 to 8 glasses of water a day. Water is the most essential nutrient for life. Without it, a person can only live a few days. Water assists in the digestion and absorption of food. It helps with the elimination of waste. Through perspiration, water also helps maintain normal body temperature. Maintaining enough fluid in our bodies is necessary for good health. Fluid balance is discussed more in chapter 14 and later in this chapter.

The fluids we drink—water, juice, soda, coffee, tea, and milk—provide most of the water our bodies use. Some foods are also sources of water, including celery, lettuce, apples, peaches, meat, chicken, and fish.

2. List the six food groups on the USDA Food Guide Pyramid

Most foods contain several nutrients, but no one food contains all the nutrients that are necessary to maintain a healthy body. Therefore, it is important that we eat a daily diet that is well-balanced. Our diet should contain several foods selected from each of the food groups listed below.

The U.S. Department of Agriculture (USDA) has divided the foods that we eat into six groups:

1. Grains, including cereals, bread, rice, and pasta
2. Fruits
3. Vegetables
4. Milk and milk products
5. Meat, poultry, fish, eggs, dry beans, and nuts
6. Fats, oils, and sweets

MINERAL	SOURCE	FUNCTION
Iron	egg yolks, green leafy vegetables, breads, cereals, and organ meats	necessary for the red blood cells to carry oxygen, helps in the formation of enzymes
Sodium	almost all foods and table salt	important for maintaining fluid balance (helps the body retain water)
Calcium	milk and milk products such as cheese, ice cream, and yogurt; green leafy vegetables such as collards, kale, mustard, dandelion, and turnip greens; and canned fish with soft bones, such as salmon	important for the formation of teeth and bones, the clotting of blood, muscle contraction, and heart and nerve function
Potassium	fruits and vegetables, cereals, coffee, and meats	essential for nerve and heart function and muscle contraction
Phosphorus	milk, milk products, meat, fish, poultry, nuts, and eggs	needed for the formation of bones and teeth and nerve and heart function; important for the body's utilization of proteins, fats, and carbohydrates

Table 22-2. Source and function of essential minerals.

These six groups have been arranged into the **Food Guide Pyramid** (Fig. 22-4). Foods close to the bottom of the pyramid should make up most of our diet. Foods closer to the top should be eaten in smaller quantities.

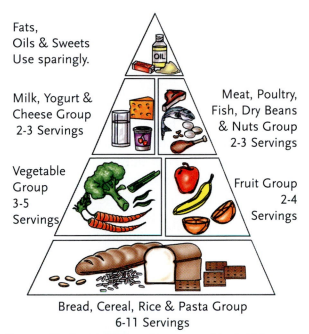

Fats,
Oils & Sweets
Use sparingly.

Milk, Yogurt &
Cheese Group
2-3 Servings

Meat, Poultry,
Fish, Dry Beans
& Nuts Group
2-3 Servings

Vegetable
Group
3-5
Servings

Fruit Group
2-4
Servings

Bread, Cereal, Rice & Pasta Group
6-11 Servings

Fig. 22-4. The Food Guide Pyramid was created by the U.S. Department of Agriculture to show the six food groups. Together, they form a healthy diet.

Grains. Grains are found in cereal, bread, rice, and pasta. Grains are a great source of carbohydrates. The Food Guide Pyramid recommends eating between six and eleven servings from the grain group each day. A **serving** is an individual portion or helping of food or drink. Examples of one serving include one slice of bread, one cup of dry cereal, or 1/2 cup of cooked cereal, pasta, or rice.

Foods containing complex carbohydrates take longer to break down. Therefore, they provide longer-lasting energy than foods containing simple carbohydrates. Whole-grain foods, such as whole-wheat breads, bran cereals, brown rice, and whole-wheat pastas, contain more complex carbohydrates than white breads, rice, pastas, and processed cereals. Whole-grain foods also contain more vitamins, protein, and energy.

Vegetables. Vegetables are excellent sources of vitamins and fiber. Choose from green leafy vegetables, including lettuce, spinach, and kale; tomatoes, green beans, peas, corn, cabbage, cauliflower, broccoli, and other vegetables. Vegetable sources of vitamin C include brussels sprouts, green or red peppers, and broccoli. The Food Guide Pyramid recommends eating three to five servings from the vegetable group each day. One serving from this group consists of one cup of raw, leafy vegetables, 1/2 cup of other vegetables, cooked or chopped, or 3/4 cup of vegetable juice.

Fruits. Fruits are good sources of complex carbohydrates, vitamins, and fiber. Fruits are one of the best sources of vitamin C, a nutrient we should eat each day. Good sources of vitamin C include oranges and orange juice, grapefruit and grapefruit juice, strawberries, mango, papaya, and cantaloupe. The Food Guide Pyramid recommends eating two to four servings from the fruit group each day. One serving from this group could include one medium-sized apple, orange, or banana; 3/4 cup of fruit juice; or 1/2 cup of chopped, cooked, or canned fruit.

Dairy Products. Milk and milk products, such as cheese and yogurt, are important sources of calcium (Fig. 22-5). We need calcium for healthy bones and teeth. Milk products also contain other minerals, protein, and vitamins. Other milk products are buttermilk, evaporated milk, and cottage cheese. Whole milk, cheese, and other products made with whole milk contain a lot of saturated fat. Most adults should eat low-fat or nonfat milk and milk products. Adults should have two to three servings from the dairy group each day. A serving of milk equals one cup. Other serving sizes include one cup of yogurt, one-and-a-half ounces of natural cheese, or two ounces of processed cheese.

Milk can be incorporated into foods, such as pudding, milkshakes, cereal, and cream soups, for people who dislike milk. Powdered milk can be used in cooking and baking as an economic alternative to regular milk. For clients who need extra protein and nourishment, powdered skim milk can be mixed with milk rather than water for puddings and milkshakes.

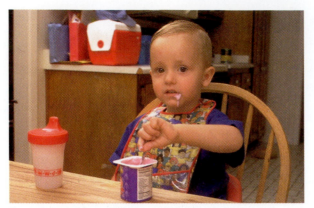

Fig. 22-5. Yogurt is a good source of calcium.

Meat, Poultry, Fish, Dry Beans, Eggs, and Nuts. These foods provide protein, minerals, and vitamins. In addition, meat is a good source of iron. Lower-fat choices from this group include most fish, chicken or turkey breast, lean cuts of meat, and dry beans. The Food Guide Pyramid recommends eating two to three servings from this group each day. One serving from this group equals two to three ounces of cooked lean meat, poultry or fish, one egg, 1/2 cup cooked dry beans, or 1/3 cup of nuts.

Fats, Oils, and Sweets. Fats and oils help the body absorb fat-soluble vitamins. They also provide flavor and make us feel full. Fats are needed by the body in very small quantities. Most adults eat more fat than their bodies need. Fats have more than twice as many calories per gram as carbohydrates or proteins. The body stores excess fat as fatty tissue. The best kinds of fats to use in a healthy diet are vegetable oils, including olive oil, canola oil, and corn oil (Fig. 22-6).

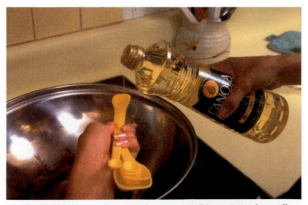

Fig. 22-6. Substitute olive, canola, or corn oil in recipes that call for less healthful oils.

Sweets, including candy, cookies, cakes, pies, and ice cream, contain large quantities of fat and/or sugar and should be eaten sparingly. In general, sweets provide no nutritional value. Eating too many sweets will cause weight gain. Some clients, particularly those with diabetes, must avoid sweets altogether.

3. Identify ways to assist clients in maintaining fluid balance

Most clients should be encouraged to drink at least eight glasses, or 64 ounces, of water a day. Remember that water is an essential nutrient for life. The sense of thirst can diminish as people age. Remind your elderly clients to drink fluids often (Fig. 22-7). However, some clients may have an order to force fluids (FF) or restrict fluids (RF) because of medical conditions. Follow your client's care plan.

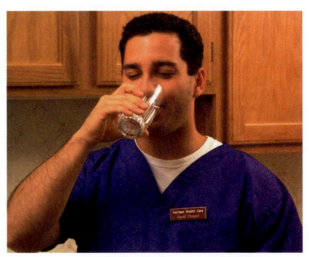

Fig. 22-7. Remember, drinking plenty of water is good for you, too!

Dehydration (*dee-high-DRAY-shun*) occurs when a person does not have enough fluid in the body. Dehydration is a serious condition. People can become dehydrated if they do not drink enough or if they have diarrhea or are vomiting.

OBSERVING AND REPORTING
Dehydration

Report any of the following immediately:

- if a client drinks less than eight eight-ounce glasses of liquid per day

- if a client needs help drinking from a cup
- if a client has trouble swallowing liquids
- if a client experiences frequent vomiting, diarrhea, or fever
- if client is easily confused or tired

Report if the client has any of the following:

- dry mouth
- cracked lips
- sunken eyes
- dark urine
- strong-smelling urine

Preventing Dehydration

- Report observations and warning signs to your supervisor immediately.
- Encourage your clients to drink every time you see them (Fig. 22-8).
- Offer fresh water or other fluids often.
- Record fluid intake and output.
- Ice chips, frozen flavored ice sticks, and gelatin are also forms of liquids. Offer them often. Do not offer ice chips or sticks if a client has a swallowing problem.
- If appropriate, offer sips of liquid between bites of food at meals and snacks.
- Make sure a pitcher and cup are near enough and light enough for a client to lift.
- Offer assistance if a client cannot drink without help. Use adaptive cups as needed.

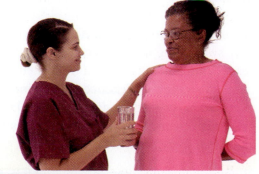

Fig. 22-8. Encouraging your clients to drink every time you see them can help prevent dehydration.

Fluid overload occurs when the body is unable to handle the amount of fluid consumed. This condition often affects people with heart or kidney disease.

Fluid Overload

Report any of the following to your supervisor:

- swelling/edema of extremities (ankles, feet, fingers, hands)
- weight gain (daily weight gain of one to two pounds)
- decreased urine output
- shortness of breath
- increased heart rate
- skin that appears tight, smooth, and shiny

Fluid balance is taking in and eliminating equal amounts of fluid. It can be measured by monitoring a client's intake and output. Chapter 14 describes how to do this. If you suspect a client is experiencing either dehydration or fluid overload, contact your supervisor immediately.

4. Identify nutritional problems of the elderly or ill

Aging and illness can lead to emotional and physical problems that affect the intake of food. For example, people who are lonely or who suffer from illnesses that affect their ability to chew and swallow may have little interest in food. Special care must be taken in meal planning and preparation to ensure adequate nutrition.

Clients who have small appetites may eat more if they are fed five or six small meals a day. If you are concerned that a client is not getting enough nutrients, talk with your supervisor about preparing high-calorie, high-protein foods and beverages. Food should look, taste, and smell good, particularly since the person may have a poor sense of taste and smell.

Unintended weight loss is a serious problem for the elderly. Weight loss can mean the client

has a serious medical condition. It can lead to skin breakdown, which leads to pressure sores. It is very important to report any weight loss you notice, no matter how small (Fig. 22-9). If a client has diabetes, chronic obstructive pulmonary disease, cancer, HIV, or other diseases, he is at a greater risk for malnutrition.

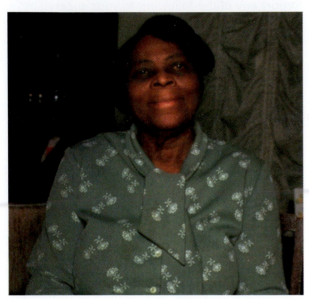

Fig. 22-9. Observing your clients for weight loss is an important part of your job.

OBSERVING AND REPORTING
Unintended Weight Loss

Report any of the following immediately:

- if a client needs help eating or drinking
- if a client eats less than half of meals/snacks served
- if client has mouth pain
- if a client has dentures that do not fit properly
- if client has any difficulty chewing or swallowing
- if a client coughs or chokes while eating
- if a client is sad, has crying spells, or withdraws from others
- if a client is confused, wanders, or paces

GUIDELINES
Preventing Unintended Weight Loss

- Report observations and warning signs to your supervisor.
- Encourage clients to eat.
- Honor clients' food likes and dislikes.
- Offer many different kinds of foods and beverages.
- Help clients who have trouble feeding themselves.
- Allow enough time for clients to finish eating.
- Notify your supervisor if clients have trouble using utensils.
- Record the meal/snack intake.
- Provide oral care before and after meals.
- Position clients sitting upright for feeding.
- If a client has had a loss of appetite and/or seems sad, ask about it.

Certain medications or limited activity cause constipation. Constipation often interferes with appetite. Fiber, fluids, and exercise can improve this common problem. Many illnesses require restrictions in fluids, proteins, certain minerals, or calories. Always check with your supervisor before changing a client's diet.

In addition, clients who are ill are often fatigued, nauseated, or in pain. Make sure these clients get plenty of rest and take prescribed medications. Some medications must be taken with food. Others must be taken before meals. These instructions are important both for reminding clients to take medications and for limiting nausea and upset stomach caused by medications. People who are nauseated may tolerate cold foods better than warm foods, because cold foods have less aroma. Eating small amounts of food throughout the day and eating slowly may also help.

Clients who have had strokes may have difficulty swallowing liquids because of facial weakness. Liquids that have been thickened may be easier to swallow. Thickened liquids include milk shakes, pureed foods, sherbet, gelatin, thin hot cereal, cream soups, and fruit juices that have been frozen to a slushy consistency.

When the digestive system does not function properly, **intravenous hyperalimentation**

(*in-tra-VEE-nus high-per-al-ih-men-TAY-shun*), or **IVH**, may be necessary. A solution of nutrients that can be administered directly into the bloodstream is infused into the client's veins. Home health aides are not responsible for IVH. You may be assigned to take the person's temperature or assemble supplies for a sterile dressing change. In addition, you should observe, report, and document any observation of changes in the client or problems with the feeding.

Clients are sometimes fed through a tube. This tube can travel through the nose and esophagus into the stomach. This is called a **nasogastric tube**. It can also be placed through the skin directly into the stomach. This is called a **gastrostomy** (Fig. 22-10). Tube feedings are used when residents cannot swallow but can digest food. Conditions that may prevent clients from swallowing include coma, cancer, stroke, refusal to eat, or extreme weakness.

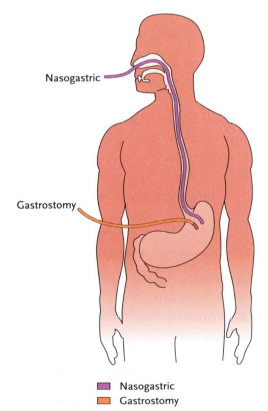

Nasogastric

Gastrostomy

■ Nasogastric
■ Gastrostomy

Fig. 22-10.

Home health aides never insert tubes, do the feeding, or irrigate (clean) the tubes. However, you may assemble equipment and supplies and hand them to the nurse. You may position the client for feeding. You may also dispose of used equipment and supplies, or clean and store reusable equipment and supplies. Check to make sure that the tubing is not kinked and make sure the client is not resting on the tubing. If you see any redness or drainage around the opening, report it.

5. Demonstrate awareness of regional, cultural, and religious food preferences

Culture, ethnicity, income, education, religion, and geography affect attitudes about nutrition. Food preferences may be formed by what you ate as a child, by what tastes good, or by personal beliefs about what should be eaten (Fig. 22-11). For instance, some people choose not to eat any animals or animal products, such as steak, chicken, butter, or eggs. These people are called vegetarians or vegans.

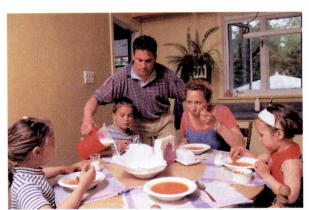

Fig. 22-11. Food likes and dislikes are influenced by what you ate as a child.

The region or culture you grow up in often influences your food preference. For example, people from the southwestern US may like spicy foods. "Southern cooking" may include fried foods, like fried chicken or fried okra. Ethnic groups often have certain foods that are common to them. These may be eaten at certain times of the year or all the time. Religious beliefs influence diet, too. For example, some Muslims and Jewish people do not eat any pork. Mormons may not drink alcohol, tea, or coffee.

When planning meals and cooking for your clients, know their food preferences. Some of these may be listed in the care plan. You will also need to find out more before planning meals. Ask the client or a family member to tell you about food preferences, or suggest some sample menus and ask for reactions. Pay attention to what is eaten when you serve meals. If a client never finishes her chicken, it may mean that she prefers other kinds of meats. Cost may also be a factor in choosing foods. Protein-rich foods are generally the most expensive, but also the most important for the healing process. You will learn to consider all these aspects of meal planning in chapter 23.

6. List and define common health claims on food labels

Food packages often make claims about the health benefits of the food they contain. Remember that food labels are advertising designed to convince you to buy a product. Although some regulations exist about what labels can claim, read health claims carefully before making a decision to buy.

Key Claims in Food Label Advertising

Low-fat, nonfat, fat-free, reduced fat, or light. If a product is labeled low-fat or nonfat, it usually does not contain much fat. One exception to this is 2% milk, which is often labeled low-fat, but actually gets more than 30% of its calories from fat. Always read the label anyway to determine the fat content of the food.

Products labeled "reduced fat" or "light" contain less fat than other versions of the same product. For example, salad dressing labeled "reduced fat" should contain 25% less fat than regular salad dressing. But it may still be high in fat. Salad dressing labeled "light" should contain 50% less fat than regular. Read the label to determine fat content. Some foods labeled low-fat, nonfat, or reduced fat may contain fat substitutes. In general, the best food and dollar value is found in products that do not contain these substitutes.

Cookies, cakes, and other treats labeled "fat-free" or "reduced fat" usually contain a lot of sugar and calories. Remember that all sweets should be used sparingly, as they provide little or no food value. Also remember that extra calories, especially sugars, are quickly converted to fat by the body.

Low-sodium, sodium-free, or no salt added. For clients who must reduce their sodium or salt intake, foods labeled "low-sodium" or "sodium-free" are important. Most foods naturally contain some sodium. Avoid foods that list salt or sodium as added ingredients. In general, canned foods and prepared foods like soups and frozen dinners usually have a lot of added salt and should be avoided.

Cholesterol-free. Cholesterol-free foods may be useful for those clients who must restrict their cholesterol intake. However, the best way to limit cholesterol is to avoid foods containing animal fats, such as butter, cheese, whole milk, eggs, red meats, and organ meats.

Sugar-free or no sugar added. Clients who must restrict their weight or who are diabetic must be very careful about consuming any sugar. Sugar-free products can be helpful, but you must read the labels carefully. Sugar-free products may contain artificial sweeteners, such as saccharin or aspartame. These have no food value and should be used sparingly. Foods sweetened with fruit juice may still contain a lot of calories. Diabetics may need to avoid fruit-juice-sweetened products as well as sugar-sweetened ones.

Organic. Organic food is produced without using most conventional pesticides, fertilizers made with synthetic ingredients or sewage sludge, bioengineering, or ionizing radiation. Organic meat, poultry, eggs, and dairy products come from animals that are given no antibiotics or growth hormones. Before a product can be labeled "organic," a government-approved certifier inspects the farm where the food is grown to make sure the farmer is following all the rules to meet USDA organic standards. Companies that handle or process organic food before it gets to the supermarket or restaurant

must be certified, too. Organic food differs from conventionally produced food in the way it is grown, handled, and processed (Fig. 22-12).

Natural, healthy, or good for you. These claims may have little or no meaning. Buy whole, unprocessed grains, fresh fruits and vegetables, and lean meats, poultry and fish, and you will know you are buying food that is healthful and nutritious. Don't be swayed by the advertising you see on labels; check the facts before you buy.

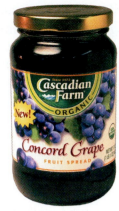

Fig. 22-12. One kind of organic food.

7. Explain the information on the FDA-required Nutrition Facts label

The Food and Drug Administration (FDA) requires that all packaged foods contain a standardized nutrition label, called "Nutrition Facts." This label contains information about the nutritional content of food. Because the label is in the same format on all foods, it is easy to compare different products (Fig. 22-13).

Regular Frozen Lasagna

Nutrition Facts
Serving size 1 Package (10.75 oz.)

Amount Per Serving

Calories 360	Calories from Fat 120

	% Daily Value
Total Fat 13g	20%
Saturated Fat 7g	35%
Cholesterol 35mg	11%
Sodium 960mg	40%
Total Carbohydrate 40g	14%
Dietary Fiber 6g	23%
Sugars 10g	
Protein 21g	
Calcium	35%
Vitamin A	10%
Vitamin C	10%
Iron	6%

Fig. 22-13. The FDA-required Nutrition Facts label contains standard nutritional information that makes it easier to compare different products.

The Nutrition Facts label gives you the following information:

Serving size and number of servings per container: Check the size of the serving. Remember that a serving may be a different amount than what a client actually eats.

Calories per serving and calories from fat per serving: The number of calories per serving tells you how much food energy a serving contains. It does not tell you how much nutritional value the food has. A candy bar is high in calories, providing quick energy, but has very few nutrients and lots of fat and sugar.

The number of calories from fat tells you a lot about the fat content of a food. In general, no more than one-third, or roughly 30%, of the total calories should come from fat. Thus, potato chips containing 110 calories per ounce and 80 calories from fat per ounce are not a good food choice. With more than two-thirds of their calories from fat, they are a high-fat food.

Amounts and % daily totals: For each of the following items, the label tells you two things. First, how much a serving contains, and second, what percent of the recommended daily total a serving contains. For example, crackers that contain three grams of fat per serving contain 5% of the recommended daily total of fat. These recommended daily totals are based on a 2,000-calorie diet. Someone who eats fewer than 2,000 calories per day should have less fat each day. Someone who eats more than 2,000 calories per day can have more fat. The label provides information on total fat and saturated fat, cholesterol, sodium, total carbohydrates, dietary fiber, sugars, and protein. The FDA-required label gives amounts and daily totals for the percentage (%) of the daily recommended amount one serving of the food provides.

Vitamins and minerals: The label lists the percentages of the recommended daily total for certain vitamins and minerals. If the label says one serving contains 50% of the vitamin C needed each day, you know this food is a good source of vitamin C.

22

Clients' Nutritional Needs

8. Explain special or modified diets

A doctor sometimes places clients who have certain illnesses on special diets. These diets are known as **therapeutic**, **modified**, or **special diets**. Certain nutrients or fluids may be restricted or eliminated. Some medications may also interact with certain foods, which then must be restricted. Clients who do not eat enough may be placed on a special supplementary diet. Diets are also prescribed for weight control and food allergies.

You will play an important role in helping clients follow their modified diets. Several types of modified diets are available for different illnesses. Some clients may be on a combination of restricted diets. The care plan should specify any special diet the client is on. It should also explain any eating problems that a client may have and how the client's eating habits can be improved (Fig. 22-14). Never modify a client's diet. Therapeutic diets can only be prescribed by doctors and planned by dietitians. Follow the client's diet plan without making judgments. Report observations to your supervisor.

NUTRITION	Diet Order:	Low fat		
✔	Meal Preparation			
	Assist with Feeding			
✔	Limit/Encourage Fluids			
	Grocery Shopping			
	Wash Clothes			

Fig. 22-14. The care plan specifies special diets or dietary restrictions.

Sodium-Restricted Diet (Low-Sodium Diet)

People are most familiar with sodium as one of the two ingredients of salt. Salt is the first food to be restricted in a low-sodium diet because it is high in sodium.

Excess sodium causes the body to retain more water in tissues and in the circulatory system than is necessary. This causes the heart to pump harder. This is harmful for clients who have high blood pressure, coronary artery disease, or kidney disease. A modified fluid intake may also be required for people with these conditions, because too much fluid can lead to congestive heart failure.

The human body needs 1,500 to 2,500 milligrams of sodium a day. On average, we consume twice that amount. Excess sodium is excreted in the urine and over the years can erode the kidneys, leading to hypertension and kidney disease.

Foods high in sodium include the following:

- cured meats: ham, bacon, lunch meat, sausage, salt pork, and hot dogs

- salty or smoked fish: herring, salted cod, sardines, anchovies, caviar, smoked salmon or lox

- processed cheese

- canned and dried soups

- vegetables preserved in brine: pickles, sauerkraut, olives, relishes

- salted foods: nuts, dips, and spreads

- sauces with high concentrations of salt: Worcestershire, barbecue, chili, and soy sauces; ketchup and mustard

- canned foods

- some cereals

- over-the-counter medications and drugs (Fig. 22-15)

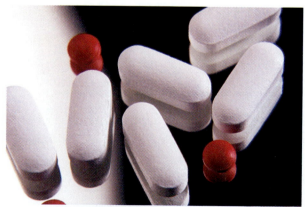

Fig. 22-15. Over-the-counter medications may be high in sodium.

Read product labels to determine if they contain salt or sodium in any form. A common form of sodium is **monosodium glutamate** (*GLOO-ta-mayt*), often added to meat tenderizers, season-

ings, and prepared foods to enhance flavor. Another common form is **sodium nitrate**, a salt used to preserve lunch meats and other cured meats.

You can make low-sodium meals more flavorful by adding lemon, herbs, dry mustard, pepper, paprika, orange rind, onion, and garlic to recipes. The flavor of meats can also be enhanced by the addition of fruits and jellies. Salt substitutes should only be used with the approval of the client's doctor. These seasonings might be high in potassium, which can be harmful to people with certain illnesses, such as kidney disease.

Fluid-Restricted Diets

The amount of fluid consumed through food and fluids must equal the amount of fluid that leaves the body through perspiration, stool, urine, and expiration. This is **fluid balance**. When fluid intake is greater than fluid output, body tissues become swollen with excess fluid. In addition, people with severe heart disease and kidney disease may have difficulty processing large volumes of fluid. To prevent further heart and kidney damage, doctors may restrict a client's fluid intake. For clients on fluid restriction, you will need to measure and document exact amounts of fluid intake. Report excesses to your supervisor.

High-Potassium Diets (K+)

Some clients are on **diuretics** (*dye-you-RET-iks*), which are medications that reduce fluid volume, or on blood pressure medications. These clients may be excreting so much fluid that their bodies could be depleted of potassium. Other clients may be placed on a high-potassium diet for different reasons.

Foods high in potassium include bananas, grapefruit, oranges, orange juice, prune juice, prunes, dried apricots, figs, raisins, dates, cantaloupes, tomatoes, potatoes with skins, sweet potatoes and yams, winter squash, legumes, avocados, and unsalted nuts.

Low-Protein Diet

In addition to restricted dietary intake of fluids, sodium, and potassium, people who have kidney disease may also be on low-protein diets. Protein is restricted because it breaks down into compounds that may lead to further kidney damage. The extent of the restrictions depends on the stage of the disease and whether the client is on dialysis.

Exchange lists show foods that can be exchanged for one another on a meal plan. They are used extensively in special diets for people with diabetes. Exchange lists have also been developed for clients on diets modified for protein, potassium, and sodium. Follow the instructions for these diets carefully and ask for help whenever you need it.

Low-Fat/Low-Cholesterol Diet

People who have high levels of cholesterol in their blood are at risk for heart attacks and heart disease. People with gallbladder disease, diseases that interfere with fat digestion, and liver disease are also placed on low-fat/low-cholesterol diets.

Low-fat/low-cholesterol diets permit skim milk, low-fat cottage cheese, fish, white meat of turkey and chicken, veal, and vegetable fats (especially monounsaturated fats such as olive, canola, and peanut oils). Clients may be advised to limit their diets in the following ways:

- Eat lean cuts of meat including lamb, beef, and pork, and eat these only three times a week.
- Limit egg yolks to three or four per week (including eggs used in baking).
- Avoid organ meats, shellfish, fatty meats, cream, butter, lard, meat drippings, coconut and palm oils, and desserts and soups made with whole milk.
- Avoid fried foods and sweets.

People who have gallbladder disease or other digestive problems may be placed on a diet that restricts all fats.

22

Clients' Nutritional Needs

Modified Calorie Diet for Weight Management

Some clients may need to reduce calories to lose weight or prevent additional weight gain. Other clients may need to gain weight and increase calories because of malnutrition, surgery, illness, or fever. Clients with certain conditions need more protein to promote growth and repair of tissue and regulation of body functions.

Dietary Management of Ulcers

Gastric and duodenal (doo-a-DEE-nal) ulcers can be irritated by foods that produce or increase levels of acid in the stomach. People who have ulcers usually know the foods that cause them discomfort. Doctors will advise them to avoid these foods as well as the following: alcohol; beverages containing caffeine, such as coffee, tea, and soft drinks; and spicy seasonings such as black pepper, cayenne, and chili pepper. Three meals or more a day are usually advised. If alcohol is allowed, it should be drunk with meals.

Dietary Management of Diabetes Mellitus

Calories and carbohydrates are carefully regulated in the dietary management of diabetic clients. Protein and fats are also regulated. The types of foods and the amounts are determined by the client's nutritional and energy requirements. See chapter 20 for more information on diabetes. Two types of diets can manage diabetes mellitus:

1. **Non-concentrated Sweets Diet**. This diet is a regular, well-balanced diet that excludes concentrated sweets, such as sugars, honey, syrup, jellies, jams, preserves, candy, and cranberry sauce. The diet also eliminates cakes, pastries, cookies, puddings, ice cream, gelatin, sweetened fruit juices and beverages, sugar-coated cereals, condensed milk, and candied or glazed fruits and vegetables.

2. **Exchange List Diets**. Exchange list diets are described in more detail in chapter 20. This type of diet is more restricted than the non-concentrated sweets diet, because it involves more than just the elimination of concentrated sweets. Meals are carefully planned based on exact amounts of food from the six food groups. Exchange lists are then used to determine foods and the exact serving sizes that may be eaten to follow the meal plan. Foods are measured and must be eaten completely at certain times. Eating the necessary carbohydrates, which are found in dairy and bread groups, is very important if the client is too ill to tolerate the other foods. Any variation in eating patterns and routine must be reported to the doctor or nurse.

Chapter Review

1. List the six basic nutrients. For each nutrient describe one way a client can get that nutrient.

2. Why is whole-wheat bread more nutritious than white bread?

3. How many servings of vegetables should a person eat each day?

4. Why should most adults eat low-fat dairy products?

5. What does meat provide in addition to protein, minerals, and vitamins?

6. What are the healthiest kinds of fats to eat?

7. List five signs to report immediately about dehydration.

8. List four signs to report about fluid overload.

9. Describe five ways to prevent dehydration.

10. Why is it important to report any weight loss you notice, no matter how small?

11. Name three reasons an elderly or ill client may have nutritional problems.

12. What are two ways a client may be fed if he has a digestive system that does not function properly or he cannot swallow?

13. In what ways can you learn the food preferences of your clients?

True or False. Mark each statement with a "T" for true and a an "F" for false.

14. ___ Nonfat sweets are nutritious foods.

15. ___ Diabetics may not be able to eat fruit-juice-sweetened products.

16. ___ If a package is labeled "all natural" it may still be bad for you.

17. ___ For a steak to be called "organic," it has to come from a cow that was not given antibiotics or growth hormones.

18. ___ Many canned and prepared foods are high in sodium.

19. ___ The best way to limit cholesterol is to limit intake of all fats.

20. What information can you learn by looking at the number of calories from fat in a food?

21. Why is it important to check serving size on a food label?

22. Choose one of the diets listed in learning objective 8. Describe a meal that would be appropriate for a client on that diet.

23

Meal Planning, Shopping, Preparation, and Storage

1. Explain how to prepare a basic food plan and list food shopping guidelines

It is very important to plan meals for a week or at least several days before shopping. When planning, take into account the client's dietary restrictions, food preferences, number of family members present at meals, and the client's budget.

On a large sheet of paper write out the days for which you will shop. Leave space under each day for meals and snacks. You may end up serving the meals in a different order. However, by planning for each day, you will plan the right number of meals and buy the right amount of food (Fig. 23-1).

Fill in breakfasts, lunches, dinners, and snacks for each day. Ask the client or family for ideas or look in cookbooks. Plan to have leftovers that can be easily reheated on days you will not be in the home. Plan plenty of nutritious snacks; clients may need as many as three snacks a day. Remember to list beverages as well.

	MONDAY	TUESDAY	WEDNESDAY	THURSDAY	FRIDAY
BREAKFAST	Oatmeal w/Raisins Toast Juice	Scrambled eggs Orange Coffee	WAFFLES BANANAS JUICE	POACHED EGG ½ GRAPEFRUIT COFFEE	CORN FLAKES STRAWBERRIES OJ
SNACK	PEARS CHEESE	BRAN MUFFIN MILK	SLICED PEACH TOAST MILK	BRAN MUFFIN MILK	PEARS CHEESE
LUNCH	TOSSED SALAD w/ TURKEY, TOMATO, + CUCUMBER	CHICKEN SOUP SOURDOUGH BREAD ICED TEA	ROAST BEEF SANDWICH APPLESAUCE	TOMATO SOUP HAM SANDWICH	CHICKEN SALAD SANDWICH TOMATO SLICES
SNACK	BRAN MUFFIN MILK	APPLE SLICES CHEDDAR CHEESE	ENGLISH MUFFIN HOT TEA	APPLE SLICES CHEDDAR CHEESE	BANANA BREAD MILK
DINNER	ROAST BEEF POTATOES CARROTS APPLESAUCE	SMOKED HAM MASHED POTATOES GRAVY GREEN BEANS	BAKED POTATO w/ BROCCOLI AND CHEESE SOURDOUGH BREAD	BAKED CHICKEN PEAS + CARROTS CANTALOUPE	TUNA CASSEROLE SOURDOUGH BREAD PEACHES + YOGURT
SNACK	HOT COCOA ENGLISH MUFFIN	GRAHAM CRACKERS MILK	CORN MUFFIN MILK	BANANA BREAD ~~BLUEBERRY MUFFIN~~ MILK	CORN MUFFIN MILK

Fig. 23-1. A meal plan will help you know what kinds and quantities of food to buy for a week.

When your meal plan is completed, make your shopping list. On another large sheet of paper, write down categories including produce, meats, canned goods, frozen foods, dairy, and other. Leave space under each category to list the foods you need to buy. Listing items by category will save you time in the grocery store. Go through your plan meal by meal. Write down all of the ingredients you will need for each meal. Remember to include beverages. Check the refrigerator, cabinets, and pantry for ingredients. Many ingredients you need may already be in the home.

Keep a shopping list going all the time so family members, clients, and you can write down things you run out of during the week.

Meals that Make Good Leftovers

beef stew

chili

spaghetti with sauce

casseroles

red beans and rice

split pea soup

lentil soup

chicken soup

macaroni and cheese

lasagna

meat loaf

pot roast

Nutritious Snacks

Take into account the client's dietary needs when planning snacks.

- low-salt pretzels and tomato juice or vegetable juice
- celery with peanut butter or cream cheese and milk
- graham crackers and milk
- rice cakes with peanut butter and milk
- cereal and milk
- yogurt
- baked tortilla chips with salsa
- carrot or celery sticks with salsa
- crackers and cheese
- gelatin with fruit
- bran muffin and milk
- raisins, dates, figs, prunes, or dried apricots
- trail mix
- "milk shakes" made with yogurt, milk, and fruit blended together
- fresh fruit
- apple with peanut butter
- apple with cheese

GUIDELINES
Shopping for Clients

- Use coupons. If your client receives a newspaper, scan it for coupons from stores or manufacturers. Clip and use only those coupons for items you have already planned to buy.

- Check store circulars for advertised specials. Compare foods by reading the unit price tags that are on the shelves in front of the product (Fig. 23-2). Store brands are usually cheaper than advertised brands.

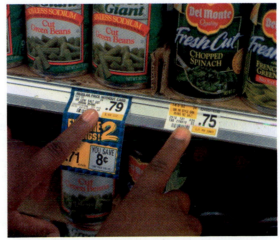

Fig. 23-2. Compare foods by reading the unit price tag.

- Buy fresh foods that are in season, when they are at peak flavor and inexpensive.

23

Meal Planning, Shopping, Preparation & Storage

g Buy in quantity. Large amounts or larger sizes are usually more economical, but do not buy more than you can store.

g Shop from your list. Don't be tempted by items that are not on your list.

g Avoid processed, already-mixed, or ready-made foods. They are usually more expensive and less nutritious. When time allows, buy staples, or basic items.

g Buy a cheaper brand when appearance is not important. For example, store brand mushroom bits are fine to use in a casserole and cheaper than name-brand mushroom pieces.

g Read labels to be sure you are getting the kind of product and the quantity you want. Read labels for ingredients that may be harmful to your client, for example, excessive salt or sodium.

g Estimate the cost per serving before buying. Divide the total cost by the number of servings to determine the cost per serving.

g Consider the amount of waste in bones and fat when buying cheaper cuts of meat. Some cuts of less expensive meats yield only half of what leaner cuts yield per pound. For clients on low-fat/low-cholesterol diets, pick lean meats and take the skin off chicken and turkey parts. The skin holds much of the fat.

Inexpensive Meals

pasta dishes

baked stuffed potatoes

rice and beans

tuna casserole

chicken thighs or legs

hamburger casserole

pot roast

stews

lentil soup

split pea soup

lasagna

When deciding what to buy, keep these four factors in mind:

1. **Nutritional value**. Does this food contain essential nutrients, vitamins, and minerals? Is it unprocessed, without added salt or sugar?

2. **Quality**. Is this food fresh and in good condition? Fruits, vegetables, and meats should look fresh. Canned goods should not be dented or rusted. Milk and dairy products should not have passed their expiration dates.

3. **Price**. Is this the most economical choice? If it costs more, is it worth it?

4. **Preference**. Will my client like this food? Can I make an appealing meal using this food?

2. List guidelines for safe food preparation

Food-borne illnesses affect up to 100 million people each year. Elderly people are at increased risk partly because they may not see, smell, or taste that food is spoiled. They also may not have the energy to prepare and store food safely. For people who have weakened immune systems because of AIDS or cancer, a food-borne illness can be deadly.

GUIDELINES
Safe Food Preparation

g Wash hands frequently. Wash your hands thoroughly before beginning any food preparation. Wash your hands after handling raw meat, poultry, or fish.

g Keep everything clean. Clean and disinfect countertops and other surfaces before, during (as necessary), and after food preparation.

g Handle raw meat, poultry and fish carefully. Use an antibacterial kitchen cleaner or a dilute bleach solution to clean any countertops on which meat juices were spilled. Wrap paper or packaging containing meat juices in plastic and discard immediately.

🄖 Once you have used a knife or cutting board to cut fresh meat, do not use it for anything else until it has been washed in the dishwasher or in very hot, soapy water containing bleach. Use plastic cutting boards for raw meat, wooden ones for vegetables and other foods (Fig. 23-3).

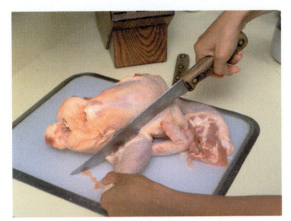

Fig. 23-3. Carefully wash areas used to cut raw meat.

🄖 Change dishcloths, sponges and towels frequently. Sponges may be washed in the dishwasher to disinfect them.

🄖 Defrost frozen foods in the refrigerator, not on the countertop. Do not remove meats or dairy products from the refrigerator until just before use.

🄖 Wash fruits and vegetables thoroughly in running water to remove pesticides and bacteria.

🄖 Cook meats, poultry, and fish thoroughly to kill any harmful microorganisms they may contain. Heat leftovers thoroughly. Never leave food out for over two hours. Keep cold foods cold and hot foods hot.

3. Identify methods of food preparation

The following basic methods of food preparation will allow you to prepare a variety of healthy meals:

Boiling: Food is cooked in boiling water until tender or done. This is the best method for cooking pasta, noodles, rice, and hard- or soft-boiled eggs (Fig. 23-4).

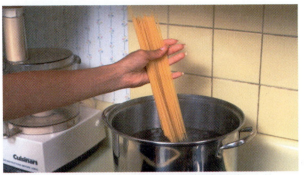

Fig. 23-4. Boiling works well for pasta and other grains.

Steaming: Steaming is a healthy way to prepare vegetables. A small amount of water is boiled in the bottom of a saucepan and food is set over it on a rack (Fig. 23-5). The pan is tightly covered to keep the steam in.

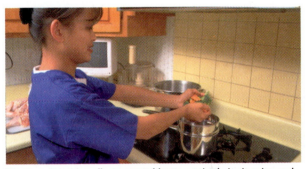

Fig. 23-5. Steaming allows vegetables to retain their vitamins and flavor.

Poaching: Fish or eggs may be cooked by poaching in barely boiling water or other liquid. Eggs are cracked and shells discarded before poaching. Fish may be poached in milk or broth, on top of the stove or in the oven in a baking dish (Fig. 23-6).

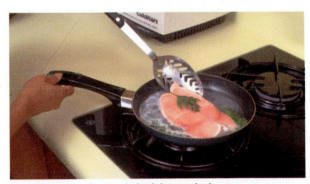

Fig. 23-6. Fish and eggs can both be poached.

Roasting: Used for meats and poultry or some vegetables, roasting is a simple way to cook. Dry heat roasting means food is roasted in an open

pan in the oven (Fig. 23-7). Meats and poultry are **basted**, or coated with juices or other liquid, during roasting.

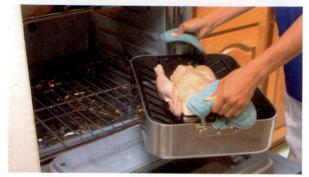

Fig. 23-7. Meats roast well at high temperatures (450°) but may need to be basted. Vegetables can also be roasted.

Moist heat roasting is used for lean cuts of beef such as pot roast. Liquid such as broth, wine, or tomato sauce is poured over and around the meat and the pot is covered. Moist heat roasting may be done in the oven or on the stove top.

Baking: Baking is used for many foods, including breads, poultry, fish, and vegetables. Baking is done at moderate heat, 350°F to 400°F. Vegetables such as potatoes and winter squash bake very well (Fig. 23-8).

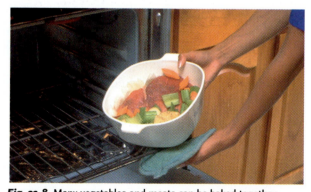

Fig. 23-8. Many vegetables and meats can be baked together.

Broiling: Used primarily for meats, broiling involves cooking food close to the source of heat at a high temperature for a short time (Fig. 23-9). Meat must be tender to be broiled successfully; inexpensive and lean cuts are often better cooked using moist heat. The "broil" setting on the oven can also be used to melt cheese or brown the top of a casserole. Leave the oven door ajar when broiling and never leave the kitchen: things can burn very fast.

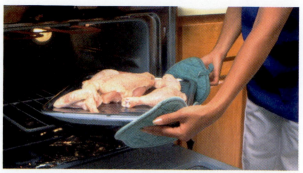

Fig. 23-9. Broiling involves cooking at a very high temperature.

Sautéing or stir-frying: These are quick cooking methods for vegetables and meats. Use a small amount of oil in a frying pan or wok over high heat (Fig. 23-10).

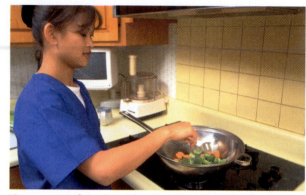

Fig. 23-10. Stir frying is quick and uses very little fat. Food must be stirred constantly to prevent it from sticking.

Microwaving: Microwave ovens are safe to use for defrosting, reheating, and cooking. However "cold spots" can occur in microwaved foods because of the irregular way the microwaves enter the oven and are absorbed by the food. If food does not cook evenly, bacteria may survive and cause food-borne illness.

To minimize cold spots, stir and rotate the food once or twice during cooking. Arranging foods uniformly in a covered dish and turning large foods upside down during cooking also help.

When defrosting food in the microwave, remove food from store wrap first. Foam trays and plastic wraps may melt and cause chemicals to migrate into the food. Place food in a microwave-safe bowl instead.

Foods being reheated in the microwave should be steaming and hot to the touch, or at least

165°F. Cover foods. Stir them from the outside in to encourage safe, even heating.

To insure that meat is properly cooked, use a meat thermometer or the oven's temperature probe. This verifies that the food has reached a safe temperature. Check in several places to be sure red meat is 160°F and poultry 180°F. Check for visual signs of doneness. Juices should run clear and meat should not be pink.

Never place metal thermometers or any metal object in the microwave oven. Be aware that some clients cannot be near a microwave during operation.

Frying: Frying uses a lot of fat and is the least healthy way to cook. Avoid frying foods for clients (Fig. 23-11).

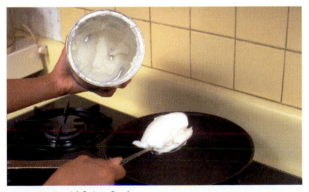

Fig. 23-11. Avoid frying foods.

Fresh, uncooked foods: Many fruits and vegetables have the most nutrients when eaten fresh, as in salads (Fig. 23-12). However, fresh fruits and vegetables may be difficult for some clients to chew or digest. Wash fruits and vegetables well to remove any chemicals or pesticides.

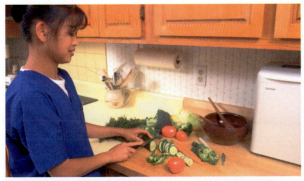

Fig. 23-12. Many fruits and vegetables have the most nutrients when eaten uncooked and fresh.

4. Identify four methods of low-fat food preparation

1. **Cook lean**. Boiling, steaming, broiling, and roasting are all methods of cooking that require little or no added fat. Broiling also allows fats in meat to drip out before food is consumed. This lowers the fat content even more.

2. **Drain fat**. When using ground meat, brown it first. Then drain it on paper towels to remove excess fat.

3. **Plan lean**. Choosing foods with lower fat content to begin with will make low-fat cooking easier. Planning meals around grains will help cut the fat content. Low-fat meals based on grains include pasta dishes, rice and beans, baked or stuffed potatoes, and soups.

4. **Substitute or cut down**. Sometimes high-fat ingredients can be left out or replaced to lower the fat content of a recipe. Leave out or cut down the amount of cheese used on sandwiches or to top casseroles. Substitute plain nonfat yogurt for mayonnaise or sour cream. Nonfat cottage cheese can also be used. Try it on a baked potato instead of sour cream.

5. List four guidelines for safe food storage

1. **Buy cold food last; get it home fast**. After shopping, put away refrigerated foods first.

2. **Keep it safe; refrigerate**. Maintain refrigerator temperature between 36°F and 40°F. Maintain freezer temperature at 0°F. Refrigerated items that spoil easily should be kept in the rear of the refrigerator, not the door. Look on the jar or package to determine if food requires refrigeration once it has been opened (Fig. 23-13). Do not refreeze items after they have been thawed.

3. **Use small containers that seal tightly**. Foods cool more quickly when stored in smaller containers. Store with enough room around them for air circulation. Never leave foods out for

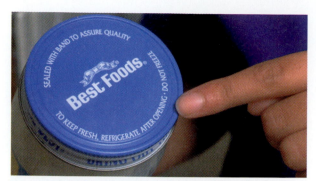

Fig. 23-13. Look for refrigeration guidelines on food labels.

more than two hours. Tightly cover all foods. To prevent dry foods, such as cornmeal and flour, from becoming infested with insects, store these items in tightly-sealed containers. If you find items that are already infested, discard them. Use a clean container to store a fresh supply. Check dry storage areas periodically for signs of insects and rodents.

4. **When in doubt, throw it out**! If you are not sure whether food is spoiled, don't take any chances. Discard it. Check the expiration dates on foods, especially perishables. Check the refrigerator often for spoiled foods. Discard any you find.

6. Describe guidelines for assisting with eating

Clients who must be fed are often embarrassed and depressed about their dependence on another person. Be aware of this. Only give assistance as specified, when necessary, or when the client requests it. Encourage clients to do whatever they can for themselves. For example, if a client can hold and use a napkin, he should.

GUIDELINES
Assisting a Client with Eating

- Never treat the client like a child. This is embarrassing and disrespectful. It is difficult for many people to accept help with feeding. Be as supportive and encouraging as you can.

- Sit at the client's eye level.

- Check the temperature at your wrist before offering a bite of food.

- Cut foods and pour liquids as needed.

- Ask the client which food he prefers to eat first. Allow him to make the choice, even if he wants to eat dessert first.

- Do not rush the meal. Appear relaxed.

- Be social and friendly. Make simple conversation if the client wishes to do so (Fig. 23-14). Try not to ask questions that require answers.

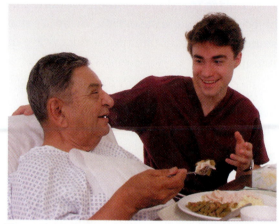

Fig. 23-14. Be pleasant and friendly while a client is eating.

- Give the client your full attention while he or she is eating.

- Alternate offering food and drink.

Assisting a Client with Eating

Equipment: meal, eating utensils, clothing protector if appropriate, 1-2 napkins or washcloths

1. Wash your hands.

2. Explain the procedure to the client, speaking clearly, slowly, and directly, maintaining face-to-face contact whenever possible.

3. Assist the client to wash her hands if client cannot do it on her own.

4. Before assisting with feeding the client, see that client is in an upright sitting position (at a 90-degree angle).

5. Assist client to put on clothing protector, if desired.

6. Sit next to the client at the client's eye level (Fig. 23-15). Sit on the stronger side if the client has one-sided weakness.

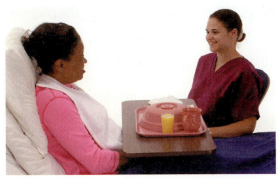

Fig. 23-15.

7. Check temperature of food. Offer the food in bite-sized pieces (Fig. 23-16). Alternate types of food offered, allowing for client's preferences. (Do not feed all of one type before offering another type.) Make sure the client's mouth is empty before offering the next bite of food or sip of drink.

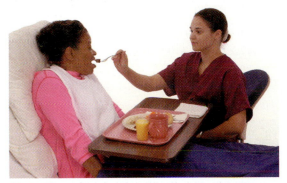

Fig. 23-16.

8. Offer drinks throughout the meal. If you are holding the cup, touch it the client's lips before you tip it. Give small frequent sips. Use a straw or adaptive cup as necessary or as the client requests it.

9. Wipe food from the client's mouth and hands as necessary during the meal. Wipe again at the end of the meal (Fig. 23-17).

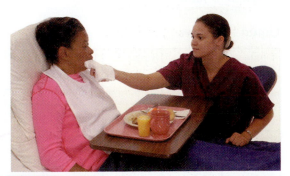

Fig. 23-17.

10. Talk with the client during meal. It makes mealtime more enjoyable. Do not rush the client.

11. When the client is done eating, remove the clothing protector if used. Remove the tray or dishes.

12. Wash your hands.

13. Assist the client to a comfortable position.

14. Document the client's intake, if required, and any observations. How did the client tolerate being upright for the meal? Did the client eat well? What foods did the client eat or not eat? Report any swallowing difficulties to your supervisor.

7. Describe eating and swallowing problems a client may have

Clients may have conditions that make eating or swallowing difficult. A stroke, or CVA, can cause weakness on one side of the body and paralysis. Nerve and muscle damage from head and neck cancer, multiple sclerosis, Parkinson's or Alzheimer's disease may also be present. If a client has difficulty swallowing, you will probably serve soft foods and thickened liquids. A straw or special cup will help make swallowing easier.

Swallowing problems put clients at high risk for choking on food or drink. Inhaling food or drink into the lungs is called **aspiration**. Aspiration can cause pneumonia or death. Alert your supervisor immediately if any problems occur while feeding a client.

GUIDELINES
Preventing Aspiration

🅖 Position client properly. He or she must sit in a straight, upright position. Do not try to feed a client in a reclining position.

🅖 Offer small pieces of food or small spoonfuls of pureed food.

🅖 Feed the client slowly.

🅖 Place food in the non-paralyzed or unaffected side of the mouth.

23

Meal Planning, Shopping, Preparation & Storage

g Make sure the mouth is empty before offering the next bite of food or sip of drink.

When a person is completely unable to swallow, he or she may be fed through a special tube. A **nasogastric tube** is inserted into the nose and goes to the stomach. A **gastrostomy tube** is inserted through the abdomen, directly into the stomach. If a person's digestive system does not function properly, **hyperalimentation** (*high-per-al-ih-men-TAY-shun*) or **total parenteral nutrition** (TPN) may be necessary. With TPN a client receives nutrients directly into the bloodstream. It bypasses the digestive system.

Home health aides are not responsible for these types of artificial feeding. However, you must make sure that the tubing is not kinked or pulled in any way. Observe, report, and document any changes in the client or problems with the equipment.

Chapter Review

1. Create a meal plan for yourself for two days. Include breakfast, lunch, and dinner.

2. Why is more expensive meat sometimes a better deal?

3. Why are processed or ready-made foods not as desirable as food made from scratch?

4. What is the longest period of time you should leave cooked food out of the refrigerator?

5. How can you remove pesticides from fresh fruits and vegetables?

6. How can you disinfect a sponge?

True or False. Mark each statement with either a "T" for true or "F" for false.

7. ___ If fried foods are your client's favorite, you should fry for him/her often.

8. ___ Boiling is a good way to prepare pasta.

9. ___ Fish can be poached in the oven or on the stove.

10. ___ Broiling is very time-consuming.

11. ___ Steaming is a healthy way to prepare vegetables.

12. You have browned ground beef to make soft tacos for your client. What should you do before adding the seasoning?

13. What makes the healthiest base for a chicken stir-fry: brown rice, white rice, or crunchy fried noodles?

14. Can you think of low-fat substitutions in addition to those listed in the text?

15. When it is acceptable to refreeze an item?

16. Give an example of an item that requires refrigeration after opening.

17. What should you do if you find insects in the flour?

18. Why might a client who must be fed be embarrassed or depressed?

19. Why do you think it is important to encourage a client to do whatever she can for herself while eating?

20. How should a client be positioned to prevent aspiration?

21. What is your responsibility with tube feedings or intravenous feedings?

Conversion Tables

Liquid Measures

1 gal=	4 qt=	8 pt=	16 cups=	128 fl oz
1/2 gal=	2 qt=	4 pt=	8 cups=	64 fl oz
1/4 gal=	1 qt=	2 pt=	4 cups=	32 fl oz
	1/2 qt=	1 pt=	2 cups=	16 fl oz
	1/4 qt=	1/2 pt=	1 cup=	8 fl oz

Dry Measures

1 cup=	8 fl oz=	16 tbsp=	48 tsp=
3/4 cup=	6 fl oz=	12 tbsp=	36 tsp=
2/3 cup=	5 1/3 fl oz=	10 2/3 tbsp=	32 tsp=
1/2 cup=	4 fl oz=	8 tbsp=	24 tsp=
1/3 cup=	2 2/3 fl oz=	5 1/3 tbsp=	16 tsp=
1/4 cup=	2 fl oz=	4 tbsp=	12 tsp=
1/8 cup=	1 fl oz=	2 tbsp=	6 tsp=
		1 tbsp=	3 tsp=

Emergency Substitutions

Emergency substitutions can sometimes be made, although it's best to use the ingredients called for in recipes.

VEGETABLES	
Ingredient	**Substitute**
1 cup canned tomatoes	1 1/3 cups cut-up fresh tomatoes, simmered 10 minutes
1/2 lb. fresh mushrooms	4-oz. can mushrooms
Legumes	With the exception of lentils, dry beans can be used interchangeably to suit personal preference.

HERBS, SPICES, SEASONINGS	
Ingredient	**Substitute**
1 tbsp. snipped fresh herbs	1 tsp. same herb, dried, or 1/4 tsp. powdered or ground
1 tsp. dry mustard	2 tsp. prepared mustard
1 tsp. pumpkin pie spice	1/2 tsp. cinnamon, 1/2 tsp. ginger, 1/8 tsp. ground allspice, 1/8 tsp. nutmeg

THICKENERS	
Ingredient	**Substitute**
1 tbsp. cornstarch	2 tbsp. flour, or 1 1/3 tbsp. quick-cooking tapioca
1 tbsp. flour	1/2 tbsp. cornstarch, or 2 tsp. quick-cooking tapioca, or two egg yolks
1 tbsp. tapioca	1 1/2 tbsp flour

BAKING	
Ingredient	**Substitute**
1 tsp. baking powder	1/4 tsp. baking soda plus 1/2 tsp. cream of tartar
1 pkg. active dry yeast	1 tbsp. dry yeast
1 cup oil	1/2 lb. butter or margarine
1 cup brown sugar	1 cup granulated sugar

23

Meal Planning, Shopping, Preparation & Storage

24

Managing Time, Energy, and Money

1. Explain three ways to work more efficiently

Taking care of the client and other family members who need assistance and support is your most important responsibility. For this to be accomplished, you must maintain an orderly and clean environment. To balance these responsibilities, you must manage your time and energy efficiently. The following are ways to be sure your work schedule is as efficient as possible:

Distribute Tasks. Look at the client care plan and your assignments. Note the assigned housekeeping tasks. Divide the tasks and schedule them for the week and the month. Make sure all your assignments can be completed in the time you have. Some tasks are best accomplished together. For example, it is most efficient to do all the laundry on one day. Then you are able to do larger loads and fold and iron all at once. Plan one morning or afternoon to do the laundry. For more efficiency, plan other tasks to do while loads are in the washer or dryer.

Prioritize Tasks. Prioritizing your tasks is an important time and energy management skill. Think about the jobs you want to complete throughout the day. Which ones must be done immediately? Which ones must be done at a certain time? Which activities are not absolutely essential and could be put off? Spend time on activities that are most important first.

Simplify Tasks. Learn to simplify your tasks. Take time to think about how you will go about doing a task. Try to eliminate a few steps but still get the same result. For example, when baking a cake, can you mix everything in one bowl? When you clean up, can you stack everything on a tray and take it all to the sink at one time?

Finally, **be realistic**. You may not be able to get everything done even if you plan carefully. Reassess your schedule during the day. Have you finished what you planned or are you behind? When tasks take longer than you expected, or unexpected tasks need to be done, be realistic about what you can do. Do not be afraid to change your plan. It is better to accomplish the highest-priority tasks and let others go unfinished than to do everything half way. The key to success is to be flexible.

Simple Ways to Conserve Time and Energy

Energize. Use good body mechanics. Take occasional breaks to restore your energy. Alternate longer tasks with shorter tasks, and high-energy tasks with low-energy ones. Take care of yourself—eat right, exercise, and get plenty of rest.

Organize. At the beginning of the day, do a mental run-down of the tasks that must be done and rearrange your schedule if necessary. Plan what must be done and do it. Store frequently used items in convenient places near the work area. Assemble your equipment and

materials before you begin a task. Keep clutter in control and work in good light. Think about how to organize activities and equipment to avoid unnecessary work. Make and use shopping lists.

Economize. Save time and energy by doing a little extra ahead of time. Use trays, baskets, or carts to carry several things at once. Prepare often-used food items ahead of time and freeze them. Cook in quantity and freeze meal-size portions. Cook more than one item in the oven at a time.

Minimize. Look for ways to make tasks shorter and easier. Modify your workspace to make your work more comfortable and easier.

Specialize. Use the right tool for each task. For example, a vegetable peeler is more efficient than a knife for peeling carrots. Take pride in what you are doing. Finally, be sure to thank family members who have picked up, cleaned up, or participated in household chores.

2. Describe how to follow an established work plan with the client and family

The client care plan and your assignments will tell you what tasks are required. You can develop your own work plan. This will allow you to finish all your assigned tasks as quickly and efficiently as possible. For each day or block of time you will spend in a home, list all the tasks you must complete. Then, prioritize them. Mark the most important as "1" and the next most important as "2," and so on. Finally, write out a schedule for the day, filling in the highest priority tasks first. If there are tasks that must be done at a certain time, put those tasks on the schedule at the appropriate time.

Remember to distribute tasks, so that you are not trying to do all the housecleaning on one afternoon and end up with no time to bathe or care for a client. Simplify tasks whenever possible to allow you to accomplish more.

Following an established work plan will allow you to get more done in less time. It will also allow your clients and families to know what to expect of you. You may even want to discuss the plan with a client or family member as you are making it up or when it is finished. Some people appreciate knowing what will be happening in their homes at any given time.

3. Discuss ways to handle inappropriate requests

Occasionally, you may be asked to do something that is not in the care plan or your assignments. Because each client's situation is unique, you will not be assigned to the same tasks for every client. For example, the care plan may specify grocery shopping for Mrs. Singer, who lives alone and cannot drive. But if another client who lives with family members asks you to run to the store, you have to say no if it is not in the care plan or your assignments.

Several things will help you handle requests that you must refuse. First, explain that you are only allowed to do tasks assigned in the care plan. Explain that nurses familiar with the client's condition give you your assignments. Emphasize that you would like to help, but you are limited to the tasks outlined in the care plan and your assignments. After explaining this to the client, contact your supervisor and discuss the request. Your supervisor may add the task requested by the client to your assignments. It is possible it was left out of your assignments by mistake. Be sure to document the client's request and the actions you took to address it.

Establishing a work schedule will also help you handle inappropriate requests. If a client and family know what to expect of you, they may not be tempted to ask you to do other tasks. Sharing a schedule of everything you must accomplish in a visit may help the client understand your job. If inappropriate requests continue, refer clients or family members to your supervisor.

4. List five money-saving homemaking tips

1. Check store circulars for advertised specials. Plan your menus around foods that are a good value; for example, raw foods are less expensive than prepared ones. Chapter 23 discusses more ways to plan economical meals.

2. Use coupons. If your client receives a newspaper, scan it for coupons from stores or manufacturers (Fig. 24-1).

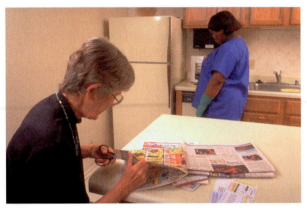

Fig. 24-1. Clipping coupons can save your client money. Some clients may enjoy doing this task themselves.

3. Shop from your list. Don't be tempted by items that are not on your list, even if they are on sale.

4. Avoid convenience stores. Shopping at large supermarkets or discount stores usually guarantees you will get the best prices.

5. Plan ahead. Knowing what you need before you run out will save you money. Planning will also save you time and energy. For example, you won't have to make a special trip when you discover you've run out of laundry detergent.

5. List guidelines for handling a client's money

Different states and employers have different regulations and policies regarding healthcare employees handling clients' money. Find out from your employer whether you will be expected to handle clients' money. If you are not allowed to handle money, never agree to do so,

even occasionally. You could get yourself and your employer into serious trouble.

If your state and your employer permit you to handle clients' money, there are several guidelines you must follow in doing so.

GUIDELINES
Handling a Client's Money

g Never use a client's money for your own needs, even if you plan to pay it back. This is considered stealing. You could lose your job and/or be arrested.

g Estimate the amount of money you will need before requesting it. If you are making a trip to the grocery store, show the client your list and ask how much he or she is willing to spend on groceries, or how much is budgeted. You may need to take things off your list or estimate the total bill as you go along in the store to stay within the money allotted (Fig. 24-2).

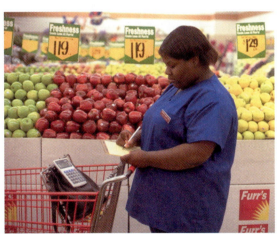

Fig. 24-2. Taking a calculator to the grocery store helps you to stay within the client's budget.

g Take checks rather than cash, when possible. Have the client or family member fill out the name of the store. A signed check that is not made out is as good as cash. If you lose cash or a signed bank check, you may be responsible for paying back the amount.

g Get a receipt for every purchase. This proves how much you spent and provides a record for you and the client.

g Return receipts and change to client or family member immediately. Don't wait until the

end of the day or week to settle up. Do it right away while everything is fresh in your mind. Forgetting to return change could be viewed by the client or a family member as stealing.

ⓖ Keep a record of money you've spent. Follow your agency's policies and procedures for documenting money issues. Write down how much you spent and where. Note any change returned to client. The better record you have, the smaller the chance of any misunderstanding.

ⓖ Keep a client's cash separate from yours. If you must use the client's cash, don't put it in your own wallet. Keep it in a separate, safe place. Do the same with change. This will prevent confusion.

ⓖ Never offer money advice to a client. You should not even refer a client to others regarding their financial matters.

ⓖ Remember, your clients' financial matters are private. Never discuss your clients' money matters with anyone.

Chapter Review

1. List the ways to work efficiently.

2. What does it mean to "prioritize" tasks?

3. How might you help your client and his/her family understand your job? How could this help reduce inappropriate requests?

4. Do you have any money-saving homemaking tips of your own? What are they?

5. Write a scenario that demonstrates why you and your employer could get into trouble if you are not allowed to handle a client's money but do it anyway.

6. Why is it important to get a receipt for anything you purchase with a client's money?

7. Why might it be useful to take a calculator to the store with you when you shop for a client?

25

Caring for Yourself and Your Career

1. Explain how to conduct a job search

You may soon be looking for a job. To find a job, you must first find potential employers. Then you must contact them to find out about job opportunities. To find potential employers, use the newspaper, telephone book, the Internet, or personal contacts. Try these resources:

- Classified or employment sections of the newspaper list jobs currently available. Circle ads for home health aide positions. Make a list of names and phone numbers to contact (Fig. 25-1).

- Look in the yellow pages under "Home Health Services" for a list of agencies.

- Call the state or local Department of Social Services. Many states hire or place home health aides.

- Ask your instructor for potential employers. Some schools maintain a list of employers seeking home health aides.

- Check the Internet (Fig. 25-2). One good web site is www.carecareers.net. Other good ones are www.jobsearch.org and www.monster.com. You can also visit a search engine: www.google.com or www.yahoo.com. Type in "home health aide" and your city. See what employment opportunities are there.

CNA's & HHA's/Whether you are just starting out in the healthcare field or you are an experienced professional seeking new challenges, we invite you to join one of the country's leading providers of home health care. Because our HHAs are the backbone of our quality care, we provide a competitive salary, attendance, bonus program and benefits package, as well as opportunities to advance your career. For consideration, apply in person at our downtown facility, 120 Main St., (555) 291-3333. Pre-employment drug screening and criminal background check required. EOE Home Health America

Home Health Aides/Part-time or full-time. 3pm–11pm & 4pm–9pm. CNA or 1 year experience. Send resume to: Las Portales Village, 555 North Cottonwood Pl, City, 87555

Home Health Aides or CNAs with a minimum of 1 year experience as an aide needed immediately for part-time home care positions throughout city and surrounding areas. Must have proof of current comprehensive/liability auto insurance. Individuals with valid CPR certification preferred. Bilingual a plus. Contact Josh at (555) 293-6598 for application info.

Home Health Aide to work as an independent contractor, providing care for elderly patient. Personal care, bathing, meals, LT, housekeeping, certification required. PT hours, incl. overnight, 289-0224

Fig. 25-1. Newspaper ads are one way to identify potential employers.

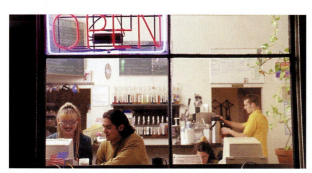

Fig. 25-2. Searching the Internet is one good way to find a job.

Once you have a list of potential employers, you need to contact them about job opportunities. Phoning first, unless they mention not to do so, is a good way to find out what opportunities are available. Ask how to apply for a job with each potential employer.

Making Contact with Potential Employers

When you call an employer, ask to speak to someone in the personnel or human resources department.

"Hello, I am calling about employment opportunities as a home health aide. May I speak to someone in the personnel department please?"

When you get someone in personnel, the first thing to say is who you are and why you are calling.

"Hello, my name is Gina Graham and I am a graduate of Kingston Vocational Centers' home health aide training program. I am looking for work as a home health aide."

If you are calling an employer who advertised in the paper, you know there is a job opening. After introducing yourself, you can say,

"I saw your ad in the paper. Can you tell me about job opportunities available?"

If you are calling a potential employer that has not advertised a job, be more general.

"Can you tell me about job opportunities you might have?"

If there are jobs available, ask for an appointment to come in and speak to someone. Be sure to write down the time and date of the appointment. Ask where the agency is located and what office to go to.

2. Identify documents that may be required when applying for a job

You may need several documents in order to apply for a job. When making an appointment, ask what information to bring with you. Make sure you have this information with you when you go. Some of these documents include the following:

- Identification: driver's license, social security card, birth certificate, passport, or other official form of identification to prove who you are

- Proof of your legal status in this country and proof that you are legally able to work, even if you're a U.S.-born citizen. All employers must have files showing that all employees are legally allowed to work in this country. Do not be offended by this request.

- High school diploma or equivalency, school transcripts, and diploma or certificate from your home health aide training course. Take the name and phone number of your instructor with you as well.

- References are people who can be called to recommend you as an employee. They include former employers or former teachers, or your minister. Do not use relatives or friends as references. You can ask your references beforehand to write general letters for you, addressed "To whom it may concern," explaining how they know you and describing your skills, qualities, and habits. Take copies of these with you for employers to keep.

3. Demonstrate completing an effective job application

On one sheet of paper, write down the general information you will need to complete an application. Take it with you. This will save time and avoid mistakes.

Include the following information:

- your address and phone number
- your birth date

- your social security number
- the name of the school or program where you were trained and the date you completed your training, as well as your certification number from a certification card, if you have one
- the names and addresses of your previous employers, and the dates you worked there
- the names and phone numbers of your references
- the days and hours you are available to work
- a brief statement of why you are changing jobs or why you want to work as a home health aide

Fill out the application carefully and neatly (Fig. 25-3). Never lie on a job application. Before you write anything, read it all the way through once. If you are not sure what is being asked, find out before filling in that space.

Employment Application

Personal Information

Name: Rosie Ferguson
Date: 1/15/04
Social Security Number: 555-99-9999
Home Address: 8529-A Indian School Rd. NE
City, state, Zip: Albuquerque, NM 87112
Home Phone: 505-291-1274
Business Phone: N/A
US Citizen? Yes
If Not Give Visa No. & expiration:

Position Applying For

Title: Home Health Aide
Salary Desired: $8.50/hr
Referred By: Ms. McClain, Instructor, HHA Training Center
Date Available: 1/15/04

Education

High School (Name, City, State): Laguna High School, Albuquerque, NM
Graduation Date: December 2003
Technical or Undergraduate School: HHA Training Center, Albuquerque, NM
Dates Attended: July – Dec. 2003
Degree Major:

References

Mr. Robert Castro, Instructor, HHA Training Center, 505-291-1284
Ms. Scott, Health Occupations, Laguna HS, 505-555-6255
Kate Crawford, Instructor, HHA Training Center, 505-291-1294

Fig. 25-3. A sample job application.

By law, your employer must perform a criminal background check on all new aides hired. You may be asked to sign a form granting the agency permission to do this. Don't take it personally; it is a law intended to protect patients, clients, and residents.

4. Demonstrate competence in job interview techniques

To make the best impression at a job interview, be professional:

- Dress neatly and appropriately.
- Shower or bathe and use deodorant or antiperspirant.
- Wear only simple makeup and jewelry or none at all.
- Arrive 10 or 15 minutes early.
- Introduce yourself, smile, and shake hands (Fig. 25-4).

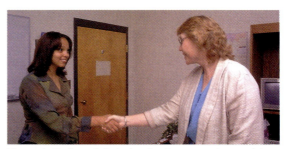

Fig. 25-4. Smile and shake hands when you arrive at a job interview.

- Answer questions clearly and completely.
- Make eye contact to show you are sincere (Fig. 25-5)

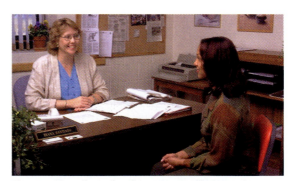

Fig. 25-5. Be polite and make eye contact during an interview.

- Avoid using slang words or expressions.
- Never eat, drink, chew gum, or smoke in an interview.
- Sit up or stand up straight, and look happy to be there.

- Do not bring friends or children to the interview with you.

Be positive when answering questions. Emphasize what you enjoy or think you will enjoy about being an aide. Do not complain about any previous jobs you held. Make it clear that you are hard-working and willing to work with all kinds of clients.

The following are some questions you can expect to be asked:

- Why did you become a home health aide?

- What do you like about working as an aide?

- What don't you like? (If this is your first job, you may be asked what you expect to like or dislike.)

- What are your best qualities? What are your weaknesses?

- Why did you leave your last job?

- What kinds of clients do you prefer to work with?

Usually interviewers will ask if you have any questions. Have some prepared and written down so you do not forget things you really want to know. Questions you may want to ask include the following:

- What hours would I work?

- What benefits does the job include? Is health insurance available? Would I get paid sick days or holidays?

- How much traveling would I have to do between clients? Do I need a car? Would I be paid for mileage or travel time?

- What orientation or training is provided?

- How much contact would I have with my supervisor?

Later in the interview, you may want to ask about salary or wages if you have not already been given this information.

Listen carefully to the answers to your questions. Take notes if needed. At the end of the interview, you will probably be told when you can

expect to hear from the employer. Do not expect to be offered a job at the interview. When the interview is over, stand up, shake hands again, and say something like, "Thank you for taking the time to meet with me today. I look forward to hearing from you."

Send a letter to the employer after the interview to say thank you and to express your continued interest in a job (Fig. 25-6). If you have not heard anything from the employer within the time frame you discussed with your interviewer, call and ask whether the job was filled.

August 18, 2004

Marilyn Michaels
4356 12th St.
Rio Grande, TX 74568
505 291-1274

Nancy Proust, Personnel Manager
HomeHelp, Inc.
332 S. Main
Rio Grande, TX 74568

Dear Ms. Proust:

Thank you for taking the time to interview me last week for a home health aide position with HomeHelp, Inc. It was a pleasure to talk to you and to learn more about your agency. I look forward to hearing from you soon regarding the home health aide openings listed in the newspaper.

Sincerely,

Marilyn Michaels

Fig. 25-6. After a job interview send a professional thank you letter.

5. Discuss appropriate responses to criticism

Handling criticism is difficult for most of us. Being able to accept criticism and learn from it is important in all relationships, including employment. From time to time you will receive evaluations from your employer. These evaluations contain ideas to help you improve your job performance. Here are some ideas for handling criticism and using it to your benefit:

- Listen to the message that is being sent. Do not get so upset that you are unable to understand the message.

- Hostile criticism and constructive criticism are not the same. Hostile criticism is angry and negative. Examples are, "You are useless!" or "You are lazy and slow." Hostile criticism should not come from your employer or supervisor. You may experience hostile criticism from clients, family members, or others. The best response is to say something like, "I'm sorry you are so disappointed," and nothing more. Give the person a chance to calm down before trying to discuss their comments.

- Constructive criticism may come from your employer, supervisor, or other people. Constructive criticism is intended to help you improve. Examples are, "You really need to be more accurate in your charting," or "You are late too often. You'll have to make more of an effort to be on time." Listening and acting on constructive criticism can help you be more successful in your job, so pay attention to it (Fig. 25-7).

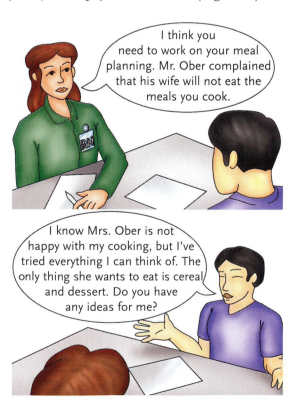

Fig. 25-7. Ask for suggestions when receiving constructive criticism.

- If you aren't sure how to avoid a mistake you have made, always ask the person criticizing you for suggestions on improving your performance.

- Apologize and move on. If you have made a mistake, apologize as needed (Fig. 25-8). This may be to your supervisor, your client, or others. Learn what you can from the incident and put it behind you. Don't dwell on it or hold a grudge. Being able to respond professionally to criticism is important for success in any job.

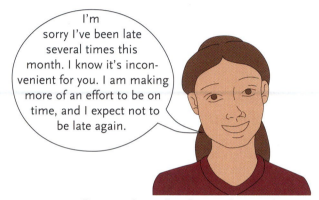

Fig. 25-8. Be willing to apologize if you have made a mistake.

6. Identify effective ways to make a complaint to an employer or supervisor

Sometimes you will need to make a complaint or voice a concern about some part of your job. Do not be afraid to do this, but do it carefully.

Think about the problem. Some major problems must be reported right away. For example, if a client, family member, or coworker threatens you, report this to your supervisor immediately. Other problems may work themselves out in time. If a new client seems rude, it is possible that he or she feels uncomfortable with new people or doesn't understand your role. You may want to wait several days or weeks to see if things improve before making a complaint. Know which problems should be reported immediately to your supervisor.

Plan what you will say. Think through and even write out what you will say to your supervisor.

This will help you present your complaint clearly and completely.

HHA: *Ms. Greene, I have a concern about the daughter of my client, Mrs. Paulsen. Last week she asked me to cut her mother's toenails. I explained I was not allowed to do that procedure and she would have to wait for the nurse to come. On Monday she wanted me to take her car out and fill the gas tank while she visited with her mother. I told her that was not in the care plan. Yesterday she dropped a glass and told me to clean up my mess or she would have me fired. I cleaned up the glass, but I think this woman has a problem with me. I wanted to let you know what had happened and ask if you could help me solve this problem.*

Don't get emotional. Some situations may be very upsetting. However, you will be more effective in communicating and problem-solving if you can keep your emotions out of it. Share your feelings about a situation—whether you are mad, hurt, or annoyed—with a friend. Tell your supervisor the facts.

Do not hesitate to communicate situations that you feel are important or that may put you or a client at risk. One common problem in home care is aides not reporting when they feel unsafe at a particular client's home. In this case, not complaining can prove dangerous for you and the client. Always report to your supervisor any situation in which you feel you or the client is at risk of harm, even if the situation involves the client's family or friends.

7. Identify guidelines for making job changes

If you decide to change jobs, be responsible. Always give your employer at least two weeks' written notice that you will be leaving. Otherwise, assignments may be left uncovered, or other aides may have to work more until the agency fills your spot. In addition, future employers may talk with past supervisors. People who change jobs too often or who do not give notice before leaving are less likely to be hired.

8. List your state's requirements for maintaining certification

Each state has slightly different requirements for maintaining certification. Be familiar with the requirements. Follow them exactly or you will not be able to keep working as an aide. Ask your instructor or employer for the requirements in your state. You should know how many hours of in-service education are required per year. You also need to know how long an absence from working is allowed without retraining or recertification.

Some states do not have a registry for home health aides like the ones they maintain for certified nursing assistants (CNAs). If, for example, you have taken the certification exam for CNAs and are on the state registry, you may need to work a certain number of hours in a long-term care facility to remain on the registry. As a home health aide, ask your employer how best to maintain your certification.

9. Describe continuing education for home health aides

The federal government requires that home health aides have 12 hours of continuing education each year. Some states may require more. "In-service" continuing education courses help you keep your knowledge and skills fresh. Classes may also provide you with more information about certain conditions, challenges that you face in working with clients, or regulation changes. You need to be up-to-date on the latest that is expected of you.

If you need more instruction in a particular area, speak to your supervisor. Perhaps he or she can arrange for an in-service continuing education class to be offered on that topic.

Your employer may be responsible for offering continuing education courses. However, you are responsible for attending and completing them. Specifically, you must do the following:

- Sign up for the course or find out where it is offered (Fig. 25-9).

- Attend all class sessions.

- Pay attention and complete all the class requirements.

- Make the most of your time in in-service programs. Participate!

- Keep original copies of all certificates and records of your successful attendance so you can prove you took the class.

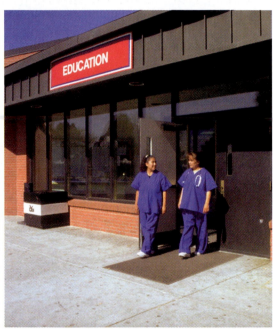

Fig. 25-9. You may want to go outside the in-service programs offered by your employer to take some continuing education courses.

10. Define stress and stressors, and list examples

Stress is the state of being frightened, excited, confused, in danger, or irritated. We usually think only bad things cause stress. However, positive situations can cause stress, too. For example, getting married or having a new baby are usually positive situations. But both can cause enormous stress because of the changes they bring to our lives.

You may be thrilled when you get a new job as a home health aide. But starting work may also cause you stress. You may be afraid of making

mistakes, excited about earning money or helping people, or confused about how to perform your new duties. Learning how to recognize stress and what causes it is helpful. Then you can master a few simple techniques for relaxing, and learn to manage stress.

A **stressor** is something that causes stress. Anything can be a stressor if it causes you stress. Some examples include the following:

- divorce

- marriage

- a new baby

- children growing up

- children leaving home

- losing a job

- starting a new job

- problems at work

- new responsibilities at work

- supervisors

- co-workers

- clients

- illness

- finances

11. Explain ways to manage stress

Stress is not only an emotional response. It is also a physical response. When we experience stress, changes occur in our bodies. The endocrine system produces more of the hormone **adrenaline** (*a-DREH-na-lin*). This can increase nervous system response, heart rate, respiratory rate, and blood pressure. This is why, in stressful situations, your heart beats fast, you breathe hard, and you feel warm or perspire.

Each of us has a different tolerance level for stress. In other words, what one person would find overwhelming might not bother another person. Your tolerance of stress depends on your personality, life experiences, and physical health.

Managing Stress

- ⓖ To manage the stress in your life, develop healthy habits of diet, exercise, and lifestyle.

- ⓖ Eat nutritious foods.

- ⓖ Exercise regularly (Fig. 25-10).

- ⓖ Get enough sleep.

- ⓖ Drink only in moderation.

- ⓖ Do not smoke.

- ⓖ Find time at least a few times a week to do something relaxing, such as taking a walk, reading a book, or sewing.

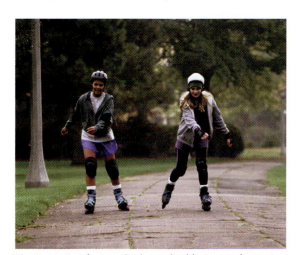

Fig. 25-10. Regular exercise is one healthy way to decrease stress.

Not managing stress can cause many problems. Some of these problems affect how well you do your job. Signs that you are not managing stress include the following:

- showing anger or being abusive toward clients

- arguing with your supervisor about your assignments

- having poor relationships with co-workers and clients

- complaining about your job and your responsibilities

- feeling work-related burn-out

- feeling tired even when you are rested

- having a difficult time focusing on clients and procedures

Stress can seem overwhelming when you try to handle it yourself. Often just talking about stress can help you manage it better. Sometimes another person can offer helpful suggestions for managing stress. Sometimes you will think of new ways to handle stress just by talking it through with another person.

Where can you turn for help managing stress? Try the following:

- your supervisor or another member of the care team for work-related stress

- your family

- your friends

- your place of worship

- your physician

- a local mental health agency

- any phone hotline that deals with related problems (check your local yellow pages)

It is not appropriate to turn to your clients or their family members to help you manage personal or job-related stress.

12. Demonstrate two effective relaxation techniques

Sometimes when you need a break, a relaxation exercise can help you feel refreshed and relaxed in only a short time. The following are two simple relaxation exercises. Try them out and see if either one helps you feel more relaxed.

The body scan. Close your eyes. Pay attention to your breathing and posture. Be sure you are comfortable. Starting at the balls of your feet, concentrate on your feet. Discover any tension hidden in the feet, and try to relax and release the tension. Continue very slowly. Take a breath between each body part. Move up from the feet, focusing on and relaxing the legs, knees, thighs, hips, stomach, back, shoulders, neck, jaw, eyes, forehead, and scalp. Take a few very deep breaths and open your eyes.

The waterfall. Breathe deeply and imagine you

are under a waterfall. The force of the water is washing away your tension. Imagine the tension is being washed away, one body part at a time, from the head through the soles of the feet. Visualize the tension being washed far away by the rushing water.

Either of these relaxation techniques takes only about two minutes. If one is helpful for you, try it the next time you need a break, whether at work or at home.

13. Describe how to develop a personal stress management plan

One of the best ways to manage stress is to develop a plan for managing stress. The plan can include things you will do every day and things to do in stressful situations. When you think about a plan, you first need to answer the following questions:

- What are the sources of stress in my life?

- When do I most often experience stress?

- What effects of stress do I see in my life?

- What can I change to decrease the stress I feel?

- What do I have to learn to cope with because I cannot change it?

When you have answered these questions, you will have a clearer picture of the challenges you face. Then you can try to come up with strategies for managing stress. Following are some examples:

Situation #1. Anita is a home health aide and a single mother. After work, she picks up her two children at day care and heads home. She is tired, the children are hungry, and dinner isn't ready. Sometimes she gets so stressed out she wants to yell at her children to get their own supper. What can she do?

Response: Planning and preparing ahead of time can make the after work/before dinner time go more smoothly. If Anita can plan and prepare suppers ahead of time for every night

she works, she will feel less stress. Keeping made-ahead meals in the refrigerator or freezer is a good way to eliminate stress (Fig. 25-11).

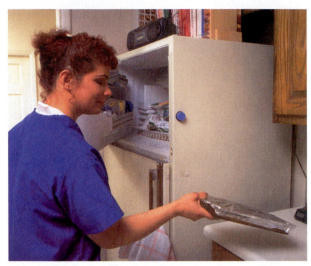

Fig. 25-11. Making and freezing meals is a good way to eliminate a stressor.

Situation #2. Martha is a home health aide and a mother and grandmother. Her husband, Chuck, lost his job so she must support them both. Last year Martha decided she had a stress problem and started going to a nursing assistant support group. She feels much better since she started, and would like to get more control in other areas of her life to reduce her stress level.

Response: Martha wrote a personal stress management plan for herself:

Every day:

Eat breakfast, take an apple and a granola bar or other healthy snacks with me to work. Take two or three breaks to stretch, sit down, and relax for several minutes.

Monday, Wednesday, Friday:

Go for a walk after supper. Invite Chuck to go with me.

Tuesday, Saturday:

Go to support group (Fig. 25-12).

Sunday:

Go to church. Visit grandchildren. Plan menus for

the week. Clip coupons from the paper and go grocery shopping.

Every week:

Do one thing I want to do, like see a movie, take a bubble bath, read a magazine.

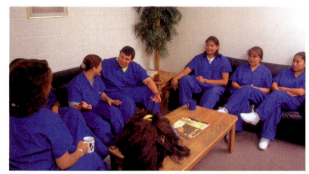

Fig. 25-12. Support groups can help you deal with stress of different types.

Martha's plan is a great start in managing stress. It helps her fit in all the things she wants to do each week. It includes healthy habits like eating breakfast and nutritious snacks, walking regularly, and taking breaks. She may not stick to her plan exactly every week, but it gives her goals to work towards.

14. List five guidelines for managing time

Many of the ideas for managing time on the job can be used to manage your personal time as well. The following are five basic strategies for managing time:

1. **Plan ahead**. Planning is the single best way to help you manage your time better. Sometimes you may feel you don't even have the time to plan, but take five minutes to sit down and list everything you have to do. Often just making the list will help you feel better. It will get you focused on accomplishing what you need to do.

2. **Prioritize**. Identify the most important things to get done. Do these first.

3. **Make a schedule**. Write out the hours of the day and fill in when you will do what. This will

help you be realistic. If you only have 20 minutes between getting off work and picking up your children, you will not be able to get the grocery shopping done. Schedule that activity for later.

4. **Combine activities**. Can you read the paper while you're on the bus? Can you prepare tomorrow's dinner while the laundry is in the dryer? Or help your son with his homework while you do the dishes? Work more efficiently when you can (Fig. 25-13).

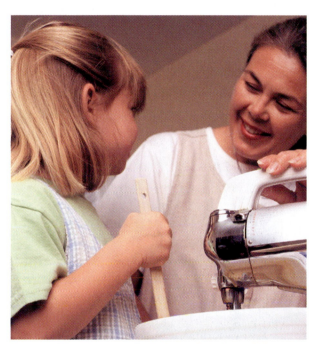

Fig. 25-13. Managing time effectively may include combining activities, such as baking while catching up with your child.

5. **Get help**. It is not reasonable for you to do everything. If children are old enough to help, give them chores to do. If other family members are available, make a plan for who will cook or clean up each night. If you have no one to help you, give yourself a break. You cannot do everything. Some things just may not get done.

15. Demonstrate an understanding of the basics of money management

Money can be a real source of stress. Not being able to buy the things we need or want, getting into debt, or facing emergencies without a cash

reserve can be very difficult. Understanding a little bit about money management can help you avoid money problems.

Make a budget. Making a personal or household budget is not complicated. It is helps you start solving money problems. To make a budget, you need to know total income and total expenses. Expenses include rent or mortgage, transportation, utilities, insurance, debts, food, clothing, medical and dental, entertainment, and miscellaneous. Expenses may be calculated on a weekly, monthly, or annual basis.

Reduce or avoid debts. When you owe money, whether to a bank, a mortgage company, or a credit card company, you pay interest. Interest is the money you pay for the right to use someone else's money. When you can avoid borrowing money, you avoid paying interest. Whenever you can, save the money to buy something instead of borrowing it.

Most people must borrow money for major purchases, like a house or a car. In these situations paying interest is unavoidable. But whenever you can avoid borrowing money, do so. If you have debts already, pay them off as soon as possible. Furthermore, when you apply for a loan to buy a house or a car, you will have to show that you can handle debt responsibly. If you have too much debt, you may not be able to get a loan for a house or a car.

When you apply for a mortgage or car loan, the bank or lender will check your credit report. A credit report is a document that lists all of the loans or debts you have ever had and shows how you paid them off. If you were ever late paying bills, this will appear on your credit report. You are legally entitled to see your credit report and have it corrected if it is wrong.

Credit cards can make it especially hard to manage money well. It is easy to get and use a credit card, so many of us buy things we do not need or could wait and save for. The interest charged on credit card debt is often the highest interest

charged on any loan. If you have trouble controlling what you buy with credit cards, consider getting rid of them altogether.

Save as much as you can. No matter how small your income or how great your expenses, always try to save some amount every time you get a check. Ten percent is a good savings goal, but if you can only save one percent of your check, do it. Open a savings account at your bank. When you take your check to cash or deposit, deposit your savings in the savings account.

There are many advantages to saving. You can avoid debt if you save rather than borrow. Also, the bank pays you interest on the money you save while it is in the bank. The more you save, the more interest you get.

Another important reason to save is that having savings allows you to face emergencies. If your car breaks down, or you have unexpected medical bills, or your work hours are cut, having savings means you have a safety net to fall back on. Get into the habit of saving. It can mean the difference between financial independence and financial disaster.

Control miscellaneous expenses. Sometimes we get to the end of the week or month and wonder, "Where did all my money go?" If this happens to you, you may be spending too much on miscellaneous items. Examples include snacks, coffee, lottery tickets, unnecessary items at the grocery store, or eating out when your budget cannot support it. Cash cards make it easy to get cash, which makes it easier to spend more.

Try writing down what you spend money on each day. A cup of coffee and a donut, a lottery ticket, a candy bar, and two sodas can add up to more than $5.00. That may not seem like a lot, but if you spend that every day for five days, that's $25.00 a week. Can your budget support that? Consider eliminating these kinds of expenses by bringing coffee and other snacks from home and skipping the lottery tickets.

Set a cash allowance for the week and stick to it. Figure out how much cash you need in a week. Count bus fare, gas, children's lunch money, any other regular expenses, and include some emergency cash. Withdraw this amount at the beginning of the week and make it last. Use your cash card for emergencies only.

Be proud of your efforts to manage money. Very few people manage their money well. Many people have too much debt, buy more than they need, and don't save enough money. It is hard to be responsible and control expenses. If you manage your money, you and your family will be better off financially and better able to face emergencies. You can also help yourself become wealthier by saving. You can live a more comfortable life, and get satisfaction from knowing that your belongings are paid for. Research shows that people who manage their money are happier than people who do not.

16. Demonstrate an understanding that money matters are emotional

Money problems are the number one cause of family and marital arguments. Money carries great meaning for most people. Money is necessary to live, but it has also come to represent value. We may think the more money we have, the better people we are.

We try to make ourselves feel better by buying something we cannot afford. The images shown on television, in the movies, or in magazines make us feel we ought to have certain possessions. Many of us feel we deserve certain things, even when we really cannot afford them. All these emotions come into play whenever we think about or talk about money matters (Fig. 25-14).

Money also equals security for many of us. When we cannot pay our bills, or when debts get too high, we feel a lot of anxiety. The best way to avoid this anxiety is to budget, plan, and manage money matters wisely. But in order to manage our money well, most of us need to spend less and save more. Look at your finan-

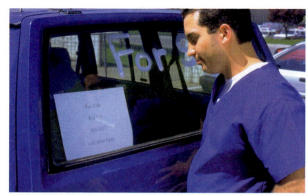

Fig. 25-14. Money matters are emotional.

cial situation realistically. Decide what you will and will not spend your money on. Separating emotions from realities about money will help you make good decisions and stick to them. You can get even greater satisfaction from being responsible and independent (Fig. 25-15).

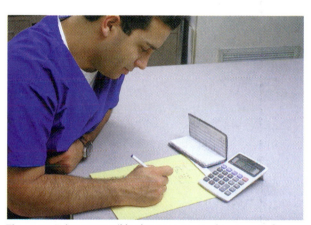

Fig. 25-15. Being responsible about money can be very satisfying.

17. List ways to remind yourself that your work is important, valuable, and meaningful

Look back over all you have learned in this program. Your work as a home health aide is very important. Every day may be different and challenging. In a hundred ways every week you will offer help that only a caring person like you can provide.

Do not forget to value the work you have chosen to do. It is important. For your clients, your work can mean the difference between living at home and living in an institution. It can mean living with independence and dignity versus liv-

ing without. The difference you make is sometimes life versus death. Look in the face of each of your clients and know that you are doing important work. Look in a mirror when you get home and be proud of how you make your living (Fig. 25-16).

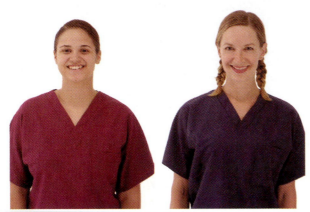

Fig. 25-16. Be proud of the work you have chosen to do. It's important.

An important life skill is being able to reflect on how you spend your time. Learn ways to fully appreciate that what you do has great meaning. Few jobs have the challenges and rewards of home health care. Congratulate yourself for choosing a path that includes helping others along the way.

Chapter Review

1. What is a good way to find out about job opportunities with a potential employer?

2. List three documents you may need to take with you when applying for a job.

3. What should you do before writing anything on a job application?

4. How can you follow up on a job interview?

5. List three things you can do to show a potential employer your professionalism during an interview.

6. What is the difference between hostile and constructive criticism?

7. What kind of problem should you report right away to a supervisor?

8. Why would an employer not hire a person who has changed jobs often?

9. Does your state have a registry for home health aides?

10. How many hours of continuing education does the federal government require that home health aides have each year?

11. What can you do to get the most out of continuing education?

12. Give three examples of stressors you've experienced in the last year. How did you respond to them?

13. What steps can you take to manage stress in your life?

14. Try both the body scan and the waterfall for relaxation. Describe how you felt after doing them.

15. Look at Situation #1 in learning objective 13. Write a stress management plan similar to the one shown in Situation #2.

16. In which of the five guidelines for managing time do you have the most room for improvement? What can you do to improve?

17. List four guidelines to manage money more effectively.

18. Have you ever bought something just to make yourself feel better? Did it work? Why or why not?

19. What do you think you will like best about being a home health aide?

INDEX

guidelines 170–171
one-sided weakness 277–278

DRGs
see diagnostic related groups

droplet precautions
see also infection control, isolation
precautions 64

drug abuse
see also substance abuse 228

drug misuse **228**

drugs
see medications

duodenal ulcer **326**

dying
see also death
grieving and 132
postmortem care 134
related care 133–134
stages 131

dyspnea **89**

E

ear
see also nervous system: sense organs
common disorders 105
observing and reporting 106
structure and function 105

eating
assisting with 334–335
client with stroke 277–278
problems 335
in adolescence 120

eating disorders **120**
see also anorexia, bulimia

education
see home health aide (HHA)
continuing 347

egg crate mattress **218**

elder
see aging

elder abuse
see also abuse 129
signs and symptoms 129

elimination
see also toileting 110

emergency supplies **94**

emergency(ies)
burns 90–91
choking 87–88
client assessment 84
controlling bleeding 89–90
CPR 85
documenting 85
fainting 92
falls 93
first aid 85
heart attack 89
Heimlich manuever 87
HHA role 84–85
medications 227
nosebleed 92–93
obstructed airway 87–88
poisoning 90
reporting 84
seizures 91–92
shock 88

emesis
see also nausea, vomiting

care after 197
observing and reporting 198

emotional abuse
child 119

emotional problems
AIDS and 286

emotions
money and 353

empathetic **32**

empathize **99**

empathy **33**

emphysema
respiratory system disorder 108

employer responsibilities
infection control 69–70
to HHA 33–34

employers
contacting potential 342–343

employment
changing jobs 347
interview questions 345
interview techniques 344–345
job application 343–344
maintaining certification 347
making complaints 346–347
required documents 343
responding to criticism 345–346

employment applications **343–344**

endocrine system
care guidelines for aging client 126
common disorders 112
normal changes of aging 126
observing and reporting 113
structure and function 112

epilepsy
nervous system disorder 104

epistaxis
see emergency(ies) or nosebleed 92

esophagus **110**

ethical behavior **36**

ethics **36**

evacuation **93**

exchange lists
diabetes and 275

exercise
stress and 349

expiration **107**

exposure report
infection control and 68

extension **211, 212**

external catheter
see condom catheter

external rotation **211, 212**

eye
see also nervous system: sense organs
common disorders 105
observing and reporting 106
structure and function 105

eye shield **61**

F

face mask
see mask

facilities **17**

fallacy **121**

falling client **141**

falls
emergency care for 93
prevention of 75

family(ies)
adjustments to illness/disability 98
community resources 99
emotional needs 99
establishing a work plan 339
functions 97
housekeeping 299

family assistance
client with cancer 271

family contact
of HHA 22

family roles
health care 97

family support **26**

farsightedness **240**

fats
basic nutrient 315
food group 316

fat-soluble **315**

feces **111**

feeding
client with stroke 278
infants 254

female reproductive system
see reproductive system

fiber **314**

fire
see also safety: fire 79

fire extinguishers
see safety: fire

flexibility
of HHA 23

flexion **211, 212**

flossing
procedure 173–174

flotation pads **218**

fluid
conversion tables 196

fluid balance
defined 196
see also urinary system 109
assisting with 318–319
importance of 196

fluid overload
observing and reporting 319

fluid retention
see nephritis

food
planning and shopping 328–330
pricing 329
purchasing 330
storage 333–334

food additives
cancer and 268

Food and Drug Administration (FDA) **323**

food groups **316–318**

food guide pyramid **317**

H